Skin-Related Neglected Tropical Diseases (Skin-NTDs)

Skin-Related Neglected Tropical Diseases (Skin-NTDs)

A New Challenge

Special Issue Editors

Roderick J. Hay
Kingsley Asiedu

MDPI • Basel • Beijing • Wuhan • Barcelona • Belgrade

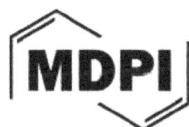

MDPI

Special Issue Editors
Roderick J. Hay
The International Foundation for Dermatology
UK

Kingsley Asiedu
World Health Organization
Switzerland

Editorial Office
MDPI
St. Alban-Anlage 66
4052 Basel, Switzerland

This is a reprint of articles from the Special Issue published online in the open access journal *Tropical Medicine and Infectious Disease* (ISSN 2414-6366) from 2018 to 2019 (available at: https://www.mdpi.com/journal/tropicalmed/special_issues/Skin_NTDs).

For citation purposes, cite each article independently as indicated on the article page online and as indicated below:

LastName, A.A.; LastName, B.B.; LastName, C.C. Article Title. *Journal Name* **Year**, *Article Number*, Page Range.

ISBN 978-3-03921-253-8 (Pbk)
ISBN 978-3-03921-254-5 (PDF)

Cover image courtesy of Daniel Mason.

Contents

About the Special Issue Editors

Roderick J. Hay is Emeritus Professor of Cutaneous Infection, Kings College London, and of Dermatology, Queens University Belfast, and is currently Consultant Dermatologist at the London Bridge Hospital. He is a graduate of Oxford University and Guy's Hospital, where he did his early training before working at the Centers for Disease Control, Atlanta, and the London School of Hygiene and Tropical Medicine. His clinical and research interests are in infectious and tropical diseases of the skin, with a focus on fungal infections. For over 30 years, Hay ran a skin infection clinic in London. He is a former Dean of the St Johns Institute of Dermatology, London. From 2002 to 2007, he was Head of the School of Medicine and Dentistry and Dean of the Faculty of Medicine and Health Sciences, Queens University Belfast.

Kingsley Asiedu, Dr., received his medical degree from the Kwame Nkrumah University of Science and Technology Kumasi, Ghana, in 1990. After completing his rotations in pediatrics, obstetrics, and genecology and surgery at the Komfo Anokye Teaching Hospital in Kumasi, he then started his career in public health in 1993 in the remote rural district of Amansie West, one of the country's most deprived areas. As the district medical officer as well as the medical officer in charge of the district hospital, St Martin's Catholic Hospital, he managed public health activities and curative services for a population of over 100,000 people. In 1997, he earned his Masters in Public Health with a focus on health policy and management at the Rollins School of Public Health, Emory University, Atlanta, United States of America. He joined WHO in 1998 as a Medical Officer responsible for Buruli ulcer. In 2007, he took up the additional responsibility of the eradication of yaws. Since 2015, he has been coordinating the cross-disciplinary departmental work on integrating the control and management of a number of NTDs with skin presentations. His main interest is in the control of tropical diseases, district health systems, the role of community health workers in service delivery, and operational research.

Preface to "Skin-Related Neglected Tropical Diseases (Skin-NTDs)—A New Challenge"

The skin of the patient is the first and most visible structure of the body that any healthcare worker encounters in the course of an examination. It is also highly visible, and any disease that affects it is both noticeable and will have an impact on a patient's personal and social wellbeing. It is therefore an important entry point for diagnosis, disease mapping, and integrated management. Many of the major neglected tropical diseases produce changes in the skin, often the first indicator of illness that patients will notice. Changes to the skin often re-enforce feelings of isolation and stigma experienced by patients with NTDs, but they also provide opportunities for simplifying diagnosis and developing an integrated and strategic approach to care.

A key challenge in taking the common feature of skin involvement in NTDs to a higher level is that skin disease, in general, is very common, particularly in resource-poor settings, and seeking solutions to the first without addressing the commonality of skin disease is not an option.

Roderick J. Hay, Kingsley Asiedu
Special Issue Editors

Tropical Medicine and Infectious Disease

MDPI

Editorial

Skin-Related Neglected Tropical Diseases (Skin NTDs)—A New Challenge

Roderick J. Hay [1,*] and Kingsley Asiedu [2]

[1] The International Foundation for Dermatology, London W1P 5HQ, UK
[2] Department of Control of Neglected Tropical Diseases, World Health Organization, 1202 Geneva, Switzerland; asieduk@who.int
* Correspondence: roderick.hay@ifd.org

Received: 21 December 2018; Accepted: 22 December 2018; Published: 25 December 2018

Medical teaching has emphasised over many years the uniqueness of disease states, valuing the rare skills on which the art of diagnosis is based and the intricacies of individual patient-centred management. Yet with the growing appreciation of the public health dimensions of illnesses and the shrinking of the world due to modern travel, coupled with a massive expansion in the availability of, and access to, data, it has become increasingly important to recognise that good health outcomes are often best achieved by pooling expertise and implementing collective actions. The concept of Neglected Tropical Skin Diseases (Skin NTDs) is an example of this approach. Skin NTDs are diseases that present with lesions on the skin surface which may, in turn, provide not only practical clues to the diagnosis but also a greater understanding of disease through investigation, such as mapping, as well as management by identifying common pathways for therapeutic interventions [1,2]. Adopting strategies based on this idea opens access to a reservoir of skills and knowledge that shows how one disease can contribute to a better understanding of others; the integration and exploitation of areas of commonality are both key to initiatives in public health. As an example, the use of mass drug administration (MDA) has also highlighted what NTDs, and their management pathways, have in common rather than what separates them. The use of ivermectin, for example, in control programmes for lymphatic filariasis and onchocerciasis has produced unintentional, but major impacts on the prevalence of other common diseases from soil helminth infections to scabies [3]. This has provided an incentive to pursue the control of these diseases in other regions, as was seen in the recent clinical trial of ivermectin in Fiji for the control of scabies [4]. The use of azithromycin for both yaws and trachoma is a further example [5].

A patient's skin is accessible and easy to examine, after basic training, by any health care worker. It is therefore a common starting point for disease recognition. It is equally important to appreciate that skin diseases in general are very common, accounting for between 10 and 30% of all health worker/patient encounters depending on location, climate, genetic predisposition, underlying health and local prevalence of transmissible disorders. Therefore, while the skin may provide an entry point for the recognition of NTDs, it is also the focus of a number of very common conditions. Navigating this milieu involves recognising the clues that may lead a) to the identification of NTDs usually through examination and further simple investigations coupled with b) the provision of simple schemes for the management of the most common skin disorders. The development of a simple framework for accomplishing this strategy is an achievable goal. For instance, the World Health Organization (WHO) has recently published a training guide for the recognition of NTDs and common skin problems [6].

This issue takes this approach a step further by exploring the use of other techniques such as distance consultation using Telederm or Whatsapp, and simple training pathways for providing support to field workers as well as the introduction of a downloadable app for the recognition of skin diseases. Problems in diagnosis remain where there is a range of clinical manifestations that may lead to a single diagnosis (e.g., mycetoma), or where the presentation of disease states is camouflaged

Trop. Med. Infect. Dis. **2019**, *4*, 4

by inappropriate treatments such as cheap and easily available corticosteroids. The operation of community-based schemes for diagnosis and management is explored further as is the potential for new diagnostic interventions. The use of these interventions, adapted however to local conditions, is critical, an issue which is also explored in this series. In addition, the skin is highly visible to the patient or family member, and any disease that affects it is both noticeable and will have an impact on personal and social wellbeing. Changes to the skin often re-enforce feelings of social isolation and stigma experienced by patients with NTDs, and addressing these diseases must form a central plank of any control strategy.

Identifying a common ground is critical for the successful control and management of a number of neglected diseases, particularly for reasons of practicability in implementing operations in the field. Grouping some of these together as skin NTDs will advance this cause. This strategy also produces different impacts on different diseases in different ways. For example, in the case of leprosy, despite the introduction of post-exposure prophylaxis, the identification of cases through recognition of the signs on the skin remains at the heart of effective control. The same is true of other neglected diseases from mycetoma to Buruli ulcer. Ensuring that patients can be identified is also critical for those diseases that are amenable to mass drug administration, because the detection of the remaining cases will be a key element of the task of completing elimination. There will be areas where MDA cover has been incomplete or where finding "missed" cases forms a key to preventing resurgences in the future or recognizing the emergence of drug resistance. Seizing a common ground in the management of disease disability is also crucial as, for instance, the care, rehabilitation and protection of peripheral limbs is a key strategy for leprosy, podoconiosis, mycetoma and lymphatic filariasis as it is in diabetic foot [7–9]. These arguments for an integrated approach extend even further through interdependence and the promotion of community education, the relief of stigma, disease mapping, as well as research and training.

Funding: This research received no external funding.

Conflicts of Interest: The authors declare no conflict of interest.

References

1. Engelman, D.; Fuller, L.C.; Solomon, A.W.; McCarthy, J.S.; Hay, R.J.; Lammie, P.J.; Steer, A.C. Opportunities for Integrated Control of Neglected Tropical Diseases That Affect the Skin. *Trends Parasitol.* **2016**, *32*, 843–854. [CrossRef] [PubMed]
2. Mitjà, O.; Marks, M.; Bertran, L.; Kollie, K.; Argaw, D.; Fahal, A.H.; Fitzpatrick, C.; Fuller, L.C.; Izquierdo, B.G.; Hay, R.; et al. Integrated control and management of neglected tropical skin diseases. *PLoS Negl. Trop. Dis.* **2017**, *11*, e0005136. [CrossRef] [PubMed]
3. Ottesen, E.A.; Hooper, P.J.; Bradley, M.; Biswas, G. The Global Programme to Eliminate Lymphatic Filariasis: Health Impact after 8 Years. *PLoS Negl. Trop. Dis.* **2008**, *2*, e317. [CrossRef] [PubMed]
4. Romani, L.; Whitfeld, M.J.; Koroivueta, J.; Kama, M.; Wand, H.; Tikoduadua, L.; Tuicakau, M.; Koroi, A.; Andrews, R.; Kaldor, J.M.; et al. Mass Drug Administration for Scabies Control in a Population with Endemic Disease. *N. Engl. J. Med.* **2015**, *373*, 2305–2313. [CrossRef] [PubMed]
5. Marks, M.; Vahi, V.; Sokana, O.; Chi, K.H.; Puiahi, E.; Kilua, G.; Pillay, A.; Dalipanda, T.; Bottomley, C.; Solomon, A.W.; et al. Impact of Community Mass Treatment with Azithromycin for Trachoma Elimination on the Prevalence of Yaws. *PLoS Negl. Trop. Dis.* **2015**, *9*, e0003988. [CrossRef] [PubMed]
6. World Health Organization. Recognizing Neglected Tropical Diseases Through Changes on the Skin. A Training Guide for Front-Line Health Workers. 2018. Available online: https://www.who.int/neglected_diseases/resources/9789241513531/en/ (accessed on 11 December 2018).
7. World Health Organization Wound and Lymphoedema Integrated management 2010. Available online: Whqlibdoc.who.int/publications/2010/9789241599139_eng.pdf (accessed on 11 December 2018).
8. Stocks, M.; Freeman, M.C.; Addiss, D.G. The Effect of Hygiene-Based Lymphedema Management in Lymphatic Filariasis-Endemic Areas: A Systematic Review and Meta-analysis. *PLoS Negl. Trop. Dis.* **2015**, *9*, e0004171. [CrossRef]

9.   Abbas, M.; Scolding, P.S.; Yosif, A.A.; Rahman, R.F.E.; EL-Amin, M.O.; Elbashir, M.K.; Groce, N.; Fahal, A.H. The disabling consequences of mycetoma. *PLoS Negl. Trop. Dis.* **2018**, *12*, e0007019. [CrossRef] [PubMed]

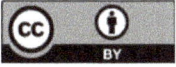

Tropical Medicine and
Infectious Disease

MDPI

Review

Potential Animal Reservoir of *Mycobacterium ulcerans*: A Systematic Review

Avishek Singh [1,*] ⬥, **William John Hannan McBride** [1] ⬥, **Brenda Govan** [2] **and Mark Pearson** [3]

1   Cairns Clinical School, College of Medicine and Dentistry, James Cook University, Cairns City, QLD 4870, Australia; john.mcbride@theiddoctor.com
2   College of Public Health, Medical & Vet Sciences, James Cook University, Townsville, QLD 4811, Australia; brenda.govan@jcu.edu.au
3   Australian Institute of Tropical Health & Medicine, James Cook University, Smithfield, QLD 4878, Australia; mark.pearson@jcu.edu.au
*   Correspondence: avishek.singh@my.jcu.edu.au; Tel.: +61-451-020-653

Received: 11 April 2018; Accepted: 24 May 2018; Published: 30 May 2018

Abstract: *Mycobacterium ulcerans* is the causative agent of Buruli ulcer, also known in Australia as Daintree ulcer or Bairnsdale ulcer. This destructive skin disease is characterized by extensive and painless necrosis of the skin and soft tissue with the formation of large ulcers, commonly on the leg or arm. To date, 33 countries with tropical, subtropical and temperate climates in Africa, the Americas, Asia and the Western Pacific have reported cases of Buruli ulcer. The disease is rarely fatal, although it may lead to permanent disability and/or disfigurement if not treated appropriately or in time. It is the third most common mycobacterial infection in the world after tuberculosis and leprosy. The precise mode of transmission of *M. ulcerans* is yet to be elucidated. Nevertheless, it is possible that the mode of transmission varies with different geographical areas and epidemiological settings. The knowledge about the possible routes of transmission and potential animal reservoirs of *M. ulcerans* is poorly understood and still remains patchy. Infectious diseases arise from the interaction of agent, host and environment. The majority of emerging or remerging infectious disease in human populations is spread by animals: either wildlife, livestock or pets. Animals may act as hosts or reservoirs and subsequently spread the organism to the environment or directly to the human population. The reservoirs may or may not be the direct source of infection for the hosts; however, they play a major role in maintenance of the organism in the environment, and in the mode of transmission. This remains valid for *M. ulcerans*. Possums have been suggested as one of the reservoir of *M. ulcerans* in south-eastern Australia, where possums ingest *M. ulcerans* from the environment, amplify them and shed the organism through their faeces. We conducted a systematic review with selected key words on PubMed and INFORMIT databases to aggregate available published data on animal reservoirs of *M. ulcerans* around the world. After certain inclusion and exclusion criteria were implemented, a total of 17 studies was included in the review. A variety of animals around the world e.g., rodents, shrews, possums (ringtail and brushtail), horses, dogs, alpacas, koalas and Indian flap-shelled turtles have been recorded as being infected with *M. ulcerans*. The majority of studies included in this review identified animal reservoirs as predisposing to the emergence and reemergence of *M. ulcerans* infection. Taken together, from the selected studies in this systematic review, it is clear that exotic wildlife and native mammals play a significant role as reservoirs for *M. ulcerans*.

Keywords: *Mycobacterium ulcerans*; animal reservoir; transmission

---

1. Introduction

Sir Albert Cook, a British missionary doctor appointed at the Mengo Hospital in Kampala, Uganda, first noted the skin ulcer caused by *Mycobacterium ulcerans* in 1896. Later, in the late 1930s, two general practitioners, Drs. J. R. Searl and D. G. Alsop, working in rural Victoria, Australia, noticed a group of cases of mysterious skin ulcers around the town of Bairnsdale [1]. The cases were not published in the literature at the time and the causative organism was not identified or characterized. Professor Peter MacCallum and his colleagues first provided the detailed description of the disease in 1948, using presentation data of six patients in the Bairnsdale district, near Melbourne. They were the first to isolate *M. ulcerans* as the causative organism of the mysterious skin ulcer [2]. The first large cluster of *M. ulcerans* infection was identified in the Buruli County of Uganda (now called Nakasongola District) in the 1960s and the disease was termed 'Buruli ulcer' (BU) thereafter [3].

There have been several known outbreaks of Buruli ulcer around the world and each outbreak has its own unique characteristics in terms of epidemiology and the animals reported to be involved in transmission [4,5]. The World Health Organization (WHO) has classified BU as a neglected tropical disease [6]. Presently, BU has been reported (but not always microbiologically confirmed) in more than 30 countries spread over Africa, the Americas, Asia, and Oceania [7]. Australia is the only developed country with significant local transmission of BU, with foci of infection in tropical Far North Queensland [8,9], the Capricorn Coast region of central Queensland [10], the Northern Territory [11] and temperate coastal Victoria [10]. Non-human cases of *M. ulcerans* are prevalent in Australia only, where several cases of BU have been described in both native wildlife and domestic mammal species such as koalas (*Phascolarctos cinereus*) [12,13], common ringtail possums (*Pseudocheirus peregrinus*) [14,15], a mountain brushtail possum (*Trichosurus cunninghami*) [5,14,15], two horses [16], an alpaca [17], four dogs [18] and a cat [19]. Recent research in Victoria, Australia, has suggested the transmission of infection by mosquitoes, and possums with chronic BU as an important environmental reservoir of *M. ulcerans* in Victoria [14].

2. Materials and Methods

The PRISMA guidelines developed by the Centre for Review Dissemination (CRD) were used as the methodology for the systematic review [20]. A review protocol was registered with PROSPERO international prospective register of systematic reviews, which can be viewed online [21]. The systematic literature review was conducted using online databases MEDLINE and INFORMIT to aggregate all the published literature. Initially, MEDLINE was used to retrieve all the scientific information concerning the research topic. INFORMIT was searched with same search strategies adopted for MEDLINE. The following key words were chosen after a series of trial searches in order to ensure an adequate number of relevant articles were reviewed: (Buruli OR '*Mycobacterium ulcerans*') AND (Host OR Vector OR Reservoir OR Animal), accessed on 6 May 2018. The title and abstract of each of the articles were initially scanned to ensure that the included articles met the aim and scope of the systematic review. Articles that were deemed irrelevant to the aim of this systematic review or out of the research scope were excluded. For those articles that were not clear by the title and abstract, the full text was retrieved and further analyzed in order to determine if they met the inclusion and exclusion criteria below. The studies that reported only experimental or laboratory exposure of *M. ulcerans* in animals were excluded. The search strategy exclusively focused on potential animal reservoirs, not the vectors. The detection of the causative agent had to be confirmed by culture of bacteria and/or PCR. To be considered positive a sample needed to be confirmed either by culture of bacteria or positive for IS 2404 and reconfirmed by KR and IS 2606. Undoubtedly, PCR targeting IS 2404 is highly specific for detecting *M. ulcerans* in clinical specimen [22]. However, for detecting *M. ulcerans* from environmental samples, confirmatory PCR targeting two additional insertion sequences, IS 2606 and the ketoreductase B domain (KR), is essential to differentiate *M. ulcerans* from other environmental mycobacteria that may carry IS 2404 and other non-mycolactone-producing mycobacteria [22]. Thus, IS 2404-PCR used in conjunction with IS 2606 and KR-PCR confirms that the detected organism is *M.*

ulcerans. There were no language restrictions. Risk of bias was assessed by one reviewer on the basis of independent factors such as sample size, location and nature of infection.

3. Results

3.1. Results of the Literature Search and Method of Inclusion

The total number of discovered articles in MEDLINE database was 351. Three hundred and fourteen articles were excluded after reading the title and abstracts as they were not relevant to the research question. Full texts of thirty-seven studies were retrieved in portable document format (PDF) for further analysis. Of these remaining 37 studies, 19 were excluded as they clearly did not meet inclusion criteria (i.e., they were review articles, focused on vectors rather than on animal reservoirs, or pertained to laboratory or experimental exposure). One additional duplicate article was excluded as well. The remaining 17 studies from the PubMed database were included for systematic review. There were no additional articles in INFORMIT that did not appear in the initial MEDLINE search results. The flow chart for study selection process is shown in Figure 1.

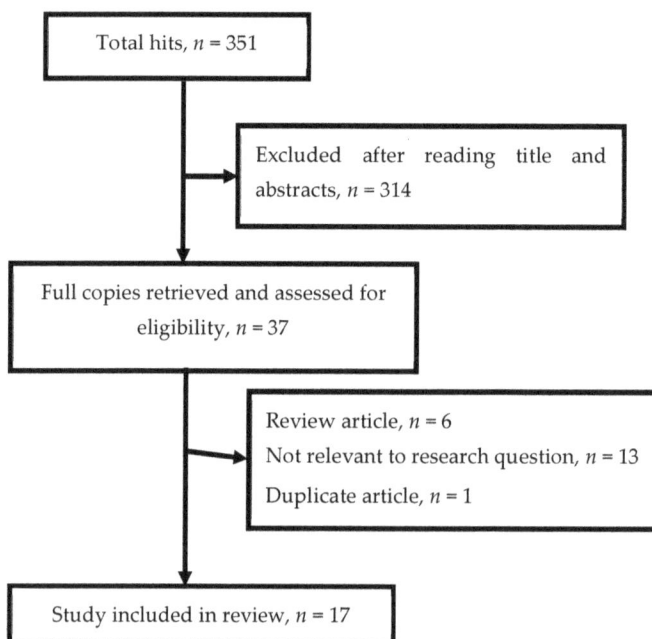

Figure 1. Flow chart of study selection process.

3.2. Basic Characteristics of Selected Studies

Out of the 17 included studies, ten were conducted in Australia, two in Ghana and one was conducted in each of Ivory Coast, North America, United States, Benin and Japan. The basic characteristics of selected studies for review are shown in Table 1 below.

Table 1. Basic characteristics of selected studies on occurrence of *Mycobacterium ulcerans*.

Author and Year	Sample and Sample Size	Collection Year, Location and Setting	Detection Method, Result or *M. ulcerans* Positive Signal
Rohlgen, Pluschke, Johnson, & Fyfe, 2017 [9]	102 environmental samples: 55 from soil/vegetation; 35 from insects or small insects pool and 12 from animal excreta	September 2013 Northern Queensland, Australia	RT-PCR IS 2404 positive: 1 soil specimen: 2 bandicoot faeces, one individual mosquito and 1 pool of 2 mosquitoes IS 2606 and KR (ketoreductase) positive: 2 bandicoot faeces and pool of two mosquitoes
Tobias et al., 2016 [23]	180 faecal specimens from dominant domestic animals (ovine, porcine, avian, reptiles, canine)	September 2013 4 BU-endemic and one non-endemic villages of Ghana, West Africa	RT-PCR IS 2404 positive: 2/86 ovine; 1/69 avian: 1/16 reptiles IS 2606 and KR: all negative
Tian, Niamke, Tissot-Dupont, &Drancourt, 2016 [24]	496 environmental samples: 100 from soil (endemic n = 50 and non-endemic n = 50); 200 from stagnant water (endemic n = 100 and non-endemic n = 100); 100 from plants (endemic n = 50 and non-endemic n = 50) and 96 animal faeces (*Thryonomys swinderianus* (agouti) stools) (endemic n = 48 and non-endemic n = 48)	June–October 2014 Ivory Coast, West Africa	RT-PCR 43 samples with at least one positive IS 2404 and KR Out of 43, only 10 positive for both IS2404 and KR, IS 2606 not performed: 7 water specimen; 2 *T. swinderianus* (agouti) faeces and one soil specimen
Carson et al., 2014 [5]	Fecal sample: 216 common ringtail possums and 6 common brushtail possums	Southeast Australia, State Victoria	RT-PCR targeting IS 2404, IS 2606 and KR 20 common ringtail possums and 4 common brushtail possums
O Brien et al., 2014 [15]	69 possums (ringtail and brushtail) trapped at Point Lonsdale: Faecal samples: 57; blood samples: 63; buccal swab: 67; urine sample: 16; pouch swab: 15; cloacal swab: 20 69 fecal samples from 15 mountain brushtail possums	1998–2011 Victoria, Australia	RT-PCR targeting IS 2404, IS 2606 and KR Point Lonsdale: Positive: faecal sample: 12 (25%); blood sample: 0; buccal swab: 7 (16%); urine sample: 0; pouch swab: 3 (20%) Bellbird Creek: Positive: 4 mountain brushtail possums (27%)
C. O'Brien et al., 2013 [17]	Case report: two alpacas (*Vicugna pacos*) ulcerated tissue	Case 1: September 1997 Case 2: May 2011 Victoria, Australia	RT-PCR targeting IS 2404, IS 2606 and KR positive
Willson et al., 2013 [25]	587 fish representing 13 genera and 17 species and 351 amphibians representing 10 genera: external swab	2008–2009 Ghana, West Africa	RT-PCR targeting IS 2606 and KR not performed. Not confirmed
C. R. O'Brien et al., 2011 [18]	Case report: Case 1: 14 months old female kelpie Case 2: 3 years old female kelpie Case 3: 6 years old male whippet Case 4: 3 years old male koolie	2011 Victoria, Australia	RT-PCR targeting IS 2404, IS 2606 and KR All 4 dogs positive for *M. ulcerans*
Sakaguchi et al., 2011 [26]	Case report; Indian flap-shelled turtle, *Lissemys punctata punctata*	Imported from India to aquarium in Japan	PCR assays targeting the *rpoβ* gene: unable to differentiate *M. ulcerans* from mycolactone-producing *M. marinum* (MPMM)

Table 1. *Cont.*

Author and Year	Sample and Sample Size	Collection Year, Location and Setting	Detection Method, Result or *M. ulcerans* Positive Signal
Fyfe et al., 2010 [14]	589 fecal samples from ringtail possums and 250 samples from brushtail possums. Live trapping: 42 ringtail possums and 21 brushtail possums	2007–2009 Victoria, Australia	RT-PCR targeting IS 2404, IS 2606 and KR *M. ulcerans* DNA detected in 43% of ringtail possum and 29% of brushtail possum faecal samples. 38% ringtail possum have *M. ulcerans* lesion and/or positive faeces Lower in brushtail possums: 1 with *M. ulcerans* lesion and/or positive faeces and 4 with no lesions and low *M. ulcerans* DNA in faeces.
Durnez et al., 2010 [27]	565 small mammals: 326 rodents and 222 shrews	2006 Benin, West Africa	RT-PCR: No *M. ulcerans* specific DNA detected
Van Zyl et al., 2010 [16]	2 horses: Case report Case 1: 21-year-old quarterhorse-cross Case 2: 32-year-old standard bredgelding	Case 1: May 2006 Case 2: October 2006 Southeastern Australia	RT-PCR *M. ulcerans* specific DNA detected from both horses
Elsner et al., 2008 [19]	Cat: Case report 10-year-old castrated male domestic cat	2006 Victoria, Australia	RT-PCR *M. ulcerans* specific DNA detected
Appleyard & Clark, 2002 [28]	Case report: three cats Case 1: An 8-year-old spayed female shorthair Case 2: 6-year-old spayed female shorthair Case 3: 11-year-old domestic longhair cat	2002 North America	PCR Could not differentiate *M. ulcerans* from other *Mycobacterium* spp. (a new *Mycobacterial* spp. namely '*Mycobacterium visibilis*' suggested)
Heckert, Elankumaran, Milani, &Baya, 2001 [29]	60 wild striped bass: Swab from external ulcerative dermatitis and granulomatous-like lesions in the internal organs	1997 Chesapeake Bay, USA	PCR No *M. ulcerans* specific DNA detected (a new mycobacterial spp. suggested)
Mitchell, McOrist, &Bilney, 1987 [13]	36 male and 51 female adult koalas captured	1980–1985 Raymond Island, southeastern Australia	Pathological and bacteriological examination 18 out of 87 captured koalas had skin wound 11 koalas were found positive for *M. ulcerans*
McOrist, Jerrett, Anderson, & Hayman, 1985 [12]	Case study: 2 koalas: one male and one female Ulcerated tissue	1982 Raymond Island, southeastern Australia	Pathological and bacteriological examination Both koalas suggested positive for *M. ulcerans*

4. Discussion on Possible Reservoirs and Vectors of *Mycobacterium ulcerans* by Country

This systematic review assessed the potential animal reservoir of *M. ulcerans* around the world recorded to date. This is essential for understanding the epidemiology and mode of transmission of the disease, which subsequently aids in prevention, control and elimination strategies.

4.1. Australia

Out of 17 studies included in this review, 10 were conducted in Australia. In Australia, the disease is more prevalent in the southeastern state of Victoria and in Far North Queensland. After the detection of *M. ulcerans* infection in four koalas in 1980 at Raymond Island, Australia [13], the entire island was searched for koalas in the following year. Thirty-six male and 51 female koalas were captured and examined. Of these, 18 out of 87 animals had skin wounds and 11 were found positive for *M. ulcerans*. Diagnosis was made on pathological and bacteriological examination; the PCR-based method used for the identification of *M. ulcerans* from clinical and environmental samples was only implemented in 1996 [30]. Non-human cases of *M. ulcerans* in Australia have been reported in marsupial species such as koalas [13], ringtail and brushtail possums [14,15,31], horses [16], alpacas [17], dogs [18] and cats [19]. A study conducted by Fyfe and colleagues between 2007–2009, at Point Lonsdale, a small coastal town south east of Melbourne, Australia, which is also endemic for BU, found that 43% of ringtail possum and 29% of brushtail possum faecal samples were positive for *M. ulcerans* DNA [14]. Only 1% of faecal samples from non-endemic area possums were positive for *M. ulcerans* DNA in this study, suggesting terrestrial mammals such as possums are potential reservoirs of *M. ulcerans* in southeast Australia. Several studies have identified possums (both ringtail and brushtail) as potential reservoirs since then [5,15]. In Australia, other than the southeastern state of Victoria, BU is also prevalent in Far North Queensland [8]. Inspired by the evidence of possums as potential reservoirs of *M. ulcerans* in Victoria, a study conducted by Roltgen and colleagues (2013) in northern Queensland, Australia, detected *M. ulcerans* DNA from two bandicoot faecal samples, suggesting the possibility that bandicoots are a potential reservoir of *M. ulcerans* in Far North Queensland [9].

4.2. Africa

Out of the 17 studies included in this review, four were conducted in West African countries: two in Ghana [23,25], one in the Ivory Coast [24] and one in Benin [27]. Durnez and colleagues (2006) caught 326 rodents and 222 shrews from endemic and non-endemic villages of Benin and tested for *M. ulcerans*, but no specific DNA was detected from any of their samples [27]. Despite their results, they suggested the necessity of more intensive research focusing on small mammals in Africa. Willson reported positive PCR with IS 2404 only from tadpoles and fishes from Ghana [25]. Similarly, two faecal specimens from *Thryonomys swinderianus* (agouti) were reported positive for *M. ulcerans* in a study conducted by Bi Diangoné Tian and colleagues (2014) from the Ivory Coast [24]. They suggested agouti, which are closely related to Australian possums, could be a potential reservoir of *M. ulcerans* in Africa. However, RT-PCR targeting IS 2606 was not conducted to confirm *M. ulcerans*. A faecal survey of domestic animals in rural Ghana for *M. ulcerans* conducted by Tobias and associates suggested no evidence of association between domestic animals and *M. ulcerans* in endemic and non-endemic villages in Ghana [23]. Unlike Australia, not a single study in Africa has reported the presence of *M. ulcerans*-positive DNA or cases in non-human species, suggesting that transmission dynamics may be different in Africa and Australia or, alternatively, a host animal is yet to be identified in Africa.

4.3. Other Countries

No study has reported *M. ulcerans* DNA or cases in non-human species in any country other than Australia. A study conducted by Heckert in 1997 at Chesapeake Bay, USA detected a new *Mycobacterium* species from wild striped bass [29]. This new isolate was closely related to *M. marinum*, *M. ulcerans*, and *M. tuberculosis*. Similarly, Sakaguchi and associates reported an atypical

Trop. Med. Infect. Dis. **2018**, *3*, 56

mycobacterial infection in an Indian flap-shelled turtle (*Lissemys punctata punctata*), imported from India to Japan in an aquarium [26]. A PCR assay targeting the *rpoβ* gene revealed the isolate had 89–100% homology to *M. ulcerans* and *M. marinum*. Again, this study could not differentiate *M. ulcerans* from mycolactone-producing *M. marinum* (MPMM). Appleyard and Clark (2002) reported a new *Mycobacterial* species, namely '*Mycobacterium visibilis*' from three cats initially suspected of having *M. ulcerans* infection [28].

5. Conclusions

Human cases of BU have been reported in more than 30 countries from Africa, America, Asia and Oceania. Since the implementation of PCR-based methods for the detection and identification of *M. ulcerans* from clinical and environmental samples, there has been a significant increase in overall knowledge of BU. There is no record of direct human-to-human transmission of *M. ulcerans*, unlike tuberculosis and leprosy. Australia is the only country where non-human cases of BU have been identified, with small mammals, especially possums and, to some extent, bandicoots, being implicated as potential reservoirs of *M. ulcerans*. Despite there having been several outbreaks in African countries, no non-human cases have been recorded so far and there is no evidence of any animal acting as a potential reservoir for this organism. None of the studies included in this review discussed strain variation of *M. ulcerans* in different geographical regions leading to an increase or decrease in susceptibility among animal or human population. Compared to other mycobacteria, such as *M. tuberculosis*, there is very little genetic diversity among isolates of *M. ulcerans*. Some variation among the strains of *M. ulcerans* from Africa, the Americas, Asia and the Western Pacific has been recorded; however, the linkage between these various strains and virulence in human or animal population has not been recognized so far. Remarkable differences in the type of mycolactone produced by *M. ulcerans* in different geographical location has been recorded. African strains produce more mycolactone variant A and B, whereas strains from Australia produce more mycolactone variant C. However, this variation has nothing to do with host susceptibility to *M. ulcerans*; rather, it determines cytopathogenecity and thus clinical presentation of disease.

This systematic review suggests the need for extensive laboratory and field research focusing on domestic animals and wildlife to elucidate their roles in BU-endemic countries.

Author Contributions: A.S. and W.J.H.M. designed the study. A.S. collected and analyzed the data. A.S. wrote the paper with input from all authors. All authors reviewed the final manuscript.

Funding: This research was funded by Far North Queensland Hospital Foundation, College of Medicine and Dentistry, James Cook University (JCU-QLD-730121).

Acknowledgments: The authors would like to acknowledge Janet A. Fyfe, Victorian Infectious Diseases Reference Laboratory, Melbourne, VIC 3000, Australia, for her continuous support and feedback. We would like to thank Far North Queensland Hospital Foundation and James Cook University for funding this research.

Conflicts of Interest: The authors declare no conflict of interest.

References

1. Alsop, D.G. The Bairnsdale ulcer. *Aust. N. Z. J. Surg.* **1972**, *41*, 317–319. [CrossRef] [PubMed]
2. MacCallum, P.T.J.C.; Tolhurst, J.C.; Buckle, G.; Sissons, H.A. A new mycobacterial infection in man. *J. Pathol. Bacteriol.* **1948**, *60*, 93–122. [CrossRef] [PubMed]
3. Clancey, J.; Dodge, R.; Lunn, H.F. Study of a *Mycobacterium* causing skin ulceration in Uganda. *Ann. Soc. Belg. Med. Trop.* **1920**, *42*, 585–590.
4. Johnson, P.D.; Azuolas, J.; Lavender, C.J.; Wishart, E.; Stinear, T.P.; Hayman, J.A.; Brown, L.; Jenkin, G.A.; Fyfe, J.A. *Mycobacterium ulcerans* in mosquitoes captured during outbreak of Buruli ulcer, southeastern Australia. *Emerg. Infect. Dis.* **2007**, *13*, 1653–1660. [CrossRef] [PubMed]
5. Carson, C.; Lavender, C.J.; Handasyde, K.A.; O'Brien, C.R.; Hewitt, N.; Johnson, P.D.; Fyfe, J.A. Potential wildlife sentinels for monitoring the endemic spread of human Buruli ulcer in south-east Australia. *PLoS Negl. Trop. Dis.* **2014**, *8*, e2668. [CrossRef] [PubMed]

6. World Health Organization. Neglected Tropical Diseases. 2018. Available online: http://www.who.int/neglected_diseases/diseases/en/ (accessed on 4 October 2017).
7. World Health Organization. *Distribution of Buruli Ulcer, Worldwide 2014*; WHO: Geneva, Switzerland, 2014.
8. Steffen, C.M.; Smith, M.; McBride, W.J. *Mycobacterium ulcerans* infection in North Queensland: The 'Daintree ulcer'. *ANZ J. Surg.* **2010**, *80*, 732–736. [CrossRef] [PubMed]
9. Röltgen, K.; Pluschke, G.; Johnson, P.D.; Fyfe, J. *Mycobacterium ulcerans* DNA in bandicoot excreta in Buruli ulcer-endemic area, northern Queensland, Australia. *Emerg. Infect. Dis.* **2017**, *23*, 2042–2045. [CrossRef] [PubMed]
10. Francis, G.; Whitby, M.; Woods, M. *Mycobacterium ulcerans* infection: A rediscovered focus in the Capricorn Coast region of central Queensland. *Med. J. Aust.* **2006**, *185*, 179–180. [PubMed]
11. Radford, A.J. *Mycobacterium ulcerans* in Australia. *Aust. N. Z. J. Med.* **1975**, *5*, 162–169. [CrossRef] [PubMed]
12. McOrist, S.; Jerrett, I.V.; Anderson, M.; Hayman, J. Cutaneous and respiratory tract infection with *Mycobacterium ulcerans* in two koalas (*Phascolarctos cinereus*). *J. Wildl. Dis.* **1985**, *21*, 171–173. [CrossRef] [PubMed]
13. Mitchell, P.J.; McOrist, S.; Bilney, R. Epidemiology of *Mycobacterium ulcerans* infection in koalas (*Phascolarctos cinereus*) on Raymond Island, southeastern Australia. *J. Wildl. Dis.* **1987**, *23*, 386–390. [CrossRef] [PubMed]
14. Fyfe, J.A.; Lavender, C.J.; Handasyde, K.A.; Legione, A.R.; O'Brien, C.R.; Stinear, T.P.; Pidot, S.J.; Seemann, T.; Benbow, M.E.; Wallace, J.R.; et al. A major role for mammals in the ecology of *Mycobacterium ulcerans*. *PLoS Negl. Trop. Dis.* **2010**, *4*, e791. [CrossRef] [PubMed]
15. O'Brien, C.R.; Handasyde, K.A.; Hibble, J.; Lavender, C.J.; Legione, A.R.; McCowan, C.; Globan, M.; Mitchell, A.T.; McCracken, H.E.; Johnson, P.D.; et al. Clinical, microbiological and pathological findings of *Mycobacterium ulcerans* infection in three Australian possum species. *PLoS Negl. Trop. Dis.* **2014**, *8*, e2666. [CrossRef] [PubMed]
16. van Zyl, A.; Daniel, J.; Wayne, J.; McCowan, C.; Malik, R.; Jelfs, P.; Lavender, C.J.; Fyfe, J.A. *Mycobacterium ulcerans* infections in two horses in south-eastern Australia. *Aust. Vet. J.* **2010**, *88*, 101–106. [CrossRef] [PubMed]
17. O'Brien, C.; Kuseff, G.; McMillan, E.; McCowan, C.; Lavender, C.; Globan, M.; Jerrett, I.; Oppedisano, F.; Johnson, P.; Fyfe, J. *Mycobacterium ulcerans* infection in two alpacas. *Aust. Vet. J.* **2013**, *91*, 296–300. [CrossRef] [PubMed]
18. O'Brien, C.R.; McMillan, E.; Harris, O.; O'Brien, D.P.; Lavender, C.J.; Globan, M.; Legione, A.R.; Fyfe, J.A. Localised *Mycobacterium ulcerans* infection in four dogs. *Aust. Vet. J.* **2011**, *89*, 506–510. [CrossRef] [PubMed]
19. Elsner, L.; Wayne, J.; O'Brien, C.R.; McCowan, C.; Malik, R.; Hayman, J.A.; Globan, M.; Lavender, C.J.; Fyfe, J.A. Localised *Mycobacterium ulcerans* infection in a cat in Australia. *J. Feline Med. Surg.* **2008**, *10*, 407–412. [CrossRef] [PubMed]
20. Moher, D.; Liberati, A.; Tetzlaff, J.; Altman, D.G.; Prisma Group. Preferred reporting items for systematic reviews and meta-analyses: The PRISMA statement. *Int. J. Surg.* **2010**, *8*, 336–341.
21. PROSPERO Registered Study Protocol. Available online: https://www.crd.york.ac.uk/prospero/display_record.php?RecordID=85484 (accessed on 12 January 2018).
22. Fyfe, J.A.; Lavender, C.J.; Johnson, P.D.; Globan, M.; Sievers, A.; Azuolas, J.; Stinear, T.P. Development and application of two multiplex real-time PCR assays for the detection of *Mycobacterium ulcerans* in clinical and environmental samples. *Appl. Environ. Microbiol.* **2007**, *73*, 4733–4740. [CrossRef] [PubMed]
23. Tobias, N.J.; Ammisah, N.A.; Ahortor, E.K.; Wallace, J.R.; Ablordey, A.; Stinear, T.P. Snapshot faecal survey of domestic animals in rural Ghana for *Mycobacterium ulcerans*. *PeerJ* **2016**, *4*, e2065. [CrossRef] [PubMed]
24. Tian, R.B.; Niamké, S.; Tissot-Dupont, H.; Drancourt, M. Detection of *Mycobacterium ulcerans* DNA in the environment, Ivory Coast. *PLoS ONE* **2016**, *11*, e0151567. [CrossRef] [PubMed]
25. Willson, S.J.; Kaufman, M.G.; Merritt, R.W.; Williamson, H.R.; Malakauskas, D.M.; Benbow, M.E. Fish and amphibians as potential reservoirs of *Mycobacterium ulcerans*, the causative agent of Buruli ulcer disease. *Infect. Ecol. Epidemiol.* **2013**, *3*, 19946. [CrossRef] [PubMed]
26. Sakaguchi, K.; Iima, H.; Hirayama, K.; Okamoto, M.; Matsuda, K.; Miyasho, T.; Kasamatsu, M.; Hasegawa, K.; Taniyama, H. *Mycobacterium ulcerans* infection in an Indian flap-shelled turtle (*Lissemys punctata punctata*). *J. Vet. Med. Sci.* **2011**, *73*, 1217–1220. [CrossRef] [PubMed]

27. Durnez, L.; Suykerbuyk, P.; Nicolas, V.; Barriere, P.; Verheyen, E.; Johnson, C.R.; Leirs, H.; Portaels, F. Terrestrial small mammals as reservoirs of *Mycobacterium ulcerans* in Benin. *Appl. Environ. Microbiol.* **2010**, *76*, 4574–4577. [CrossRef] [PubMed]

28. Appleyard, G.D.; Clark, E.G. Histologic and genotypic characterization of a novel *Mycobacterium* species found in three cats. *J. Clin. Microbiol.* **2002**, *40*, 2425–2430. [CrossRef] [PubMed]

29. Heckert, R.A.; Elankumaran, S.; Milani, A.; Baya, A. Detection of a new *Mycobacterium* species in wild striped bass in the Chesapeake Bay. *J. Clin. Microbiol.* **2001**, *39*, 710–715. [CrossRef] [PubMed]

30. Ross, B.C.; Marino, L.; Oppedisano, F.; Edwards, R.; Robins-Browne, R.M.; Johnson, P.D. Development of a PCR assay for rapid diagnosis of *Mycobacterium ulcerans* infection. *J. Clin. Microbiol.* **1997**, *35*, 1696–1700. [PubMed]

31. Portaels, F.; Hibble, J. *Mycobacterium ulcerans* in wild animals. *Rev. Sci. Technol.* **2001**, *20*, 252–264. [CrossRef]

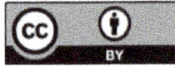

Tropical Medicine and Infectious Disease

MDPI

Case Report

Cushing Syndrome due to Inappropriate Corticosteroid Topical Treatment of Undiagnosed Scabies

Guadalupe Estrada-Chávez [1], Roberto Estrada [2], Daniel Engelman [3], Jesus Molina [4] and Guadalupe Chávez-López [5,*]

[1] Department of Dermatology and Dermato-Oncology, Instituto Estatal de Cancerología "Dr. Arturo Beltrán Ortega", Health Secretary Guerrero, Faculty of Medicine, Universidad Autónoma de Guerrero Mexico, Community Dermatology Mexico C.A., 39850 Acapulco, Guerrero, Mexico; estradaguadalupe@hotmail.com
[2] Community Dermatology Mexico C.A.; Health Secretary Guerrero, 39355 Acapulco, Guerrero, Mexico; restrada_13@hotmail.com
[3] Centre for International Child Health, University of Melbourne, Melbourne, Australia/Group A Streptococcal Research, Murdoch Children's Research Institute, 3010 Melbourne, Australia; Daniel.Engelman@rch.org.au
[4] Department of Pediatrics, Acapulco General Hospital, Health Secretary Guerrero, 39901 Acapulco, Guerrero, Mexico; molinabravo@prodigy.net.mx
[5] Department of Dermatology and Mycology Acapulco General Hospital, Health Secretary Guerrero, Community Dermatology Mexico C.A., 39355 Acapulco, Guerrero, Mexico
* Correspondence: chavezg13@live.com.mx; Tel.: +52-(744)-4865162

Received: 26 June 2018; Accepted: 24 July 2018; Published: 3 August 2018

Abstract: The uncontrolled sale of topical corticosteroids has become an important risk factor for the development of iatrogenic Cushing syndrome in children, especially in countries where medications are sold over the counter. This is exacerbated by the lack of information for both the patients and pharmacists. This report documents a series of eight cases of iatrogenic Cushing syndrome secondary to an inappropriate use of topical steroids, due to a misdiagnosis of scabies.

Keywords: scabies; Cushing syndrome; iatrogenic; topical corticosteroids

---

1. Introduction

Scabies is a highly contagious skin disease caused by the mite *Sarcoptes scabiei* var. *hominis*. Transmission mainly occurs through direct skin contact, often from family members. Scabies is estimated to affect 200 million people worldwide [1]. Reported prevalence rates vary from 0.3–46% [2], with the highest prevalence rate observed in children in tropical countries. Predisposed factors include heat, humidity, overcrowding and increased contact with exposed skin areas [3]. Common (also known as typical or classical) scabies is highly symptomatic, with an intense itch and a rash consisting of discrete to moderate disseminated papules. These are secondary to the antigen released by the parasite and subsequent immune and inflammatory reactions. Other family members frequently have similar symptoms. Crusted scabies is a rarer form of the disease, usually affecting immunosuppressed patients, and presents with hyperkeratotic skin lesions containing thousands of mites.

In Mexico, a common superstition suggests that infants can develop illness if they are not held by a person who gazes at them, as it puts the infant at risk of acquiring 'the evil eye'. Therefore, parents commonly encourage others, even complete strangers, to touch and hold their child [4]. There is also a general lack of awareness that prolonged contact with an infected person can be the cause of scabies or other infectious diseases. Instead, dogs, cats or poor quality of water are often blamed as the cause of the disease. Once a child becomes unwell, parents commonly use household remedies or medications obtained at local pharmacies, where employees may not have any medical or pharmacological training. As many inflammatory dermatological conditions will respond to topical corticosteroids, these are frequently purchased by patients without consultation with a clinician. Topical corticosteroids are known to exacerbate some conditions, particularly infections such as tinea and scabies [5,6].

Topical steroids are graded in terms of potency as either low, medium, high or very high. Whilst low potency steroids are often well tolerated, the absorption of higher potency steroids through the skin can cause Cushing syndrome due to suppression of the hypothalamic-pituitary-adrenal axis, especially if used over large areas of skin, or for prolonged periods [7,8]. In Mexico, topical steroids at all potencies are available without medical prescription over the counter. One of those most commonly sold products is a combination cream containing betamethasone (0.5%), clotrimazole, and gentamicin. The cost is approximately 1.5 USD per 25 g tube [9]. In recent times, high potency combination steroid creams have been widely promoted in Mexico on television, bus advertising, social media and on-site at pharmacies. Even though steroids are used widely in dermatology, their misuse for the treatment of scabies has become increasingly common and problematic in the last 2 to 3 years, causing severe medical problems that deserve wider recognition and prevention.

Permethrin is the most effective topical treatment for scabies, but, it is expensive, which limits its use in Mexico. Other topical treatments for scabies include benzyl benzoate (the most widely available in Mexico), sulfur cream or ointment, crotamiton and lindane [10]. Topical treatments frequently cause adverse effects, including contact dermatitis, erythema, and a worsening itch, which can lead to the early suspension of treatment, intermittent usage and a high frequency of relapse. Ivermectin is an effective oral treatment but is unavailable in many settings. Furthermore, although treatment of all close contacts is recommended, family members and other contacts may be asymptomatic or otherwise reluctant to be treated, further encouraging reinfestation [11].

2. Case Series

This report documents a series of cases involving eight infants, aged from 3 months to 1.5 years (Table A1). All patients clinical signs of Cushing syndrome, including increased adiposity, prominent cheeks, mild to moderate hirsutism on the forehead and side brows, discrete striae and telangiectasias. One patient had such significant weight gain that she lost the ability to support her own body weight. All patients also had disseminated lesions of scabies, with papules, scaling and nodules predominantly in skin folds and the soles of their feet. Two infants had the severe form of crusted scabies.

All cases had a history of continuous or discontinuous use of topical corticosteroids (betamethasone (0.5%) combined with clotrimazole and gentamicin), applied to affected lesions or used on the entire body's surface.

All scabies patients were diagnosed at the Dermatology department of the Acapulco General Hospital in Guerrero, Mexico. Diagnosis was made clinically in all patients based on the typical rash, itch and affected cohabitants. The patients with crusted scabies had extensive scaling lesions on the back, palms and soles with moderate papules and discrete nodules on the rest of the body's surface, particularly in the skin folds. Symptoms of scabies had been present for 1 to 7 months prior to diagnosis. In all cases, the mothers also had clinical lesions of scabies, and in four of eight cases, the mothers had a history that was suggestive of scabies during pregnancy. The number of family members in each household that had daily contact with the patients ranged from 3 to 12. In all cases, the use of the steroid cream was reported to have resulted in initial improvement of symptoms. However, the signs and symptoms would return and worsen whenever the usage of corticosteroid was suspended. Affected family members did not seek medical advice until symptoms worsened. None of the parents were aware that the weight gain and other physical signs of Cushing syndrome were related to the use of the steroid cream. Two patients experienced recurrent upper pulmonary infections during the use of topical steroids that required referral to a physician.

All patients were treated with sulfur cream (4%). Family contacts were treated with oral ivermectin. Twenty-four-hour urine cortisol was requested for patients, but this was often not completed in the majority of cases due to lack of financial resources. One case had the investigation performed one month after cessation of betamethasone, which was reported to be within normal limits.

Follow-up information for patients was limited by the fact that families resided in distant places. All patients were referred to the pediatric service, while two attended for a consultation, with no further complications found. The rest of the patients did not attend a consultation, possibly due to the resolution of scabies symptoms after effective treatment and cessation of steroids. A telephone contact follow-up was attempted but unsuccessful. A check of the patients' hospital files did not reveal any further visits for outpatient consultation or to the emergency department.

3. Discussion

Scabies has recently been added to the list of Neglected Tropical Diseases designated as priorities for control by the World Health Organization [12]. Organizations like the International Alliance for the Control of Scabies have focused on building the evidence base and advocacy strategy for the global control of scabies. This is because of the disease's frequency, global burden, complications and effects on already disadvantaged populations [13]. Whilst common scabies, without secondary bacterial infection, is not life threatening and can be treated simply in many patients, this case series demonstrates that the uncontrolled and chronic use of high potency steroids, including clobetasol and betamethasone, can lead to potentially harmful complications such as Cushing syndrome and other endocrine disorders as well as the development of crusted scabies [7,14]. Patients with crusted scabies have intense scaling on the palms and soles and numerous nodular lesions on axillary and inguinal folds as well as on the scrotum for boys and diaper rim on the waist [15] (Figure A3). Topical or systemic glucocorticoids should be used with caution and never as a treatment for scabies in children.

There are many factors that contribute to the development of Cushing syndrome in this case series and the many other cases we have observed in our practice. Scabies is often not accurately diagnosed, particularly as a medical opinion is not sought after by families, which leads to erroneous treatment. Scabies has recently re-emerged as a major health problem in parts of Mexico, and families are searching for effective treatments for this highly symptomatic disease. At the same time, over-the-counter creams have been promoted to pharmacies and general practitioners as low-cost treatments for a broad range of bacterial, mycotic and inflammatory skin conditions. Previously, steroid-misuse complications have been widely reported, but most reports relate to either eczema in developed countries or to skin lightening creams or fungal infections in underdeveloped countries [5,16]. Patients with scabies may consider these treatments to be cost effective due to the rapid (initial) relief of itch and desire to avoid the cost of medical consultation [17].

Parents may not recognize the rapid weight gain as one of the signs of the infant's developing health problem [4], due to the common belief that 'a fat baby is a healthy one', which leads to reassuring and positive comments on the infant's appearance from friends and family members [18,19].

The incidence of Cushing syndrome secondary from the use of topical steroids is unknown and quite likely underreported [8,20–22]. In addition to the inappropriate treatment of scabies and other skin disorders (including diaper rash, psoriasis, tineas or inflammatory diseases) causing iatrogenic Cushing syndrome, there are reports of Cushing syndrome being caused by inappropriate steroid use for ophthalmologic conditions including cataracts and glaucoma [23]. These risks reinforce the importance of reporting the steroid-related consequences and secondary effects. Further reporting and investigation of these issues may increase awareness amongst health workers and organizations which will lead to advocacy for the regulation and restriction of cortisone-containing products in Mexico and other countries experiencing this issue [24–26].

Sulfur and benzyl benzoate are the most available topical scabies treatments in Mexico. Even though they are effective if applied to the whole body for the recommended duration, they frequently cause irritation, erythema, scaling, intense pruritus or even contact dermatitis, all of which may lead to the interruption of treatment or discontinuous therapy, which ultimately reduces the effectiveness of the treatment. Alternative treatments for scabies, such as tea tree oil, are under investigation but their effectiveness is unproven [27]. Economical and effective treatments are still needed in resource-limited countries, where family income is usually reserved for food, housing and clothing which leaves non-life-threating diseases as lower priorities [28].

The education of health workers is of great importance, as they are the point of first contact. Health workers need to know how to recognize, diagnose and appropriately treat common scabies, and to avoid the use of corticosteroids, especially in children. Complicated cases, or those that do not improve with first-line treatments, should be referred for further assessment. In countries like Mexico, in which there are fewer regulations on the sale of medications, it is essential to inform the general population of the potential risks when medications are not used as intended.

We have introduced teledermatology as part of the Community Dermatology program in Mexico [29] for the education of health workers and doctors in isolated communities. This approach promotes improvements in clinical diagnosis and treatment and can be used to reduce the number of complicated cases. Greater awareness and action are needed for the widespread health problems related to the inappropriate use of steroids [30].

4. Ethical Considerations

The study protocol was approved by the Ethical Review Committee of the Community Dermatology A.C. and was supported by the Health Secretary of Guerrero State prior to the study. Informed consent was obtained from the parents or legal guardians of the minors after a detailed explanation of the study's protocol. In accordance with the ethical review committee requirements, patient information was made confidential.

Author Contributions: Conceptualization, methodology, investigation: G.E.C., R.E., G.C.L., J.M., D.E.; Writing-original draft preparation: G.E.C.; Writing-review & editing, supervision: D.E., G.E.C.

Funding: This research received no external funding.

Acknowledgments: We would like to thank the students of the Faculty of Medicine of the University of Guerrero (UAGro.) as well as the team of Telemedicine of the Acapulco General Hospital for their support in identifying and referral of some of the patients. We would like to thank Hay for his review of the manuscript.

Conflicts of Interest: The authors declare no conflict of interest.

Appendix A

Table A1. Cases of scabies and iatrogenic Cushing syndrome.

	Age (Months)	Sex	Topical Steroid Treatment			Clinical Features		
			Usage Duration	Frequency	Regularity	Adiposity	Scabies	Symptom Duration
1	5	Female	1 month	4 times a day	Continuous	+++	Crusted	1 month
2	6	Female	5 months	1–2 times a day	Intermittent	+++	Common	6 months
3	7	Male	3 months	2 times a day	Continuous	++++	Common	3 months
4	7	Male	2 months	2–3 times a day	Intermittent	+++	Common	7 months
5	8	Male	8 months	Daily	Continuous	++++	Crusted	8 months
6	9	Female	1 month	3 times a day	Continuous	++++	Common	6 months
7	16	Male	5 months	Daily	Continuous	++	Common	6 months
8	17	Female	4 months	1–2 times a day	Discontinuous	++	Common	3 months

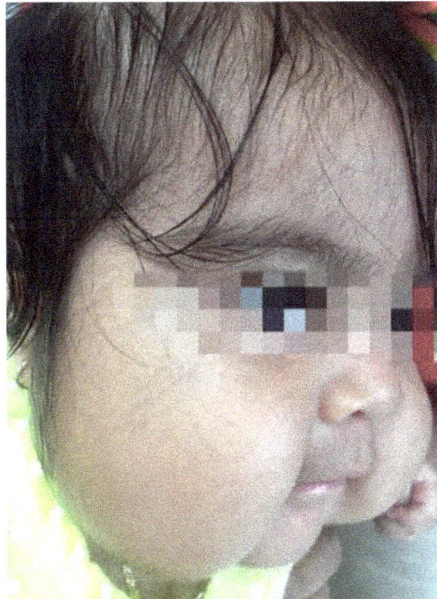

Figure A1. Infant with increased adiposity and forehead hirsutism.

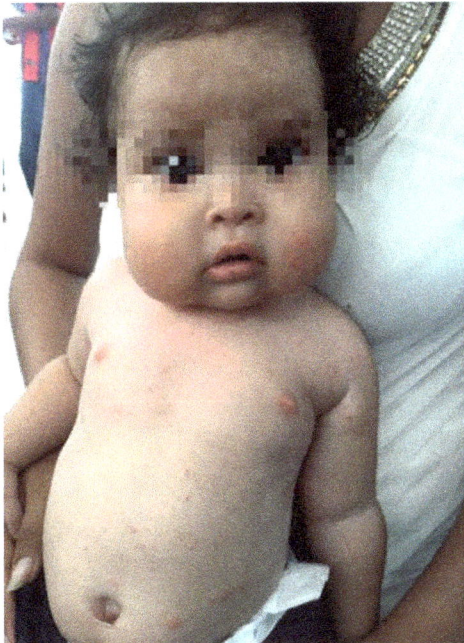

Figure A2. Prominent cheeks, mild telagiectasias and disseminated papulo-nodular lesions.

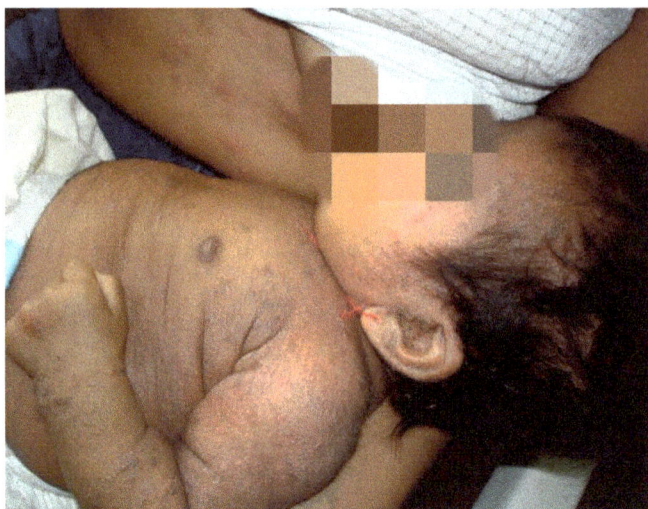

Figure A3. Crusted scabies with intense scaling and nodular lesions in child and mother with scabies.

References

1. Karimkhani, C.; Colombara, D.; Drucker, A.M.; Hay, R.; Engelman, D.; Steer, A.; Whitfield, M.; Naghavi, M.; Dellavalle, R.P. The global burden of scabies: A cross-sectional analysis from the Global Burden of Disease Study 2015. *Lancet Inf. Dis.* **2017**, *17*, 1247–1254. [CrossRef]
2. Mahe, A. Epidemiology and Management of Common Skin Diseases in Children in Developing Countries. Available online: http://whqlibdoc.who.int/hq/2005/WHO_FCH_CAH_05.12_eng.pdf (accessed on 24 July 2018).
3. Romani, L.; Steer, A.C.; Whitfield, M.J.; Kaldor, J.M. Prevalence of Scabies and impetigo worldwide: A systematic review. *Lancet Infect. Dis.* **2015**, *15*, 960–967. [CrossRef]
4. Uriostegui-Flores, A. Cultural specific syndromes treated by traditional doctors. *Rev. Salud Publica* **2015**, *17*, 277–288. [PubMed]
5. Verma, S.B.; Vasani, R. Male genital dermatophytosis- clinical features and the effects of the misuse of topical steroids and steroid combinations- an alarming problem in India. *Mycoses* **2016**, *59*, 606–614. [CrossRef] [PubMed]
6. Estrada-Chavez, G.; Estrada, R.; Chavez-López, G. Misuse of topical steroids in scabies. *Comm. Dermatol. J.* **2017**, *13*, 1–12.
7. Miller, W.L. The adrenal cortex and its disorders. In *Clinical Pediatric Endocrinology*, 4th ed.; Hindmarsh, P.C., Ed.; Oxford Blackwell Science: Oxford, UK, 2001; pp. 321–376.
8. Semiz, S.; Balci, Y.I.; Ergin, S.; Candemir, M.; Polat, A. Two cases of Cushing's syndrome due to overuse of topical steroid in the diaper area. *Pediatr. Dermatol.* **2008**, *25*, 544–547. [CrossRef] [PubMed]
9. Cómo Utilizar esta Herramienta. Available online: www.profeco.gob.mx/precios/canasta/home.aspx?th=1 (accessed on 23 February 2018).
10. Hay, R.J.; Steer, A.C.; Engelman, D.; Walton, S. Scabies in the developing world-its prevalence, complications and management. *Clin. Microbiol. Infect.* **2012**, *18*, 313–323. [CrossRef] [PubMed]
11. La-Vincente, S.; Kearns, T.; Connors, C.; Cameron, S.; Carapetis, J.; Andrews, R. Community management of endemic scabies in remote aboriginal communities of northern Australia: Low treatment uptake and high ongoing acquisition. *PLoS Negl. Trop. Dis.* **2009**, *26*, e444. [CrossRef] [PubMed]
12. Engelman, D.; Kiang, K.; Chosidow, O.; McCarthy, J.; Fuller, C.; Lammie, P.; Hay, R.; Steer, A. Members of The International Alliance For The Control of Scabies. *PLoS Negl. Trop. Dis.* **2013**, *7*, e2167.

13. Hay, R.J.; Johns, N.E.; Williams, H.C.; Bolliger, I.W.; Dellavalle, R.P.; Margolis, D.J.; Marks, R.; Naldi, L.; Weinstock, M.A.; Wulf, S.K.; et al. The global burden of skin disease in 2010: An analysis of the prevalence and impact of skin conditions. *J. Investig. Derm.* **2014**, *134*, 1527–1534. [CrossRef] [PubMed]

14. Razzaghy, A.M.; Mosalla, N.A.; Nasli, E.E. Iatrogenic Cushing's Syndrome caused by topical corticosteroid application and its life threatening complications. *J. Compr. Ped.* **2015**, *6*, e34336. [CrossRef]

15. Lima, F.C.D.R.; Cerqueira, A.M.M.; Guimaraes, M.B.S.; Padilha, C.B.S.; Craide, F.H.; Bombardelli, M. Crusted scabies due to indiscriminate use of glucocorticoid therapy in infant. *Ann. Bras. Dermatol.* **2017**, *92*, 383–385. [CrossRef] [PubMed]

16. Dlova, N.C.; Hendricks, N.E.; Martincgh, B.S. Skin-lightening creams used in Durban, South Africa. *I. J. Dermatol.* **2012**, *51* (Suppl 1), 51–53. [CrossRef] [PubMed]

17. Hay, R.J.; Estrada Castanon, R.; Alarcon Hernandez, H.; Chavez Lopez, G.; Lopez Fuentes, L.F.; Paredes Solis, S.; Andersson, N. Wastage of family income on skin disease in Mexico. *BMJ* **1994**, *309*, 848. [CrossRef] [PubMed]

18. Boscaro, M.; Giacchetti, G.; Ronconi, V. Visceral adipose tissue: Emerging role of gluco- and mineralocorticoid hormones in the setting of cardiometabolic alterations. *Ann. N. Y. Acad. Sci.* **2012**, *1264*, 87–102. [CrossRef] [PubMed]

19. Rathi, S.K.; D'Souza, P. Rational and ethical use of topical corticosteroids based on safety and efficacy. *Indian J. Dermatol.* **2012**, *57*, 251–259. [CrossRef] [PubMed]

20. Tempark, T.; Phatarakijnirund, V.; Chatproedprai, S.; Watcharasindhu, S.; Supornsilchai, V.; Wananukul, S. Exogenous Cushing's syndrome due to topical corticosteroid application: Case report and review literature. *Endocrine* **2010**, *38*, 328–334. [CrossRef] [PubMed]

21. Gen, R.; Akbay, E.; Sezer, K. Cushing syndrome caused by topical corticosteroid: A case report. *Am. J. Med. Sci.* **2007**, *333*, 173–174. [CrossRef] [PubMed]

22. Selahattin, K.; Sedat, A.; Özbek, M.N.; Ahmet, Y. Infantile Iatrogenic Cushing's Syndrome. *Indian J. Dermatol.* **2008**, *53*, 190–191.

23. Messina, M.F.; Valenzise, M.; Aversa, S.; Arrigo, T.; De-Luca, F. Iatrogenic Cushing syndrome caused by ocular glucocorticoids in a child. *BMJ Case Rep.* **2009**. [CrossRef] [PubMed]

24. West, D.P.; Micali, G. Principles of paediatric dermatological therapy. In *Textbook of Pediatric Dermatology*, 1st ed.; Harper, J., Oranje, A., Prose, N., Eds.; Blackwell Science Ltd: Oxford, UK, 2000; pp. 1731–1742.

25. Siklar, Z.; Bostancı, İ.; Atli, Ö.; Dallar, Y. An infantile Cushing syndrome due to misuse of tropical steroid. *Pediatr. Dermatol.* **2004**, *21*, 561–563. [CrossRef] [PubMed]

26. Azizi, F.; Jahed, A.; Hedayati, M.; Lankarani, M.; Bejestani, H.S.; Esfahanian, F.; Beyraghi, N.; Noroozi, A.; Kobarfard, F. Outbreak of exogenous Cushing's syndrome due to unlicensed medications. *Clin. Endocrinol.* **2008**, *69*, 921–925. [CrossRef] [PubMed]

27. Thomas, J.; Carson, C.; Peterson, G.M.; Walton, S.F.; Hammer, K.A.; Naunton, M.; Davey, R.C.; Spelman, T.; Dettwiller, P.; Kyle, G.; et al. Therapeutic potential of tea tree oil for scabies. *Am. J. Trop. Med. Hyg.* **2016**, *94*, 258–266. [CrossRef] [PubMed]

28. Hay, R.J.; Fuller, L.C. The assessment of dermatological needs in resource-poor regions. *Int. J. Dermatol.* **2012**, *50*, 552–557. [CrossRef] [PubMed]

29. Estrada, R.; Chavez-López, M.G.; Estrada-Chavez, G.; Paredes-Solis, S. specialized dermatological care for marginalized populations and education at the primary care level: Is community dermatology a feasible proposal? *Int. J. Dermatol.* **2012**, *51*, 1345–1350. [CrossRef] [PubMed]

30. Estrada-Chavez, G.E.; Estrada, C.R.; Chavez, L.G.; Paredes-Solis, S. Estudio preliminar de la prescripción indiscriminada de corticosteroides tópicos en medicina general. *Dermatol. Rev. Mex.* **2013**, *57*, 433–437.

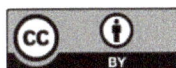

Tropical Medicine and Infectious Disease

MDPI

Article

Long-Range Diagnosis of and Support for Skin Conditions in Field Settings

Victoria Williams * and Carrie Kovarik

Department of Dermatology, Perelman School of Medicine, University of Pennsylvania,
Philadelphia, PA 19104, USA; carrie.kovarik@uphs.upenn.edu
* Correspondence: tori22@gmail.com; Tel.: +1-215-662-2737

Received: 9 July 2018; Accepted: 7 August 2018; Published: 13 August 2018

Abstract: Skin diseases are a significant cause of morbidity and mortality worldwide; however, access to dermatology services are critically limited, particularly in low- to middle-income countries (LMIC), where there is an overall shortage of physicians. Implementation of long-range technological support tools has been growing in an effort to provide quality dermatology care to even the most remote settings globally. eHealth strategies can provide realistic healthcare solutions if implemented in a feasible and sensitive way, customizing tools to address the unique needs and resource limitations of the local setting. This article summarizes the various types of telemedicine and mobile health (mHealth) tools and their practical applications and benefits for patient care. The challenges and barriers of teledermatology are discussed, as well as steps to consider when implementing a new teledermatology initiative. eHealth arguably offers one of the most flexible and realistic tools for providing critically needed access to dermatology skills in underserved LMICs.

Keywords: teledermatology; eHealth; mHealth; long range diagnosis; dermatology; telepathology; technology; skin disease

1. Introduction

Skin diseases are a significant cause of morbidity and mortality worldwide; however, access to dermatology services are critically limited, particularly in low- to middle-income countries (LMICs), where there is an overall shortage of physicians [1]. The World Health Organization (WHO) has estimated that there is a worldwide shortage of 4.3 million physicians and nurses, and countries with the lowest density of healthcare workers such as sub-Saharan Africa, have the highest level of disease burden [2–4]. When an estimated 1 billion people across the world do not have access to a trained healthcare worker, access to specialty services like dermatology care is very rare [3,4]. Many regions completely lack a dermatology specialist or have dermatologists that live only in urban areas, leaving remote populations without access to care [5,6]. Skin diseases are reported to be the 4th leading cause of disability worldwide, but with the limited number and distribution of dermatologists, it is nearly impossible to provide adequate care to everyone in need using traditional methods [7]. Thus, the implementation of long-range technological support tools has been growing in an effort to provide quality dermatology care to even the most remote settings globally. eHealth strategies can provide realistic healthcare solutions if implemented in a feasible and sensitive way, customizing tools to address the unique needs and resource limitations of the local setting.

The WHO defines eHealth as the overall use of information and communication technology for health, which can broadly apply to all parts of the healthcare system from electronic medical record systems, education, research, clinical care, and hospital information systems [8]. There are numerous subsets of eHealth that can augment the delivery of healthcare; however, when looking to improve the diagnosis and management of skin diseases in remote field settings, mobile health (mHealth) and more specifically mobile telemedicine tools can provide flexible and innovative solutions.

Telemedicine is a subset of eHealth that encompasses the use of electronic communications technology to exchange medical information for the purposes of health and education. Dermatology is uniquely suited for telemedicine because of the largely visual component involved in diagnosis. Teledermatology can be delivered using either store and forward or live methods. Store and forward (SAF) methods, which are the most commonly utilized, involve gathering data that is then sent to a distant provider to be reviewed at a later time. Live telemedicine utilizes videoconference technology to connect a patient or provider in real time with a distant provider for consultation. Live telemedicine is infrequently used in the developing world due to the difficulty in sustaining a live connection.

Mobile health encompasses the use of mobile devices to support healthcare practices via various applications. The estimated penetration of unique mobile subscribers worldwide reached 66% (5.0 billion) in 2017, and is expected to be 71% (5.9 billion) by 2025 [9]. The majority of the world's cell phone subscriptions are now in the developing world, and mobile phones offer an accessible healthcare tool that can be utilized even in the most remote settings. The type of healthcare that can be delivered through mHealth depends on the device and network connectivity. In 2017, smartphones as a percentage of mobile phone penetration were 34% in sub-Saharan Africa, and are projected to be 68% in 2025. Including 3G, mobile broadband network coverage reached 83% globally in 2016 [9]. As the connectivity advances in LMIC, the opportunities for mHealth expand.

2. Types of Mobile Health (mHealth) and Telemedicine Tools

eHealth tools come in a variety of formats that may be customized depending on the needs of the users. Table 1 outlines the various platforms that can be leveraged to practice teledermatology and summarizes their associated advantages and disadvantages. Formal telemedicine platforms utilize programs that have been specially designed to transmit secure healthcare information between providers. Traditionally, SAF teledermatology platforms were created solely for desktop use and required uploading photographs to a web-based program, which could prove challenging for providers with low computer literacy, limited internet access, and poor computer resources. In recent years, most web-based teledermatology platforms have also developed an associated mobile application that functions in parallel to the web-based program and allows for easier data collection and flexible connectivity over mobile networks or wifi. Providers can work directly from their mobile smartphones to transmit photos and patient information to remote consultants.

Formal SAF teledermatology platforms require each user to be registered in the program and are tailored to collect a predetermined set of information. A customized dermatology template can be provided for patient data collection, which allows providers with limited dermatology knowledge to perform a thorough skin history without significant prior dermatology experience. Photos of the patient can then be attached to the consultation (Figure 1). Benefits of this type of service include secure data transmission and higher likelihood of pertinent patient information being included in consultations. Limitations include the need to individually register users and train them to use the application. Most programs will work over a mobile connection but require a strong network signal for ideal performance. Examples of successful long-term teledermatology programs using formal SAF platforms to support developing countries include the Africa Teledermatology Project [10], the Swinfen Charitable Trust [11,12], the Médecins Sans Frontières Telemedicine Network [13] and Réseau Afrique Francophone de Télémédecine (RAFT) project [14].

Informal telemedicine platforms include any method that allows the electronic SAF transmission of patient data. These tools allow for the quick and easy exchange of data without the need to individually identify, register and train all users. However, they have the drawback of not providing any formal framework for the collection or organization of data. The consultation information provided may be missing key elements and the security of transmitted information cannot be guaranteed.

Table 1. Description of teledermatology and telepathology platform types, advantages, disadvantages and examples.

Platform Type	Advantages	Disadvantages	Examples
Formal Teledermatology Platforms			
Web and/or Mobile Teledermatology Applications	secure, guides referring providers through a dermatology consult, stores a record of all consults, most applications can be used on desktop or mobile device	must identify and register all users, must train all users, cost associated with creation of application or subscription to use, most time intensive for providers to utilize, difficult for providers to ask follow up questions, usually no mechanism for long term follow-up of cases, requires wifi or strong network signal	Africa Teledermatology Project [10], Swinfen Charitable Trust [11,12], MSF [13], ClickMedix [15], Azova [16]
Informal Teledermatology Platforms			
Secure Email	can be used on desktop or mobile device, minimal training needed for users, minimally time intensive, fits into most providers daily routine, options for free access	security depends on email server, requires wifi or moderate network signal, no structure to guide consults, email accounts may have limited storage capacity, provider must identify and obtain emails of consultants to connect	free encrypted email services: Proton mail [17], Tutanota [18]
Secure Cloud Based File Sharing	can be used on desktop or mobile device, options for free access, provides a mechanism for organized storage of patient information, minimally time intensive	limited storage on free versions, requires some training for users, users must register, requires wifi or strong network signal, moderately secure, no structure to guide consults	Dropbox [19], Google Drive [20], OneDrive [21], Box [22]
Secure Direct Messaging Applications	fits into providers daily routine, least time intensive, minimal training needed, allows real time communication during patient visits, options for text/photos/videos/audio messaging, allows open communication for follow up questions and patient follow up, options for free access, secure end to end encryption, allows one-on-one or group chats, works well with low signal or wifi	provider must identify a consultant and obtain a phone number to connect, no structure to guide consults, no organized record of consults or communications	Free: WhatsApp [23,24], MedTunnel [25],Bloomtext [26] Paid: Imprivata [27], TigerConnect [28], Voalte [29], QliqSoft [30], Spok Mobile [31]
Social Networking Sites	free, low time commitment, minimal training needed, allows connection to a single provider or a global network, any provider can register and connect, works well with low signal or wifi	cannot guarantee security, difficult to guarantee credentials and expertise of consultants providing advice, no structure to guide consults, no organized record of consults or communications	Tederm.org [32], Sermo [33], Facebook [34]
Telepathology Platforms			
Virtual Slide Microscopy (VSM)	secure, highest quality images, can view any part of the slide at any magnification, creates an organized library of cases for teaching or research, least time intensive for reviewer when slides are pre-scanned	high cost to purchase, ongoing costs to maintain equipment and software, requires significant training, needs high storage capacity for images, needs consistent and high bandwidth to function, slide scanning can be time intensive for sender	Olympus VS 120 [35], Zeiss Axio Scan.Z1 [36], Leica Aperio AT2 [37]

Table 1. *Cont.*

Platform Type	Advantages	Disadvantages	Examples
Dynamic Slide Microscopy (DSM)	secure, can view any part of the slide at any magnification, potentially lower cost to implement compared to VSM	highest bandwidth requirements which may limit image quality, requires strict program compatibility for viewing, requires significant training, ongoing costs to maintain equipment and software, most time intensive to use for sender and reviewer	Leica Aperio LV1 [38], 3dHistech Panoramic DESK II DW [39]
Static Imaging	lowest cost, works with any microscope, no software requirements, does not require consistent wifi	risk of sampling error, quality of images varies based on skills of photographer, can only view areas of tissue and magnification chosen by photographer, time intensive for sender and reviewer	smartphone to eyepiece attachments: LabCam [40], Magnifi [41], Snapzoom [42]; any smartphone camera through eyepiece; any digital microscope camera

Abbreviations: MSF = Médecins Sans Frontières.

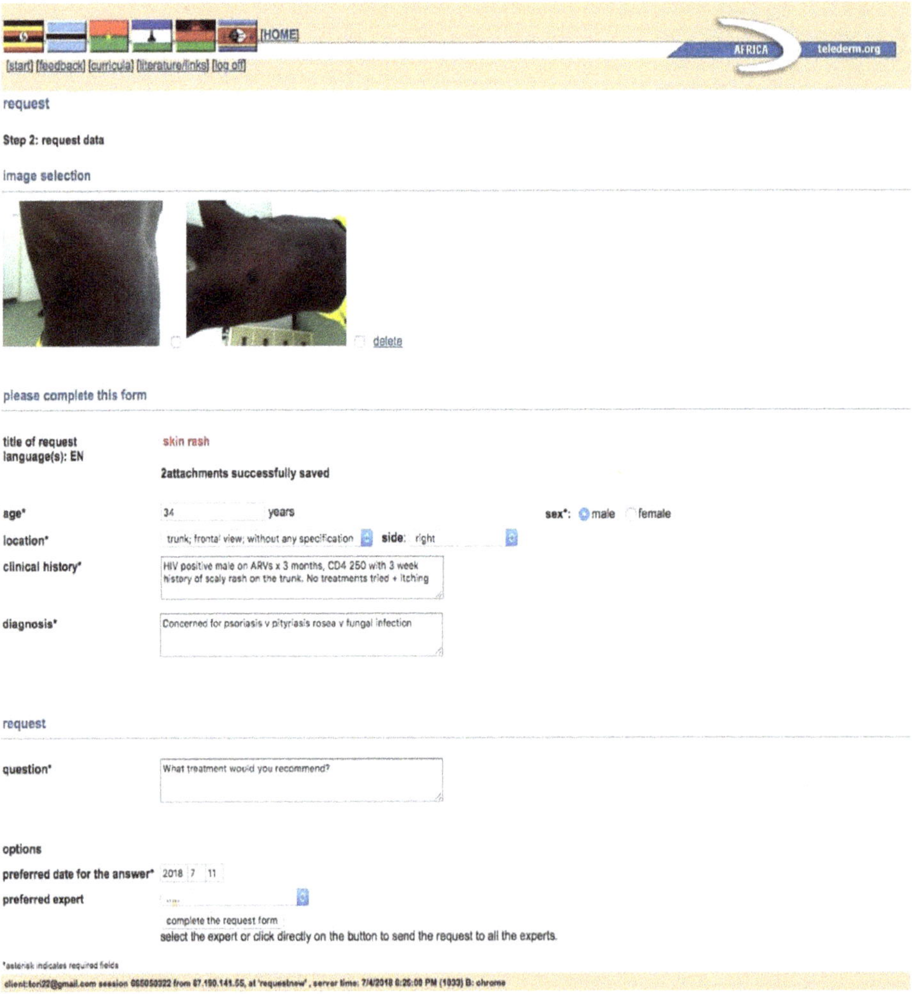

Figure 1. An example of a formal web-based teledermatology platform, the Africa Teledermatology Project, which uses a simple template to collect patient data for consultations.

Email is one of the more commonly utilized informal teledermatology platforms. Photos and pertinent patient information are included in an email message which can be sent to one provider or a group of providers for consultation. For the patient data to be secure, the sender and each recipient included must utilize a secure email service. Academic institutions with teledermatology links to developing countries via email platforms include Emory University to a teaching hospital in Kabul, Afghanistan [43]; the Medical College of Wisconsin to Hillside Healthcare International in Belize [44]; and the University of Basel, which is linked to several remote clinical sites globally [45].

Secure mobile messaging services allow the exchange of text, photos, audio, video and document files using mobile data or wifi. A widely used free mobile instant messaging application, Whatsapp, has been reported as a particularly powerful tool for teledermatology in several resource limited settings [23,24]. Because Whatsapp is already in use by more than 1 billion people in over 180 countries worldwide [46], the application can integrate seamlessly into the daily clinic routine of providers with minimal additional effort. Whatsapp can facilitate a variety of rapid patient care communications, allowing consulting physicians to learn about their patients and provide appropriate care in real time (Figure 2). Whatsapp does not require additional investments in equipment or dedicated internet access for users because it can be utilized on a provider's own smartphone with either mobile data or wifi. Most importantly, Whatsapp maintains high functionality even in areas of poor connectivity. There are several other secure mobile messaging systems that have been designed for healthcare; however, most require paid subscriptions which limit their usage in LMICs [25–31,47].

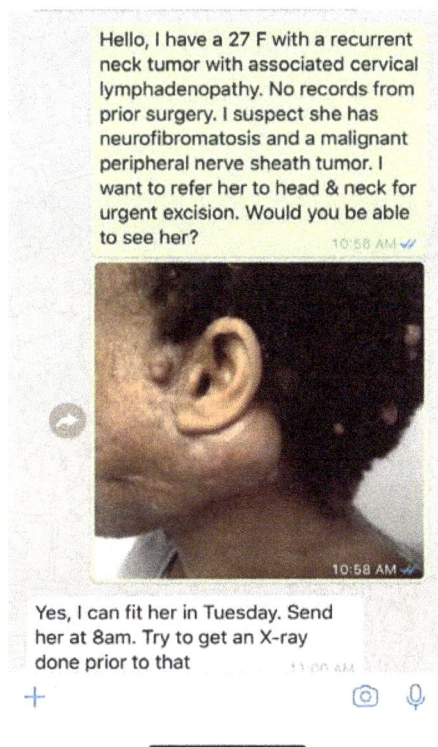

Figure 2. An example of secure direct messaging being used as a platform for teledermatology. Whatsapp is being utilized to tele-triage and coordinate care for a dermatology patient to sub-specialty care in Botswana.

Teledermatology can also be leveraged using cloud based file-hosting services that can provide a secure method for online file storage and sharing. Dropbox and Google drive are two popular cloud platforms that can facilitate Health Insurance Portability and Accountability Act (HIPAA) compliant sharing of protected patient information if utilized appropriately [19,20,48]. A recent study in Egypt, which used Dropbox for teledermatology consultation, found it to be a reliable diagnostic method with high rates of patient satisfaction [49]. Although cloud-based applications can function over mobile networks, they typically require a strong signal or wifi for optimal performance.

There has been a steady rise in the use of social networking among physicians who are starting to utilize crowdsourcing as a tool for patient care. Telederm.org is a free web-based dermatology networking platform that was started in 2002 and now has more than 2000 users [32]. After registering and creating an online profile, users can submit questions or cases to discussion forums that are divided by topic. Sermo is a similar website that connects more than 800,000 physicians of different specialties across the world via anonymous user profiles to allow the discussion of cases and other healthcare related topics [33]. Facebook, which connects users via a public profile, now has the ability to host private groups that are reportedly secure and only accessible by invitation [34]. Providers from any setting can come together to form collaborative groups in order to share challenging cases and request input from other members. Facebook groups can be tailored to specific topics of interest such as dermatopathology, tropical medicine or skin of color. Garcia-Romero et al. reported on the use of Facebook to create a teledermatology link between a rural clinic and a dermatology department at an urban general hospital in Mexico, which achieved clinical improvement in 75% of patients who received remote consultation [50]. Social media platforms have the benefit of a simple interface that requires negligible training for users and, most importantly, allows remote providers to connect with potentially thousands of dermatologists and other physicians across the world. Bandwidth requirements are low for these applications so they can be easily utilized on mobile devices in low-connectivity areas. However, there has been significant controversy about the use of social media platforms for healthcare, mainly due to the difficulty in guaranteeing patient privacy, confidentiality and security of the exchanged data. These methods should be used with caution.

Telepathology is a powerful component of teledermatology because histological analysis is vital for diagnostic confirmation in many dermatologic conditions, particularly in areas with high HIV burdens where clinical presentations are often atypical. Reliable pathology consultation services are critically needed in developing countries. Half of all fellowship trained pathologists work in the US, serving less than 5% of the global population [51]. Access to pathologists with dermatopathology experience or dermatopathology specialization is even more difficult to find in the global setting, creating an additional layer of challenges for physicians caring for skin diseases in remote settings.

Telepathology methods can also be tailored to the needs of the local community and available resources. The three methods of telepathology currently described are static imaging, dynamic imaging, and virtual slide systems (Table 1).

Static imaging is arguably the simplest telepathology method with the lowest budget requirements. The process involves taking photographs of slides at different magnifications and transmitting them to a remote dermatopathologist via any secure messaging, email or file-sharing platform. The most basic static technique utilizes a camera or smartphone to photograph a slide directly through a microscope eyepiece. Specialized adaptors and eyepiece attachments (Figure 3) have also been developed for use in combination with a smartphone to simplify the process of image capturing and improve the quality of images [52]. However, Bellina and Missoni demonstrated that quality images can be produced using any type of camera-equipped smartphone without the need for adaptors or additional technology [53], making this method ideal for low-resource settings. Digital camera attachments for microscopes are widely available and offer another simple mechanism for photographing slides. Multiple remote settings have achieved successful implementation of static telepathology programs with reported diagnostic concordance rates of up to 90.2% [45,54,55]. Major advantages of static image telepathology include minimal investment needed in equipment, training and maintenance, as well as the ability to function with unstable internet access. Static methods have the disadvantage of lower image quality, risk of sampling error and higher time requirements due to the need to select representative fields of view and take numerous pictures at different magnifications [56].

In dynamic imaging systems, slide images are examined in real time using a live microcopy viewing platform. Control of the live streaming images is either done directly by on site personnel or by the remote pathologist via robotic control of the microscope.

Live viewing systems have the advantage of allowing the pathologist to view the entire slide including different focus planes. Live view also allows cases to be discussed in real time which can increase the educational quality of consultations [57,58]. The feasibility of implementing a dynamic system has been demonstrated by the long-term use of a robotic telepathology system in a resource-limited government hospital in Botswana [59].

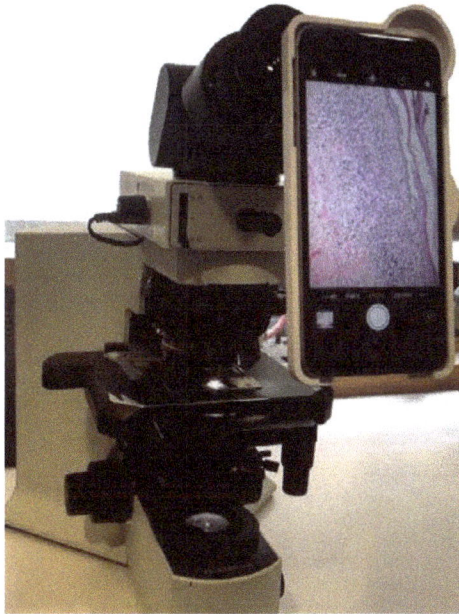

Figure 3. An example of a low-cost method for telepathology, the LabCam smartphone attachment, which allows photography of slides through the eyepiece of any microscope using an iPhone.

Virtual slide microscopy, also known as whole slide imaging systems, creates high-resolution scanned images of histology slides that can be digitally stored and then reviewed by a remote pathologist using specialized virtual slide viewing software [60]. This is also referred to as a hybrid method because it allows a pathologist to analyze the entire histology slide image dynamically by viewing selected areas digitally at higher magnification [61]. Major advantages include the ability to automate slide scanning; reduce interpretation time compared to robotic or static methods; the ability to manipulate, annotate and analyze slide images with viewing software; and the numerous educational applications that can be generated by creating a virtual 'teaching set' [61,62].

Virtual and dynamic slide telepathology systems can offer visual quality that is comparable to viewing slides in person under light microscopy, and several studies support good diagnostic concordance compared to a traditional glass slide review [63–70].

However, commercial slide-imaging systems are difficult to implement in low-resource settings due to the high cost of hardware and software, the need for skilled technicians to operate and maintain the systems locally, and the need for consistent high-bandwidth connectivity to transmit quality images [56,60,71].

In an effort to overcome the cost barriers of commercial slide-imaging systems, several low-cost interventions have been piloted utilizing innovative telepathology methods. Dudas et al. tested three low-cost telecytology systems including a Raspberry Pi attached to a webcam, an iPhone 4S with FaceTime, and an iPhone 4S with a live-streaming application [72]. All systems were able to stream live video of cytology slides to remote locations at a resolution that was suitable for a pathologist's review [72]. Meléndez-Álvarez et al. designed a telepathology prototype manufactured with plastic materials made using an open design 3D printer, a conventional optical microscope, a Celestron camera attachment, open-sourced software and electronic components that are readily available in most electronic shops [73]. The prototype had a total cost of less than $910 and the resulting images were judged to be of diagnostic quality by a pathologist [73]. Utilization of free web-based teleconferencing software such as Skype, Google Hangouts, GoToMeetings, Windows Live Messenger, Fuze, and Webex, can provide a low-cost alternative to commercial live view microscopy systems [60,74–76]. Yu et al. described the newly realized capacity of smartphones to power whole-slide imaging systems via software which splits the image digitalization process between smartphone applications and remote cloud servers [77]. An android or iOS smartphone mounted on the eyepiece of a standard optical microscope has the ability to scan whole-slide images into a virtual slide with a resulting image quality comparable to high end commercial slide-scanning systems [77,78]. This innovative smartphone technology offers the potential to bring slide scanning technology to more widespread settings in LMICs.

Implementation of any telepathology system requires careful planning and a strong partnership between local and remote providers. Additionally, it is important to note that none of these telepathology tools can overcome the need for local training and resources to perform quality skin biopsies and histopathological processing at the local site which is often the limiting factor in resource-limited settings [56]. Table 2 summarizes the advantages and disadvantages of each type of telepathology tool.

Table 2. Summary of the methods in which teledermatology can be utilized in practice, associated benefits and recommended platforms for remote providers in field settings.

Applications of Teledermatology	Benefits	Recommended Platforms for Remote Providers
Tele-Triage	appropriate and timely scheduling of patients into dermatology clinic, timely referral of dermatology patients to other specialists	secure direct messaging
Primary Care to Dermatology Consultation	diagnostic and management support, building dermatology skills over time	secure direct messaging
Specialist to Dermatology Consultation	diagnostic and management support, care coordination, building dermatology skills over time	secure direct messaging
Dermatologist to Dermatologist Consultation	second opinion, subspecialty dermatologist consultation, super specialist consultation for rare diseases, decreases isolation and burnout	formal teledermatology application, secure email, secure direct messaging, cloud based file sharing
Telepathology	expert analysis of skin biopsy specimens, improved diagnostic accuracy of skin disease, training of local pathologists	static images via smartphone or digital microscope camera
Long Term Management	allows for provider to dermatologist follow up, allows patient to dermatologist follow up, improves patient compliance and patient outcomes	secure direct messaging, secure email, cloud based file sharing
Care Coordination	allows for group chats between various providers to save time and resources	secure direct messaging, secure email, cloud based file sharing
Dermatology Education	remote access to dermatology education in any setting, builds local capacity	web based learning modules, video lectures, virtual patient encounters, email or web based access to lectures/handouts/guidelines, clinical decision support tools

In addition to supporting teledermatology functions, eHealth tools can provide access to education in many forms. The RAFT network is an example of a robust telemedicine network spanning four continents that focuses on providing medical education through a variety of low-bandwidth technologies such as interactive video lectures, virtual patient encounters, continuing medical education curriculums, tele-consults, clinical decision support tools, and web-casting of scientific conferences [14,79]. The emphasis on local involvement in coordinating and creating educational content that is most relevant to local providers has helped to make this project sustainable and successful [79].

mHealth applications are powerful educational tools because they can provide vital information to clinicians at the point of care. In recent years the number of mHealth applications has rapidly expanded to include programs to assist with disease diagnosis, management guidelines, drug reference, evidence-based medicine search tools, medical calculators, medical training tools, and clinical decision support pathways for navigating difficult clinical scenarios [80]. DynaMed, Epocrates, Medscape, Visual Dx, and UpToDate are some of the more commonly used mHealth tools, which allow clinicians to have rapid access to reference material with only a smartphone and/or mobile connection [81–85]. However, some of these applications require subscription costs, which can limit widespread usage in LMICs.

3. Benefits and Practical Applications of eHealth Tools

eHealth tools can be harnessed in a variety of different formats and combinations to benefit all levels of providers. Table 2 summarizes various methods in which teledermatology can provide solutions for the challenges of dermatology care in remote settings.

Teledermatology methods have been utilized to extend dermatologic care to developing countries since the early 1990s. The benefits of utilizing eHealth technologies are many and reports of successful programs have been published from numerous centers in Africa, Asia, and Latin America [5,10,11,44,86–89]. The growing transition to mobile teledermatology applications is supported by reports of successful implementation including satisfactory diagnosis and management of skin disease, diagnostic concordance with traditional face to face visits, patient satisfaction and provider satisfaction [23,89–96]. Utilization of tele-triage has the potential to significantly decrease the time to first evaluation of a patient by a dermatology specialist, which can in turn decrease morbidity from skin disease and increase patient satisfaction [23,97]. mHealth tools can improve the dermatology skills of front line providers who are more likely to retain knowledge because they are discussing and learning from their own patients [94]. Resident trainees in Botswana who were provided with smartphones pre-loaded with clinical decision support applications and training on how to best utilize the applications, reported multiple benefits including increased collaboration between primary care physicians and trainees, as well as increased clinician empowerment [77]. Teledermatology opens new communication and collaboration possibilities for providers and patients in isolated rural settings which can increase job satisfaction and improve care for patients with skin disease. Teledermatology can reduce healthcare costs by reducing the travel burden for patients, improving long-term follow-up and increasing successful care collaboration to improve patient outcomes [98,99]. Importantly, several studies have shown there is diagnostic concordance between teledermatology consultation and face-to-face visits, ensuring that patients are benefitting from use of the telemedicine without sacrificing quality of care [88,89,91].

4. Challenges and Barriers to Use of Teledermatology

Teledermatology is not without its challenges. Principally, sustainability becomes a key concern when setting up a program. Formal teledermatology platforms in particular require a significant amount of funding to implement, including but not limited to creation of the application, providing the necessary equipment, and training local providers. If the resources are not in place to continue the program long term, it becomes difficult to rationalize the initiation. The computer literacy of the providers being supported, local power supply, internet access, local mobile network connectivity, and availability of local technological resources all need to be carefully considered [14]. A major key to sustainability is ensuring that local clinicians are supportive of the program. Effective training on the tools being implemented can be challenging due to the often rapid provider turnover in low-resource clinical settings. Programs have a better chance of long-term success if technologies that are already in place and regularly used by local providers can be harnessed for teledermatology. Integration of the teledermatology program into the local healthcare system is essential for sustainability. Ideally the dermatologists answering the consultations are located in the country of origin of the consultee, or at the minimum, they are highly familiar with the diseases, work flow, and resources of the local healthcare system. Treatment plans being recommended must be realistic within the local socio-cultural and healthcare environment. Ideally, consultants should be available for continued collaboration and follow-up to address the common challenges that come with dermatology care in resource-limited settings. However, many teledermatology applications lack a method for long-term follow-up. Additionally, in certain cultures, teledermatology may not be an acceptable form of healthcare because patients expect face to face care or are resistant to having their skin condition photographed. Although teledermatology and mHealth applications give providers access to dermatology expertise, they do not solve the inherent challenges of local resource limitations such as medication stock outs, lack of available specialists for referral and limited diagnostic testing services.

The use of teledermatology requires a critical sensitivity to patient privacy and data security. It can be challenging to ensure that all providers participating in teledermatology are obtaining patient consent to share their information, sharing it over a secure platform, and using de-identified information to maintain patient confidentiality. Social media-based platforms must be used with caution because security settings and data-sharing policies can change rapidly and affect the ethical use of the program for patient data.

5. Practical Tips for Implementation of a New Teledermatology Initiative

The most important part of developing a new teledermatology initiative is a thorough local needs assessment of the area to be supported [12,44]. The first step in this process is evaluating the local healthcare environment. Most importantly, do local providers want to engage in teledermatology? Is there a need for or an interest in improving dermatology skills? Who would need to approve the program? Until clear need and firm local support can be secured, it is not advisable to initiate a teledermatology collaboration.

Review the current methods and workflow being used for dermatology patients. Where is the closest dermatology provider? Who cares for dermatology patients in rural areas versus urban areas? How far do most patients have to travel to see a dermatologist? How does the local healthcare system work? What is the cost of care for patients?

Then, review the locally available technological resources. Do most providers and patients use mobile phones? How prevalent are smartphones? How widespread are cellphone networks and how strong/reliable is the signal in the areas being supported? Are computers and/or wifi available in the local clinics or hospitals being supported? How technologically literate are the providers and patients being supported?

Next, identify partners that will participate in the initiative. Clearly outline the requirements and duties of all parties to be involved from the beginning to prevent problems developing later on. Have a discussion with local providers to get a firsthand understanding of their biggest concerns and the major challenges they face in caring for dermatology patients. Present your ideas for teledermatology solutions and get local feedback on the feasibility and interest in the proposed platforms. Ensure the platform can maintain patient privacy and provide a secure exchange of information.

Then, utilize the information gathered to narrow down the best options for a teledermatology platform. Identify the costs required to initiate and sustain the proposed platforms. Identify funding sources that can meet the needs of your proposal. Organize an implementation team to train all providers involved on both sides. Most importantly, identify a local means of providing ongoing training and support for the program to ensure sustainability.

If funding and resources appear to be major limitations, but local providers and leadership are supportive of developing a collaboration, consider starting with a free secure messaging application like Whatsapp. It can be integrated into even the most limited resource settings with little need for training and a low burden of time and effort for local providers to implement. If there is a robust interest in teledermatology at the local level, a strong health infrastructure that includes a dermatologist, and funding available for supplying and maintaining technological tools, a more formal teledermatology program could be feasible.

For overall success, teledermatology partnerships need to benefit both sides and need to be set up with the clear involvement of local providers. Remote dermatologists need to be willing and able to offer realistic diagnosis and treatment advice by taking into consideration local cultural norms and resource limitations. This is made possible by creating an open dialogue with local providers for exchange of information to allow both sides to learn from the interaction and improve care over time.

6. Conclusions

eHealth arguably offers one of the most flexible and realistic tools for providing critically needed access to dermatology skills in underserved LMICs. eHealth resources are ideal because they offer a wide range of customizable tools to match the needs and available resources of local providers in any setting. As the cost of mobile technology continues to decrease, the opportunities for low-cost teledermatology applications will continue to increase, making it feasible for any provider in any setting to be connected to a global community of dermatologists.

Author Contributions: V.W.: Writing-original draft preparation, C.K.: Writing-review and editing.

Funding: This research received no external funding.

Conflicts of Interest: The authors have no conflicts of interest to declare.

References

1. Karimkhani, C.; Dellavalle, R.P.; Coffeng, L.E.; Flohr, C.; Hay, R.J.; Langan, S.M.; Nsoesie, E.O.; Ferrari, A.J.; Erskine, H.E.; Silverberg, J.I.; et al. Global skin disease morbidity and mortality: An update from the Global Burden of Disease Study 2013. *JAMA Dermatol.* **2017**, *153*, 406. [CrossRef] [PubMed]
2. Evans, T.; Chen, L.; Evans, D.; Sadana, R.; Stilwell, B.; Travis, O.; Van Lerberghe, W.; Zurn, P.; Aschwanden, C. *The World Health Report 2006 - Working Together for Health*; World Health Organization: Geneva, Switzerland, 2006; ISBN 978-92-4-156317-8.
3. Chen, L.; Evans, T.; Anand, S.; Boufford, J.I.; Brown, H.; Chowdhury, M.; Cueto, M.; Dare, L.; Dussault, G.; Elzinga, G.; et al. Human resources for health: Overcoming the crisis. *Lancet* **2004**, *364*, 1984–1990. [CrossRef]
4. Crisp, N.; Chen, L. Global supply of health professionals. *N. Engl. J. Med.* **2014**, *370*, 950–957. [CrossRef] [PubMed]
5. Desai, B.; McKoy, K.; Kovarik, C. Overview of international teledermatology. *Pan Afr. Med. J.* **2010**, *6*, 3. [CrossRef] [PubMed]
6. International Foundation for Dermatology International Foundation for Dermatology. Available online: http://www.ifd.org/about2.html (accessed on 20 June 2018).
7. Hay, R.J.; Johns, N.E.; Williams, H.C.; Bolliger, I.W.; Dellavalle, R.P.; Margolis, D.J.; Marks, R.; Naldi, L.; Weinstock, M.A.; Wulf, S.K.; et al. The global burden of skin disease in 2010: An analysis of the prevalence and impact of skin conditions. *J. Investig. Dermatol.* **2014**, *134*, 1527–1534. [CrossRef] [PubMed]
8. WHO Global Observatory for eHealth. *Global Diffusion of eHealth: Making Universal Health Coverage Achievable: Report of the Third Global Survey on eHealth*; World Health Organization: Geneva, Switzerland, 2016; ISBN 978-92-4-151178-0.
9. Groupe Speciale Mobile Association. *The Mobile Economy 2014*; GSMA & International Telecomm Union: London, UK, 2014.
10. Lipoff, J.B.; Cobos, G.; Kaddu, S.; Kovarik, C.L. The Africa Teledermatology Project: A retrospective case review of 1229 consultations from sub-saharan Africa. *J. Am. Acad. Dermatol.* **2015**, *72*, 1084–1085. [CrossRef] [PubMed]
11. Wootton, R.; Geissbuhler, A.; Jethwani, K.; Kovarik, C.; Person, D.A.; Vladzymyrskyy, A.; Zanaboni, P.; Zolfo, M. Long-running telemedicine networks delivering humanitarian services: Experience, performance and scientific output. *Bull. World Health Organ.* **2012**, *90*, 341D–347D. [CrossRef] [PubMed]
12. Kaddu, S.; Kovarik, C.; Gabler, G.; Soyer, H. Teledermatology in Developing Countries. In *Telehealth in the Developing World*, Royal Society of Medicine Press/IDRC: London, UK, 2009; ISBN 978-1-85315-784.

13. Delaigue, S.; Morand, J.J.; Olson, D.; Wootton, R.; Bonnardot, L. Teledermatology in low-resource settings: The MSF experience with a multilingual tele-expertise platform. *Front. Public Health* **2014**, *2*. [CrossRef] [PubMed]
14. Bagayoko, C.O.; Müller, H.; Geissbuhler, A. Assessment of internet-based tele-medicine in Africa (the RAFT project). *Comput. Med. Imaging Graph.* **2006**, *30*, 407–416. [CrossRef] [PubMed]
15. Clickmedix. Available online: https://clickmedix.com/ (accessed on 1 July 2018).
16. Azova. Available online: http://azovahealth.com/ (accessed on 1 July 2018).
17. Proton Mail. Available online: https://protonmail.com/ (accessed on 1 July 2018).
18. Tutanota. Available online: https://tutanota.com/ (accessed on 1 July 2018).
19. Dropbox Business and HIPAA/HITECH—An Overview. Available online: https://www.dropbox.com/help/security/hipaa-hitech-overview (accessed on 20 June 2018).
20. Google Drive. Available online: https://www.google.com/drive/ (accessed on 1 July 2018).
21. Microsoft OneDrive. Available online: https://onedrive.live.com/about/en-us/ (accessed on 1 July 2018).
22. Box. Available online: https://www.box.com/home (accessed on 1 July 2018).
23. Williams, V.; Kovarik, C. WhatsApp: An innovative tool for dermatology care in limited resource settings. *Telemed. e-Health* **2018**, *24*, 464–468. [CrossRef] [PubMed]
24. Mars, M.; Scott, R.E. WhatsApp in clinical practice: A literature review. *Stud. Health Technol. Inform.* **2016**, *231*, 82–90. [PubMed]
25. Medtunnel. Available online: http://www.medtunnel.com/ (accessed on 1 July 2018).
26. Bloomtext. Available online: https://www.bloomtext.com/#/ (accessed on 1 July 2018).
27. Imprivata. Available online: https://www.imprivata.com/secure-communications (accessed on 20 June 2018).
28. Tiger Connect. Available online: https://www.tigerconnect.com/ (accessed on 20 June 2018).
29. Voalte. Available online: http://www.voalte.com/healthcare-communication-platform-2 (accessed on 20 June 2018).
30. Qliqsoft. Available online: https://www.qliqsoft.com/ (accessed on 1 July 2018).
31. Spok Mobile. Available online: https://www.spok.com/spok-mobile (accessed on 1 July 2018).
32. Telederm.org. Available online: http://www.telederm.org/ (accessed on 20 June 2018).
33. Sermo. Available online: http://www.sermo.com/ (accessed on 20 June 2018).
34. Facebook. Available online: https://www.facebook.com/ (accessed on 20 June 2018).
35. Olympus VS120-S6-W Virtual Slide Microscope. Available online: www.olympuslifescience.com/Microscopes/VC120 (accessed on 1 July 2018).
36. ZEISS Axio Scan.Z1 Digital Slide Scanner. Available online: https://www.zeiss.com/microscopy/int/products/imaging-systems/axio-scan-z1.html (accessed on 1 July 2018).
37. Leica Biosystems Aperio AT2 Telepathology Platform. Available online: https://www.leicabiosystems.com/digital-pathology/scan/aperio-at2/ (accessed on 1 July 2018).
38. Leica Biosystems Aperio LV1 Telepathology Platform. Available online: www.leicabiosystems.com/Aperio/LV1 (accessed on 1 July 2018).
39. 3DHISTECH Pannoramic DESK II DW. Available online: https://www.3dhistech.com/pannoramic_desk_II_DW (accessed on 1 July 2018).
40. Lab Cam. Available online: https://www.ilabcam.com/ (accessed on 1 July 2018).
41. Magnifi. Available online: http://www.arcturuslabs.com (accessed on 1 July 2018).
42. Snapzoom. Available online: http://snapzooms.com (accessed on 1 July 2018).
43. Ismail, A.; McMichael, J.R.; Stoff, B.K. Utility of international store-and-forward teledermatopathology among a cohort of mostly female patients at a tertiary referral center in Afghanistan. *Int. J. Womens Dermatol.* **2018**, *4*, 83–86. [CrossRef] [PubMed]
44. Bobbs, M.; Bayer, M.; Frazer, T.; Humphrey, S.; Wilson, B.; Olasz, E.; Holland, K.; Kuzminski, J. Building a global teledermatology collaboration. *Int. J. Dermatol.* **2016**, *55*, 446–449. [CrossRef] [PubMed]
45. Brauchli, K.; Jagilly, R.; Oberli, H.; Kunze, K.D.; Phillips, G.; Hurwitz, N.; Oberholzer, M. Telepathology on the Solomon Islands—two years' experience with a hybrid web- and email-based telepathology System. *J. Telemed. Telecare* **2004**, *10*, 14–17. [CrossRef] [PubMed]
46. Yueng, K. Whatsapp Passes 1 Billion Monthly Active Users. Venture Beat 2016. Available online: https://venturebeat.com/2016/02/01/whatsapp-passes-1-billion-monthly-active-users/ (accessed on 20 June 2018).

47. Monegian, B. KLAS Names Top Secure Messaging Tools. Healthcare IT News 2015. Available online: https://www.healthcareitnews.com/news/tigertext-leads-messaging-market-now (accessed on 20 June 2018).

48. Kohgadai, A. Top 5 HIPAA-Compliant Cloud Storage Services. Cloud Security Blog. Available online: https://www.skyhighnetworks.com/cloud-security-blog/top-5-hipaa-compliant-cloud-storage-services/ (accessed on 20 June 2018).

49. Saleh, N.; Abdel Hay, R.; Hegazy, R.; Hussein, M.; Gomaa, D. Can teledermatology be a useful diagnostic tool in dermatology practice in remote areas? An Egyptian experience with 600 patients. *J. Telemed. Telecare* **2017**, *23*, 233–238. [CrossRef] [PubMed]

50. Garcia-Romero, M.T.; Prado, F.; Dominguez-Cherit, J.; Hojyo-Tomomka, M.T.; Arenas, R. Teledermatology via a social networking web site: A pilot study between a general hospital and a rural clinic. *Telemed. e-Health* **2011**, *17*, 652–655. [CrossRef] [PubMed]

51. Meyer, J.; Paré, G. Telepathology Impacts and Implementation Challenges: A Scoping Review. *Arch. Pathol. Lab. Med.* **2015**, *139*, 1550–1557. [CrossRef] [PubMed]

52. Roy, S.; Pantanowitz, L.; Amin, M.; Seethala, R.R.; Ishtiaque, A.; Yousem, S.A.; Parwani, A.V.; Cucoranu, I.; Hartman, D.J. Smartphone adapters for digital photomicrography. *J. Pathol. Inform.* **2014**, *5*, 24. [CrossRef] [PubMed]

53. Bellina, L.; Missoni, E. Mobile cell-phones (M-phones) in telemicroscopy: Increasing connectivity of isolated laboratories. *Diagn. Pathol.* **2009**, *4*, 19. [CrossRef] [PubMed]

54. Abdirad, A.; Sarrafpour, B.; Ghaderi-Sohi, S. Static telepathology in Cancer Institute of Tehran University: Report of the first academic experience in Iran. *Diagn. Pathol.* **2006**, *1*, 33. [CrossRef] [PubMed]

55. Desai, S.; Patil, R.; Chinoy, R.; Kothari, A.; Ghosh, T.K.; Chavan, M.; Mohan, A.; Nene, B.M.; Dinshaw, K.A. Experience with telepathology at a tertiary cancer centre and a rural cancer hospital. *Natl. Med. J. India* **2004**, *17*, 17–19. [PubMed]

56. Evans, A.; Garcia, B.; Godin, C.; Godlewski, M.; Jansen, G.; Kabani, A.; Louahlia, S.; Manning, L.; Maung, R.; Moore, L.; et al. Guidelines from the Canadian Association of Pathologists for establishing a telepathology service for anatomic pathology using whole-slide imaging. *J. Pathol. Inform.* **2014**, *5*, 15. [CrossRef] [PubMed]

57. Kayser, K. Introduction of virtual microscopy in routine surgical pathology–a hypothesis and personal view from Europe. *Diagn. Pathol.* **2012**, *7*, 48. [CrossRef] [PubMed]

58. Weinstein, R.S.; Graham, A.R.; Richter, L.C.; Barker, G.P.; Krupinski, E.A.; Lopez, A.M.; Erps, K.A.; Bhattacharyya, A.K.; Yagi, Y.; Gilbertson, J.R. Overview of telepathology, virtual microscopy, and whole slide imaging: Prospects for the future. *Hum. Pathol.* **2009**, *40*, 1057–1069. [CrossRef] [PubMed]

59. Fischer, M.K.; Kayembe, M.K.; Scheer, A.J.; Introcaso, C.E.; Binder, S.W.; Kovarik, C.L. Establishing telepathology in Africa: Lessons from Botswana. *J. Am. Acad. Dermatol.* **2011**, *64*, 986–987. [CrossRef] [PubMed]

60. Pantanowitz, L.; Farahani, N.; Parwani, A. Whole Slide Imaging in Pathology: Advantages, Limitations, and Emerging Perspectives. *Pathol. Lab. Med. Int.* **2015**, *23*. [CrossRef]

61. Pantanowitz, L. Digital images and the future of digital pathology. *J. Pathol. Inform.* **2010**, *1*, 15. [CrossRef] [PubMed]

62. Evans, A.J.; Chetty, R.; Clarke, B.A.; Croul, S.; Ghazarian, D.M.; Kiehl, T.R.; Perez Ordonez, B.; Ilaalagan, S.; Asa, S.L. Primary frozen section diagnosis by robotic microscopy and virtual slide telepathology: The University Health Network experience. *Hum. Pathol.* **2009**, *40*, 1070–1081. [CrossRef] [PubMed]

63. Al Habeeb, A.; Ghazarian, D.; Evans, A. Virtual microscopy using whole-slide imaging as an enabler for teledermatopathology: A paired consultant validation study. *J. Pathol. Inform.* **2012**, *3*, 2. [CrossRef] [PubMed]

64. Al-Janabi, S.; Huisman, A.; Vink, A.; Leguit, R.J.; Offerhaus, G.J.A.; ten Kate, F.J.W.; van Dijk, M.R.; van Diest, P.J. Whole slide images for primary diagnostics in dermatopathology: A feasibility study. *J. Clin. Pathol.* **2012**, *65*, 152–158. [CrossRef] [PubMed]

65. Kent, M.N.; Olsen, T.G.; Feeser, T.A.; Tesno, K.C.; Moad, J.C.; Conroy, M.P.; Kendrick, M.J.; Stephenson, S.R.; Murchland, M.R.; Khan, A.U.; et al. Diagnostic accuracy of virtual pathology vs. traditional microscopy in a large dermatopathology study. *JAMA Dermatol.* **2017**, *153*, 1285. [CrossRef] [PubMed]

66. Koch, L.H.; Lampros, J.N.; Delong, L.K.; Chen, S.C.; Woosley, J.T.; Hood, A.F. Randomized comparison of virtual microscopy and traditional glass microscopy in diagnostic accuracy among dermatology and pathology residents. *Hum. Pathol.* **2009**, *40*, 662–667. [CrossRef] [PubMed]

67. Molin, J.; Thorstenson, S.; Lundström, C. Implementation of large-scale routine diagnostics using whole slide imaging in Sweden: Digital pathology experiences 2006–2013. *J. Pathol. Inform.* **2014**, *5*, 14. [CrossRef] [PubMed]

68. Nielsen, P.S.; Lindebjerg, J.; Rasmussen, J.; Starklint, H.; Waldstrøm, M.; Nielsen, B. Virtual Microscopy: An Evaluation of its Validity and Diagnostic Performance in Routine Histologic Diagnosis of Skin Tumors. *Hum. Pathol.* **2010**, *41*, 1770–1776. [CrossRef] [PubMed]

69. Shah, K.K.; Lehman, J.S.; Gibson, L.E.; Lohse, C.M.; Comfere, N.I.; Wieland, C.N. Validation of diagnostic accuracy with whole-slide imaging compared with glass slide review in dermatopathology. *J. Am. Acad. Dermatol.* **2016**, *75*, 1229–1237. [CrossRef] [PubMed]

70. Wamala, D.; Katamba, A.; Dworak, O. Feasibility and diagnostic accuracy of internet-based dynamic telepathology between Uganda and Germany. *J. Telemed. Telecare* **2011**, *17*, 222–225. [CrossRef] [PubMed]

71. Della Mea, V.; Cortolezzis, D.; Beltrami, C.A. The economics of telepathology-a case study. *J. Telemed. Telecare* **2000**, *6* (Suppl. 1), S168–S169. [PubMed]

72. Dudas, R.; VandenBussche, C.; Baras, A.; Ali, S.Z.; Olson, M.T. Inexpensive Telecytology solutions that use the Raspberry Pi and the iPhone. *J. Am. Soc. Cytopathol.* **2014**, *3*, 49–55. [CrossRef]

73. Meléndez-Álvarez, B.; Robayo, O.; Gil-Guillén, V.; Carratalá-Munuera, M. Design and validation of a low-cost telepathology system. *Telemedicine e-Health* **2017**, *23*, 976–982. [CrossRef] [PubMed]

74. Klock, C.; Gomes, R. Web conferencing systems: Skype and MSN in telepathology. *Diagn. Pathol.* **2008**, *3*, S13. [CrossRef] [PubMed]

75. Sirintrapun, S.; Cimic, A. Dynamic nonrobotic telemicroscopy via Skype: A cost effective solution to teleconsultation. *J. Pathol. Inform.* **2012**, *3*, 28. [CrossRef] [PubMed]

76. Speiser, J.J.; Hughes, I.; Mehta, V.; Wojcik, E.M.; Hutchens, K.A. Mobile teledermatopathology: Using a tablet PC as a novel and cost-efficient method to remotely diagnose dermatopathology cases. *Am. J. Dermatopathol.* **2014**, *36*, 54–57. [CrossRef] [PubMed]

77. Yu, H.; Gao, F.; Jiang, L.; Ma, S. Development of a whole slide imaging system on smartphones and evaluation with frozen section samples. *JMIR mHealth uHealth* **2017**, *5*, e132. [CrossRef] [PubMed]

78. Huang, Y.N.; Peng, X.C.; Ma, S.; Yu, H.; Jin, Y.B.; Zheng, J.; Fu, G.H. Development of whole slide imaging on smartphones and evaluation with ThinPrep cytology test samples: Follow-up study. *JMIR mHealth uHealth* **2018**, *6*, e82. [CrossRef] [PubMed]

79. Randriambelonoro, M.; Bagayoko, C.O.; Geissbuhler, A. Telemedicine as a tool for digital medical education: A 15-year journey inside the RAFT network. Digital medical education using the RAFT network. *Ann. N. Y. Acad. Sci.* **2018**. [CrossRef] [PubMed]

80. Mosa, A.S.M.; Yoo, I.; Sheets, L. A systematic review of healthcare applications for smartphones. *BMC Med. Inform. Decis. Mak.* **2012**, *12*. [CrossRef] [PubMed]

81. Dynamed. Available online: https://dynamed.com/home/ (accessed on 20 June 2018).

82. Epocrates. Available online: http://www.epocrates.com/ (accessed on 20 June 2018).

83. Medscape. Available online: www.medscape.com (accessed on 20 June 2018).

84. Visual Dx. Available online: https://www.visualdx.com/ (accessed on 20 June 2018).

85. UpToDate. Available online: https://www.uptodate.com/home (accessed on 20 June 2018).

86. Colven, R.; Shim, M.H.M.; Brock, D.; Todd, G. dermatological diagnostic acumen improves with use of a simple telemedicine system for underserved areas of South Africa. *Telemed. e-Health* **2011**, *17*, 363–369. [CrossRef] [PubMed]

87. Osei-tutu, A.; Shih, T.; Rosen, A.; Amanquah, N.; Chowdhury, M.; Nijhawan, R.I.; Siegel, D.; Kovarik, C. Mobile teledermatology in Ghana: Sending and answering consults via mobile platform. *J. Am. Acad. Dermatol.* **2013**, *69*, e90–e91. [CrossRef] [PubMed]

88. Patro, B.; Tripathy, J.; Sinha, S.; Singh, A.; De, D.; Kanwar, A. Diagnostic agreement between a primary care physician and a teledermatologist for common dermatological conditions in North India. *Indian Dermatol. Online J.* **2015**, *6*, 21. [CrossRef] [PubMed]

89. Tran, K.; Ayad, M.; Weinberg, J.; Cherng, A.; Chowdhury, M.; Monir, S.; El Hariri, M.; Kovarik, C. Mobile teledermatology in the developing world: Implications of a feasibility study on 30 Egyptian patients with common skin diseases. *J. Am. Acad. Dermatol.* **2011**, *64*, 302–309. [CrossRef] [PubMed]

90. Azfar, R.S.; Weinberg, J.L.; Cavric, G.; Lee-Keltner, I.A.; Bilker, W.B.; Gelfand, J.M.; Kovarik, C.L. HIV-positive patients in Botswana state that mobile teledermatology is an acceptable method for receiving dermatology care. *J. Telemed. Telecare* **2011**, *17*, 338–340. [CrossRef] [PubMed]

91. Azfar, R.S.; Lee, R.A.; Castelo-Soccio, L.; Greenberg, M.S.; Bilker, W.B.; Gelfand, J.M.; Kovarik, C.L. Reliability and validity of mobile teledermatology in human immunodeficiency virus–positive patients in Botswana: A pilot study. *JAMA Dermatol.* **2014**, *150*, 601. [CrossRef] [PubMed]

92. Frühauf, J.; Hofman-Wellenhof, R.; Kovarik, C.; Mulyowa, G.; Alitwala, C.; Soyer, H.; Kaddu, S. Mobile teledermatology in sub-Saharan Africa: A useful tool in supporting health workers in low-resource centres. *Acta Derm. Venereol.* **2013**, *93*, 122–123. [CrossRef] [PubMed]

93. Greisman, L.; Nguyen, T.M.; Mann, R.E.; Baganizi, M.; Jacobson, M.; Paccione, G.A.; Friedman, A.J.; Lipoff, J.B. Feasibility and cost of a medical student proxy-based mobile teledermatology consult service with Kisoro, Uganda, and Lake Atitlán, Guatemala. *Int. J. Dermatol.* **2015**, *54*, 685–692. [CrossRef] [PubMed]

94. Littman-Quinn, R.; Mibenge, C.; Antwi, C.; Chandra, A.; Kovarik, C.L. Implementation of m-Health applications in Botswana: Telemedicine and education on mobile devices in a low resource setting. *J. Telemed. Telecare* **2013**, *19*, 120–125. [CrossRef] [PubMed]

95. Mars, M.; Scott, R.E. Being spontaneous: The future of telehealth implementation? *Telemed. e-Health* **2017**. [CrossRef] [PubMed]

96. Sáenz, J.P.; Novoa, M.P.; Correal, D.; Eapen, B.R. On using a mobile application to support teledermatology: A case study in an underprivileged area in Colombia. *Int. J. Telemed. Appl.* **2018**, *2018*, 1–8. [CrossRef] [PubMed]

97. Chansky, P.B.; Simpson, C.L.; Lipoff, J.B. Implementation of a dermatology teletriage system to improve access in an underserved clinic: A retrospective study. *J. Am. Acad. Dermatol.* **2017**, *77*, 975–977. [CrossRef] [PubMed]

98. Ferrándiz, L.; Moreno-Ramírez, D.; Ruiz-de-Casas, A.; Nieto-García, A.; Moreno-Alvarez, P.; Galdeano, R.; Camacho, F.M. An economic analysis of presurgical teledermatology in patients with nonmelanoma skin cancer. *Actas Dermo-Sifiliogr.* **2008**, *99*, 795–802. [CrossRef]

99. Moreno-Ramirez, D.; Ferrandiz, L.; Ruiz-de-Casas, A.; Nieto-Garcia, A.; Moreno-Alvarez, P.; Galdeano, R.; Camacho, F.M. Economic evaluation of a store-and-forward teledermatology system for skin cancer patients. *J. Telemed. Telecare* **2009**, *15*, 40–45. [CrossRef] [PubMed]

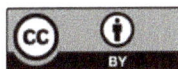

Tropical Medicine and Infectious Disease

MDPI

Review

Community Involvement in the Care of Persons Affected by Podoconiosis—A Lesson for Other Skin NTDs

Abebayehu Tora [1] , Asrat Mengiste [2], Gail Davey [3] and Maya Semrau [3,*]

1   Department of Sociology, Wolaita Sodo University, Sodo, Ethiopia; abezed@yahoo.com
2   National Podoconiosis Action Network, Addis Ababa, Ethiopia; asrat_m@napanEthiopia.org
3   Department of Global Health and Infection, Brighton and Sussex Medical School, Falmer Campus, University of Sussex, Brighton BN1 9PX, UK; G.Davey@bsms.ac.uk
*   Correspondence: M.Semrau@bsms.ac.uk; Tel.: +44-1273-872-788

Received: 20 July 2018; Accepted: 11 August 2018; Published: 16 August 2018

Abstract: Podoconiosis is a neglected tropical disease (NTD) characterized by lower-leg swelling (lymphedema), which is caused by long-term exposure to irritant red-clay soils found within tropical volcanic high-altitude environments with heavy rainfall. The condition places a substantial burden on affected people, their families and communities, including disability, economic consequences, social exclusion, and stigma; mental disorders and distress are also common. This paper focuses on community-based care of podoconiosis, and, in particular, the role that community involvement can have in the reduction of stigma against people affected by podoconiosis. We first draw on research conducted in Ethiopia for this, which has included community-based provision of care and treatment, education, and awareness-raising, and socioeconomic rehabilitation to reduce stigma. Since people affected by podoconiosis and other skin NTDs often suffer the double burden of mental-health illness, which is similarly stigmatized, we then point to examples from the mental-health field in low-resource community settings to suggest avenues for stigma reduction and increased patient engagement that may be relevant across a range of skin NTDs, though further research is needed on this.

Keywords: podoconiosis; lymphedema; neglected tropical diseases; NTDs; mental health; community engagement; patient involvement; stigma

---

1. Introduction

Podoconiosis is a neglected tropical disease (NTD), characterized by lower-leg swelling (lymphedema), which is found in highland areas of the tropics. It has often been confused with lymphatic filariasis, and is currently dealt with by the World Health Organization (WHO) under the lymphatic filariasis (LF) program (link: http://www.who.int/lymphatic_filariasis/epidemiology/podoconiosis/en/), but differs in that it is associated with long-term exposure to irritant tropical soils [1] rather than any parasite, virus, or bacterium. These red-clay soils are found in highland tropical areas, where ancient volcanic deposits have weathered [2] at high altitude (over 1000 m) under conditions of heavy rainfall (over 1000 mm/year). There is now strong evidence of underlying genetic susceptibility for podoconiosis [3], and endemic communities are usually aware that the condition clusters in families.

Countries with a high burden of podoconiosis include Ethiopia, Uganda, Cameroon, Kenya, and Tanzania [4]. Although rarely a direct cause of mortality, podoconiosis disables those affected through progressive leg swelling and repeated episodes of acute dermatolymphangioadenitis. These acute episodes occur frequently (reports vary from five [5] to 23 [6] episodes per year), and contribute substantially to the disability and social impact associated with podoconiosis [7,8]. Research has explored the enormous economic burden of podoconiosis on affected communities. In a southern Ethiopian zone of 1.5 million inhabitants, where the prevalence of podoconiosis is known to be 5.4%, the overall cost of podoconiosis was estimated to be in excess of US$16 million per year. In this zone, where the average income is less than US$100 per year, the direct costs to a patient were found to be US$143 per year [9]. In addition to its economic consequences, one of the most devastating characteristics of podoconiosis is stigma [10–12].

This article is a nonsystematic narrative review [13]. It focuses on community-based care of podoconiosis, and, in particular, the role that community involvement can have in the reduction of stigma against people affected by podoconiosis, but it also draws on other types of lymphedema, such as leprosy and LF. We start by exploring the sources and consequences of stigma among people with podoconiosis and then describe community-based approaches used to reduce stigma and provide care in Ethiopia. We then draw on examples from the field of mental health in low-resource community settings to suggest avenues for stigma reduction and increased patient engagement relevant across a range of skin NTDs. To our knowledge, this is the first review on community involvement in the care of people affected by podoconiosis, which also looks beyond NTDs to learn lessons from the mental-health field.

2. Sources and Consequences of Stigma in Podoconiosis

Stigma has commonly been defined as an undesirable or discrediting attribute that reduces an individual's status in the eyes of society [14,15]. The major sources of stigma among people affected with podoconiosis include the progressive physical disability that prevents affected individuals from making a living [9,16]; the misconceptions among community members about the causes of the disease and treatment options [7,17–19]; fear of public identification of a disease that is known to be familial [18]; and the physical disfigurement caused as the disease advances [20].

People affected by podoconiosis, as is the case for people affected by other lower-limb lymphedemas such as leprosy and LF, are stigmatized in all areas of their daily life. Overt discrimination is common during social functions, around mate selection and marriage, when seeking employment, and in relation to leadership roles. Due to deep-seated stigmatizing attitudes within the community, affected individuals also experience self-stigma, manifested in the form of low self-esteem, suicidal ideation, and avoidance of interactions with nonaffected community members [11]. The prejudice, discrimination, and self-stigma related to podoconiosis and other lymphedemas not only compromise the psychological and social wellbeing of patients and their families, but also limit their access to healthcare and adherence with treatment. This causes a vicious circle, creating further disability, illness, and reduced economic productivity. Breaking the vicious cycle of stigma related to podoconiosis has been a top priority for community organizations and researchers to improve the quality of life of patients and their families.

3. Community Interventions

Several community-based podoconiosis interventions have been implemented within Ethiopia, including provision of care and treatment, education, and socioeconomic rehabilitation. Though podoconiosis is an age-old disease, appropriate and effective means of treatment have not been understood or available until recently. Personal efforts to treat the disease using traditional knowledge have usually been counterproductive [21]. Most people affected by the disease therefore live with disfigurement and disability without receiving standardized services through the formal health system [22]. This has led to misconceptions around the possibility of cure, which, in turn, has increased the stigmatization of affected people [21].

3.1. Community-Based Care and Treatment

Over the last two decades, NGOs and faith-based organizations have played a pioneering role in providing care and treatment for people affected by the disease in vertically established outreach clinics [22,23]. In southern Ethiopia, Mossy Foot International has transformed patients who have successfully treated themselves into Community Podoconiosis Agents. Patients who have been educated to high-school completion are given full-time clinical training over a period of one week, and then become responsible for identifying patients in their own community and supporting self-care [22]. Training expert patients to provide simple, close-to-patient services is a potentially powerful solution to lack of care in countries with low formal health-services coverage. Harnessing the power of the local community to advocate for patients is likely to improve social support and diminish stigma in relation to a range of dermatologic conditions [24].

By halting the progress of disability and reducing the chances of illness related to acute attacks, the care that patients receive increases participation in community affairs and enhances their economic productivity, thereby improving their acceptance in society. Similar benefits have been documented for people affected by leprosy and LF, for example a leprosy self-care program in the 1990s and other leprosy and LF programs since then. Although the main function of the leprosy self-care groups was to encourage members to take responsibility for their own wound management, the group members reported a number of qualitative benefits, in particular improved self-respect and dignity and increased participation in society [25]. However, while these disease-specific examples are important, other studies suggest that integration of care and treatment into existing health systems may provide better opportunities to counter stigma than stand-alone vertical programs [26]. A systematic review conducted in 2016 suggested that joint approaches to reduce stigmatization across NTDs may be feasible given the similarities in causes, manifestations, and interventions against it [12]. Recent efforts to integrate podoconiosis care and treatment into government health structures alongside other types of lymphedema such as leprosy and LF are likely to play an important role in this regard [27].

3.2. Community-Based Education and Awareness

In addition to patient care and treatment, both Mossy Foot International and the International Orthodox Christian Charities (IOCC) program (in northern Ethiopia) have utilized Community Conversations or their equivalents to raise the awareness of the general population about podoconiosis causes, treatment, and prevention. These programs seek to encourage people to reflect on their place in the wider community, and to identify training, employment, and personal-development opportunities within the community sector.

The effectiveness of community-based health education run by lay people in reducing stigma has been confirmed in Ethiopia [28]. This study demonstrated that a health-education intervention that included community awareness campaigns and household skill-building activities run by lay health advisors decreased both felt and enacted stigma related to podoconiosis. In addition, awareness-raising and education amongst healthcare staff may be equally important to counter the stigmatizing attitudes and prejudices commonly held by them.

3.3. Community-Based Socioeconomic Rehabilitation

The final form of stigma reduction implemented in the context of podoconiosis is socioeconomic rehabilitation. This involves skills training (e.g., carpentry, masonry, hairdressing, shoemaking, etc.), enhancing entrepreneurship through revolving funds and loans, and providing educational opportunities [22]. Though the impact of socioeconomic rehabilitation in the context of podoconiosis has not been formally assessed, anecdotal evidences suggests that access to these services reduces stigma by increasing self-reliance, self-esteem, and financial independence, and acquiring new skills that widen opportunities for self-employment and access to public institutions. Participation in socioeconomic rehabilitation also influences the process of social integration and social acceptance through contributing to attitudinal change towards affected people [29].

4. Lessons from Community Engagement for Mental Health

Mental illness shares similar characteristics to skin NTDs in that affected persons are also heavily stigmatized and discriminated against, and are often excluded from social and economic activities [30–32]. Furthermore, rates of mental disorder (such as depression) and distress have been shown to be elevated amongst people with podoconiosis, LF, and other skin NTDs (which may both be an additional cause of stigma, as well as a consequence of the NTD-related stigma) [8,33,34]. Community engagement has been shown to be effective in addressing stigma, and thereby increasing uptake of and adherence to services, not only for NTDs such as podoconiosis and LF (as described above) but also for mental illness. It may therefore be helpful to look beyond NTDs, to learn lessons about community engagement from interventions used within the mental-health field, and how these might shape holistic interventions for stigmatized skin NTDs, particularly—but not only—for those who suffer the added burden of mental illness. However, further research on this is greatly needed.

The few studies published from low- and middle-income countries (LMICs) that have aimed to increase uptake of mental-health services by reducing stigma in the local community have included awareness-raising to change community knowledge and attitudes towards people with mental illness as their core component [35–37]. A program implemented in several states in Nigeria [35,36], for example, led to a significant increase in the use of community-based primary-care mental-health services by training voluntary lay community health workers (CHWs) to deliver positive health messages and challenge misconceptions around mental health, alongside a media campaign of radio announcements, jingles, and newspaper coverage. The program highlighted the importance of regular 'booster' training (e.g., every six months) and supervision, plus possibly other initiatives (such as incentives or paid work), to sustain CHWs' enthusiasm and the effectiveness of the program over time. Other key lessons learned from such programs have been the importance of involving and gaining buy-in from community members and leaders and health-system leaders from the start (for example, through forming of a stakeholder committee); linking raising awareness to the available services; and using 'Training of Trainers' approaches to achieve scale-up.

A further important finding from the mental-health field has been that interventions that include a social-contact element seem to be the most effective in reducing mental-health-related stigma and discrimination [38,39]. This can be either through direct contact with a patient, or indirect contact such as video testimonies, or affected persons sharing their experiences in newspapers, radio, TV, or posters. Whilst community-based awareness-raising interventions such as the ones outlined in the sections above may be essential in improving literacy of mental health and/or skin NTDs, it may therefore be valuable to explore further the inclusion of social-contact components within community-engagement interventions for skin NTDs and/or comorbid mental illness in order to increase their effectiveness. Contact interventions have indeed already shown successes in reducing leprosy-related stigma [40].

Service-user (patient) engagement is another area that may be as important for skin NTDs as for mental health, to empower and support affected people, and to facilitate self-care, and there are several good cases from the leprosy and LF field [27,41–45]. Examples of mental-health programs come from the five-year 'Emerging mental health systems in LMICs' (Emerald) program [46] and the seven-year 'PRogramme for Improving Mental health carE' (PRIME) [47], which were both implemented in countries in Africa and Asia (Ethiopia, India, Nepal, South Africa, and Uganda; plus Nigeria for Emerald). Both programs aimed to improve mental health care in these countries; whilst PRIME did so by collecting evidence on the integration and scale-up of mental health services into primary health care [47], Emerald did so by building capacity and generating evidence to enhance health-system strengthening [46]. PRIME, which also used WHO's widely-implemented mhGAP Intervention Guide [48] within primary health care, included a range of community-based interventions within its larger program, such as awareness-raising workshops, mental-health components within Community Conversation groups, information dissemination, case detection by CHWs, community mobilization, and community-based rehabilitation [49].

Both Emerald and PRIME included the engagement of mental-health patients and their families/caregivers as an important component, and acknowledged that patient involvement is essential when developing interventions and when expanding access to integrated care services within primary-care settings in LMICs [50]. A cross-country qualitative study conducted by Emerald identified the main strategies for increasing patient involvement in health-system strengthening to be patient and caregiver mobilization and empowerment; the need for capacity-building (training) of patients/caregivers and service providers; and ensuring human rights for greater involvement [51]. Alongside this, common barriers were identified that need to be tackled and that are reminiscent of skin NTDs, such as stigma, poverty, and power differentials in the health system, including lack of knowledge of services and support in the local community [50–53]. To achieve capacity-building of mental-health patients and their families/caregivers, Emerald took a country-specific multifaceted approach that aimed to include awareness-raising, stigma reduction, information, and mobilization and engagement of patients as its key ingredients; some of the main interventions used were workshops with mental-health patients and their caregivers to raise awareness and mobilize for greater advocacy and involvement, and workshops for primary-care workers and managers to support greater patient involvement [54]. The concepts of appropriateness, reciprocity, sustainability, and equality in partnerships were identified as being important and underpinned all capacity-building activities [54,55]; these may be relevant beyond the mental-health field, including within skin NTD programs.

5. Looking to the Future

While several approaches to community-based delivery of care, of education and awareness, and of socioeconomic rehabilitation have been successfully used by podoconiosis (as well as leprosy and LF) programs in Ethiopia and elsewhere, there is much potential for more. Socioeconomic community-based rehabilitation in particular is an area that warrants further research.

Looking to the experience of community-based mental health services, there are still many interventions that could potentially be applied to podoconiosis and across other stigmatized skin conditions. Holistic approaches are needed that take into account not only the physical care of skin NTDs, but also integrate mental-health components and take into account the complex interplay of physical disability, mental illness, and associated stigma. At the community level, this could include awareness-raising, not only of the implications in regards to the physical health of people affected by skin NTDs, but also the mental-health implications (for example through awareness-raising workshops, the inclusion of mental-health components within Community Conversation groups, or information dissemination). Social-contact elements may be particularly useful in this respect. Similarly, patient engagement, for example through patient groups, is vital in order to empower and support affected people, and to facilitate self-care. Services should be integrated so that patients receive care not only for their physical disabilities but also any mental distress or disorder; this can be achieved by making integrated services readily available in nearby primary healthcare facilities and/or in the community, for instance by training (and then providing regular supervision for) primary healthcare staff and/or community health workers in case detection and/or treatment of mental disorders, as well as physical healthcare. Stigma-reduction activities within this training may be important to counter any negative attitudes or prejudices. Further research is required to adapt and evaluate these programs in a range of disease and country contexts.

Author Contributions: All authors contributed to the writing of the paper, and have seen and approved the final version.

Funding: This research received no external funding. The Emerald program was funded by the European Union's Seventh Framework Programme (FP7/2007–2013) under grant agreement n° 305968. PRIME was supported by the UK Department for International Development [201446].

Trop. Med. Infect. Dis. **2018**, 3, 87

Conflicts of Interest: The authors declare no conflict of interest. The funders had no role in the design of the study; in the collection, analyses, or interpretation of data; in the writing of the manuscript; and in the decision to publish the results.

References

1. Molla, Y.; Wardrop, N.; Le Blond, J.; Baxter, P.; Newport, M.; Atkinson, P.; Davey, G. Modelling environmental factors correlated with podoconiosis: A geospatial study of non-filarial elephantiasis. *Int. J. Health Geogr.* **2014**, *13*, 24. [CrossRef] [PubMed]

2. Le Blond, J.; Cuadros, J.; Molla, Y.; Berhanu, T.; Umer, M.; Baxter, P.; Davey, G. Weathering of the Ethiopian volcanic province: A new weathering index to characterize and compare soils. *Am. Mineral.* **2015**, *100*, 2518–2532. [CrossRef]

3. Tekola Ayele, F.; Adeyemo, A.; Finan, C.; Hailu, E.; Sinnott, P.; Diaz Burlinson, N.; Aseffa, A.; Rotimi, C.; Newport, M.; Davey, G. HLA class II locus and susceptibility to podoconiosis. *N. Engl. J. Med.* **2012**, *366*, 1200–1208. [CrossRef] [PubMed]

4. Deribe, K.; Cano, J.; Trueba, M.; Newport, M.; Davey, G. Global epidemiology of podoconiosis: A systematic review. *PLoS Negl. Trop. Dis.* **2018**, *12*, e0006324. [CrossRef] [PubMed]

5. Molla, Y.; Tomczyk, S.; Amberbir, T.; Tamiru, A.; Davey, G. Podoconiosis in East and West Gojam Zones, northern Ethiopia. *PLoS. Negl. Trop. Dis.* **2012**, *6*, e1744. [CrossRef] [PubMed]

6. Bekele, K.; Deribe, K.; Amberbir, T.; Tadele, G.; Davey, G.; Samuel, A. Burden assessment of podoconiosis in Wayu Tuka Woreda, East Wollega Zone, western Ethiopia: A community-based cross-sectional study. *BMJ Open* **2016**, *6*, e012308. [CrossRef] [PubMed]

7. Molla, Y.; Tomczyk, S.; Amberbir, T.; Tamiru, A.; Davey, G. Patients' perceptions of podoconiosis causes, prevention and consequences in East and West Gojam, northern Ethiopia. *BMC Public Health* **2012**, *12*, 828. [CrossRef] [PubMed]

8. Bartlett, J.; Deribe, K.; Tamiru, A.; Amberbir, T.; Medhin, G.; Malik, M.; Hanlon, C.; Davey, G. Depression and disability in people with podoconiosis: A comparative cross-sectional study in rural northern Ethiopia. *Int. Health* **2015**, *8*, 124–131. [CrossRef] [PubMed]

9. Tekola, F.; HaileMariam, D.; Davey, G. Economic costs of endemic non-filarial elephantiasis in Wolaita Zone, Ethiopia. *Trop. Med. Int. Health* **2006**, *11*, 1136–1144. [CrossRef] [PubMed]

10. Deribe, K.; Tomczyk, S.; Mousley, E.; Tamiru, A.; Davey, G. Stigma towards a neglected tropical disease: Felt and enacted stigma scores among podoconiosis patients in northern Ethiopia. *BMC Public Health* **2013**, *13*, 1178. [CrossRef] [PubMed]

11. Tora, A.; Franklin, H.; Deribe, K.; Reda, A.; Davey, G. Extent of podoconiosis-related stigma in Wolaita Zone, southern Ethiopia: A cross-sectional study. *SpringerPlus* **2014**, *3*, 647. [CrossRef] [PubMed]

12. Hofstraat, K.; van Brakel, W. Social stigma towards neglected tropical diseases: A systematic review. *Int. Health* **2016**, *8*, i53–i70. [CrossRef] [PubMed]

13. Grant, M.; Booth, A. A typology of reviews: An analysis of 14 review types and associated methodologies. *Health Inf. Libr. J.* **2009**, *26*, 91–108. [CrossRef] [PubMed]

14. Link, B.; Phelan, J. Conceptualizing stigma. *Annu. Rev. Sociol.* **2001**, *27*, 363–385. [CrossRef]

15. Weiss, M. Stigma and the social burden of neglected tropical diseases. *PLoS Negl. Trop. Dis.* **2008**, *2*, e237. [CrossRef] [PubMed]

16. Desta, K.; Ashine, M.; Davey, G. Prevalence of podoconiosis (endemic non-filarial elephantiasis) in Wolaitta, southern Ethiopia. *Trop. Doctor* **2003**, *32*, 217–220. [CrossRef] [PubMed]

17. Yakob, B.; Deribe, K.; Davey, G. High levels of misconceptions and stigma in a community highly endemic for podoconiosis in southern Ethiopia. *Trans. R. Soc. Trop. Med. Hyg.* **2008**, *102*, 439–444. [CrossRef] [PubMed]

18. Tora, A.; Davey, G.; Tadele, G. A qualitative study on stigma and coping strategies of patients with podoconiosis in Wolaita Zone, southern Ethiopia. *Int. Health* **2011**, *3*, 176–181. [CrossRef] [PubMed]

19. Ayode, D.; McBride, C.; de Heer, D.; Watanabe, E.; Gebreyesus, T.; Tadele, G.; Tora, A.; Davey, G. The association of beliefs about heredity with preventive and interpersonal behaviors in communities affected by podoconiosis in rural Ethiopia. *Am. J. Trop. Med. Hyg.* **2012**, *87*, 623–630. [CrossRef] [PubMed]

20. Tekola, F.; Bull, S.; Farsides, B.; Newport, M.; Adeyemo, A.; Rotimi, C.; Davey, G. Impact of social stigma on the process of obtaining informed consent for genetic research on podoconiosis: A qualitative study. *BMC Med. Ethics* **2009**, *10*, 13. [CrossRef] [PubMed]

21. Tora, A.; Davey, G.; Tadele, G. Factors related to discontinued clinic attendance by patients with podoconiosis in southern Ethiopia: A qualitative study. *BMC Public Health* **2012**, *12*, 902. [CrossRef] [PubMed]

22. Davey, G.; Burridge, E. Community-based control of a neglected tropical disease: The mossy foot treatment and prevention association. *PLoS Negl. Trop. Dis.* **2009**, *3*, e424. [CrossRef] [PubMed]

23. Tomczyk, S.; Tamiru, A.; Davey, G. Addressing the neglected tropical disease podoconiosis in northern Ethiopia: Lessons learned from a new community podoconiosis program. *PLoS Negl. Trop. Dis.* **2012**, *6*, e1560. [CrossRef] [PubMed]

24. Molla, Y.; Davey, G. Podoconiosis control in rural Ethiopia: The roles of expert patients, appropriate treatment and community mobilization. *Commun. Dermatol.* **2012**, *10*, 3.

25. Benbow, C.; Temiru, T. The experience of self-care groups with people affected by leprosy: Alert, Ethiopia. *Lepr. Rev.* **2001**, *72*, 311–321. [CrossRef] [PubMed]

26. Arole, S.; Premkumar, R.; Arole, R.; Maury, M.; Saunderson, P. Social stigma: A comparative qualitative study of integrated and vertical care approaches to leprosy. *Lepr. Rev.* **2002**, *73*, 186–196. [PubMed]

27. Pryce, J.; Mableson, H.; Choudhary, R.; Pandey, B.; Aley, D.; Betts, H.; Mackenzie, C.; Kelly-Hope, L.; Cross, H. Assessing the feasibility of integration of self-care for filarial lymphoedema into existing community leprosy self-help groups in Nepal. *BMC Public Health* **2018**, *18*, 201. [CrossRef] [PubMed]

28. McBride, C.; Price, C.; Ayode, D.; Tora, A.; Farrell, D.; Davey, G. A cluster randomized intervention trial to promote shoe use by children at high risk for podoconiosis. *Int. J. Health Sci. Res.* **2015**, *5*, 518–528.

29. Ebenso, B.; Fashona, A.; Ayuba, M.; Idah, M. Impact of socio-economic rehabilitation on leprosy stigma in northern Nigeria: Findings of a retrospective study. *Asian Pac. Disabil. Rehabilit. J.* **2007**, *18*, 98–119.

30. Thornicroft, G.; Brohan, E.; Rose, D.; Sartorius, N.; Leese, M. INDIGO Study Group. Global pattern of experienced and anticipated discrimination against people with schizophrenia: A cross-sectional survey. *Lancet* **2009**, *373*, 408–415. [CrossRef]

31. Thornicroft, G.; Bakolis, I.; Evans-Lacko, S.; Gronholm, P.; Henderson, C.; Kohrt, B.; Koschorke, M.; Milenova, M.; Semrau, M.; Votruba, N.; et al. Key lessons learned from the indigo global network on mental health related stigma and discrimination. *World Psychiatry*, in press.

32. Semrau, M.; Evans-Lacko, S.; Koschorke, M.; Ashenafi, L.; Thornicroft, G. Stigma and discrimination related to mental illness in low and middle income countries. *Epidemiol. Psychiatr. Sci.* **2015**, *24*, 382–394. [CrossRef] [PubMed]

33. Mousley, E.; Deribe, K.; Tamiru, A.; Tomczyk, S.; Hanlon, C.; Davey, G. Mental distress and podoconiosis in northern Ethiopia: A comparative cross-sectional study. *Int. Health* **2015**, *7*, 16–25. [CrossRef] [PubMed]

34. Obindo, J.; Abdulmalik, J.; Nwefoh, E.; Agbir, M.; Nwoga, C.; Armiya'u, A.; Davou, F.; Maigida, K.; Otache, E.; Ebiloma, A.; et al. Prevalence of depression and associated clinical and socio-demographic factors in people living with lymphatic filariasis in Plateau State, Nigeria. *PLoS Negl. Trop. Dis.* **2017**, *6*, e0005567. [CrossRef] [PubMed]

35. Eaton, J.; Agomoh, A. Developing mental health services in Nigeria. *Soc. Psychiatry Psychiatr. Epidemiol.* **2008**, *43*, 552–558. [CrossRef] [PubMed]

36. Eaton, J.; Nwefoh, E.; Okafor, G.; Onyeonoro, U.; Nwaubani, K.; Henderson, C. Interventions to increase use of services; mental health awareness in Nigeria. *Int. J. Ment. Health Syst.* **2017**, *11*, 66. [CrossRef] [PubMed]

37. Armstrong, G.; Kermode, M.; Raja, S.; Suja, S.; Chandra, P.; Jorm, A. A mental health training program for community health workers in India: Impact on knowledge and attitudes. *Int. J. Ment. Health Syst.* **2011**, *5*, 17. [CrossRef] [PubMed]

38. Thornicroft, G.; Mehta, N.; Clement, S.; Evans-Lacko, S.; Doherty, M.; Rose, D.; Koschorke, M.; Shidhaye, R.; O'Reilly, C.; Henderson, C. Evidence for effective interventions to reduce mental-health-related stigma and discrimination. *Lancet* **2016**, *387*, 1123–1132. [CrossRef]

39. Mehta, N.; Clement, S.; Marcus, E.; Stona, A.-C.; Bezborodovs, N.; Evans-Lacko, S.; Palacios, J.; Docherty, M.; Barley, E.; Rose, D.; et al. Evidence for effective interventions to reduce mental health-related stigma and discrimination in the medium and long term: Systematic review. *Br. J. Psychiatry* **2015**, *207*, 377–384. [CrossRef] [PubMed]

40. Peters, R.; Dadun, D.; Zweekhorst, M.; Bunders, J.; Irwanto, I.; van Brakel, W. A cluster-randomized controlled intervention study to assess the effect of a contact intervention in reducing leprosy-related stigma in Indonesia. *PLoS Negl. Trop. Dis.* **2015**, 9, e0004003. [CrossRef] [PubMed]

41. Cross, H.; Chowdhary, R. Step: An intervention to address the issue of stigma related to leprosy in southern Nepal. *Lepr. Rev.* **2005**, 76, 316–324. [PubMed]

42. Sermrittirong, S.; van Brakel, W.; Bunbers-Aelen, J. How to reduce stigma in leprosy—A systematic literature review. *Lepr. Rev.* **2014**, 85, 149–157. [PubMed]

43. Peters, R.; Zweekhorst, M.; van Brakel, W.; Bunders, J.; Irwanto, I. 'People like me don't make things like that': Participatory video as a method for reducing leprosy-related stigma. *Glob. Public Health* **2016**, 11, 5–6. [CrossRef] [PubMed]

44. Lusli, M.; Peters, R.; van Brakel, W.; Zweekhorst, M.; Iancu, S.; Bunders, J.; Irwanto; Regeer, B. The impact of a rights-based counselling intervention to reduce stigma in people affected by leprosy in Indonesia. *PLoS Negl. Trop. Dis.* **2016**, 10, e0005088. [CrossRef] [PubMed]

45. Lusli, M.; Zweekhorst, M.; Miranda-Galarza, B.; Peters, R.; Cummings, S.; Seda, F.; Bunders, J.; Irwanto. Dealing with stigma: Experiences of persons affected by disabilities and leprosy. *Biomed. Res. Int.* **2015**, 2015, 261329. [CrossRef] [PubMed]

46. Semrau, M.; Evans-Lacko, S.; Alem, A.; Ayuso-Mateos, J.; Chisholm, D.; Gureje, O.; Hanlon, C.; Jordans, M.; Kigozi, F.; Lempp, H.; et al. Strengthening mental health systems in low and middle-income countries: The Emerald programme. *BMC Med.* **2015**, 13, 79. [CrossRef] [PubMed]

47. Lund, C.; Tomlinson, M.; de Silva, M.; Fekadu, A.; Shidhaye, R.; Jordans, M.; Petersen, I.; Bhana, A.; Kigozi, F.; Prince, M.; et al. PRIME: A programme to reduce the treatment gap for mental disorders in five low- and middle-income countries. *PLOS Med.* **2012**, 9, e1001359. [CrossRef] [PubMed]

48. World Health Organization (WHO). *Mhgap Intervention Guide*; WHO: Geneva, Switzerland, 2016.

49. Lund, C.; Tomlinson, M.; Patel, V. Integration of mental health into primary care in low- and middle-income countries: The PRIME mental healthcare plans. *Br. J. Psychiatry* **2016**, 208, s1–s3. [CrossRef] [PubMed]

50. Abayneh, S.; Lempp, H.; Alem, A.; Alemayehu, D.; Eshetu, T.; Lund, C.; Semrau, M.; Thornicroft, G.; Hanlon, C. Service user involvement in mental health system strengthening in a rural african setting: Qualitative study. *BMC Psychiatry* **2017**, 17, 187. [CrossRef] [PubMed]

51. Lempp, H.; Abayneh, S.; Gurung, D.; Kola, L.; Abdulmalik, J.; Evans-Lacko, S.; Semrau, M.; Alem, A.; Thornicroft, G.; Hanlon, C. Service user and caregiver involvement in mental health system strengthening in low and middle income countries: A cross-country qualitative study. *Epidemiol. Psychiatr. Sci.* **2018**, 27, 29–39. [CrossRef] [PubMed]

52. Gurung, D.; Upadhaya, N.; Magar, J.; Giri, N.; Hanlon, C.; Jordans, M. Service user and care giver involvement in mental health system strengthening in Nepal: A qualitative study on barriers and facilitating factors. *Int. J. Ment. Health Syst.* **2017**, 11, 30. [CrossRef] [PubMed]

53. Samudre, S.; Shidhaye, R.; Ahuja, S.; Nanda, S.; Khan, A.; Evans-Lacko, S.; Hanlon, C. Service user involvement for mental health system strengthening in India: A qualitative study. *BMC Psychiatry* **2016**, 16, 269. [CrossRef] [PubMed]

54. Semrau, M.; Alem, A.; Abdulmalik, J.; Docrat, S.; Evans-Lacko, S.; Gureje, O.; Kigozi, F.; Lempp, H.; Lund, C.; Petersen, I.; et al. Developing capacity-building activities for mental health system strengthening in low- and middle-income countries for service users and caregivers, service planners and researchers. *Epidemiol. Psychiatr. Sci.* **2017**, 27, 11–21. [CrossRef] [PubMed]

55. Hanlon, C.; Semrau, M.; Alem, A.; Abayneh, S.; Abdulmalik, J.; Docrat, S.; Evans-Lacko, S.; Gureje, O.; Jordans, M.; Lempp, H.; et al. Evaluating capacity-building for mental health system strengthening in low- and middle-income countries for service users and caregivers, service planners and researchers. *Epidemiol. Psychiatr. Sci.* **2017**, 27, 3–10. [CrossRef] [PubMed]

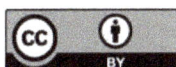

Tropical Medicine and Infectious Disease

MDPI

Article

A Teledermatology Pilot Programme for the Management of Skin Diseases in Primary Health Care Centres: Experiences from a Resource-Limited Country (Mali, West Africa)

Ousmane Faye [1,*], Cheick Oumar Bagayoko [2], Adama Dicko [1], Lamissa Cissé [1], Siritio Berthé [1], Bekaye Traoré [1], Youssouf Fofana [1], Mahamoudan Niang [2], Seydou Tidiane Traoré [2], Yamoussa Karabinta [1], Mamadou Gassama [1], Binta Guindo [1], Alimata Keita [1], Koreissi Tall [1], Somita Keita [1], Antoine Geissbuhler [4], Antoine Mahé [3] and Teledermali Team [†]

[1]   Department of Dermatology, Faculty of Medicine and Odontostomatology, Bamako, Mali;
      adadicko@yahoo.fr (A.D.); lamissa05@gmail.com (L.C.); siritio_b@yahoo.fr (S.B.); b_traore@ymail.com (B.T.);
      youssouffofana346@yahoo.fr (Y.F.); ykarabinta@yahoo.com (Y.K.); gasdiaby@yahoo.fr (M.G.);
      binta.guindo@yahoo.fr (B.G.); alimatakeita@yahoo.fr (A.K.); koreissit@yahoo.fr (K.T.);
      somitak@yahoo.fr (S.K.)
[2]   CERTES, Bamako, Mali; cob281@yahoo.fr (C.O.B.); mniang@certesmali.org (M.N.);
      trawore@keneya.net (S.T.T.)
[3]   Service de Dermatologie, Hôpital Pasteur, Colmar 68000, France; antoine.mahe@ch-colmar.fr
[4]   Département de Radiologie et Informatique médicale, Université de Genève, Genaven 1211, Switzerland;
      antoine.Geissbuhler@hcuge.ch
*   Correspondence: faye_o@yahoo.fr; Tel.: +223-6673-7149
†   Teledermali Team: Samba Ba, Dokala Diarra, Aoua Togora, Issa Koné, Modibo Traoré, Aissata Diallo, Chaka
      Koné, Drissa Traoré, Diakalia Berthé, Ousmane Cissé, Boubacar Sidiki Nanacassé, Abdoul Karim Doumbia,
      Sidi Niaré, Mamady Yattara, Bakary Traoré, Moussa Traoré.

Received: 24 July 2018; Accepted: 6 August 2018; Published: 17 August 2018

Abstract: In sub-Saharan Africa, in particular in rural areas, patients have limited access to doctors with specialist skills in skin diseases. To address this issue, a teledermatology pilot programme focused on primary health centres was set up in Mali. This study was aimed at investigating the feasibility of this programme and its impact on the management of skin diseases. The programme was based on the store-and-forward model. Health care providers from 10 primary centres were trained to manage common skin diseases, to capture images of skin lesions, and to use an e-platform to post all cases beyond their expertise for dermatologists in order to obtain diagnosis and treatment recommendations. After training, the cases of 180 patients were posted by trained health workers on the platform. Ninety-six per cent of these patients were properly managed via the responses given by dermatologists. The mean time to receive the expert's response was 32 h (range: 13 min to 20 days). Analysis of all diseases diagnosed via the platform revealed a wide range of skin disorders. Our initiative hugely improved the management of all skin diseases in the targeted health centres. In developing countries, Internet accessibility and connection quality represent the main challenges when conducting teledermatology programmes.

Keywords: teledermatology; Africa; primary health care; skin diseases; tele-expertise

---

1. Introduction

To date, there is a general agreement that skin diseases (SDs) should be considered a public issue, in particular in developing countries [1] where their management is subject to several challenges.

Prevalence studies from different continents have pointed to a high prevalence of SDs, especially in children, at an average of 30% (range 6 to 87%) [2–10]. While SDs are the fourth leading cause of consultations in health centres [11,12], patients have limited access to skin doctors with specialist skills in skin disease; these generally prefer to settle in big cities. In Africa, the situation is critical; the ratio of dermatologists to the population is extremely low, and ranges from 1 for every 500,000 to 1 million inhabitants. Mali, a country of 17 million inhabitants, had only 10 dermatologists in 2015; all were posted in the capital city. The pressure for skin care is mainly borne by front-line health facilities, and most of those personnel are swamped with other health priority programmes (immunization, malaria, tuberculosis, HIV, etc.). The capacity of such agents to manage common SDs and leprosy has been questioned [13]. The overall context of care provision in developing countries represents an additional challenge. Warm climate and overcrowded settings are likely to foster the skin infections that represent almost 70% of the skin disorders that motivate consultations [14]. Hitherto, there are no international guidelines or treatment recommendations, with the exception of leprosy, a disease that has been eliminated in most endemic countries. A previous study [15] identified the effectiveness of one-day training to improve the management of common SDs in primary health care centres. The issue remains as to how the remaining cases that need the expertise of a specialist dermatologist can be managed. The recent boom of information and communication technologies (ICTs) and their use in medicine, particularly dermatology (teledermatology), have transformed the way in which skin disorders can be properly managed in remote areas. By the year 2013, more than 560 papers were published on this subject [16] and 2000 patients were evaluated, with good kappa concordance test values ranging from 0.63 to 0.95 [17–21]. This growing awareness for teledermatology prompted us to take advantage of this technology to improve skin care in Mali through a pilot programme.

The aim of this study was to test the feasibility and the impact of a teledermatology programme on the management of skin diseases, at primary health care level.

2. Methods

2.1. Ethical Statements

The study protocol was approved by the Institutional Review Board of the National Ethical Committee for Health and Life Sciences of Mali (*Comité National d'éthique pour la santé et les sciences de la vie, CNESS*). Prior to the study, informed consent was obtained from adult participants andfrom the parents or legal guardians of minors after detailed explanation of the study protocol. In accordance with the ethical review committee requirements, patient information was made confidential. Our intervention was only focused on the health system and the management of patient care so that this could be improved in Mali. There was no new drug tested nor blood test performed in the study.

2.2. Health Care System in Mali

In Mali, as in many African countries, the health care system in the public sector comprises three levels of care. The first level, also called primary health care level, comprises community health centres (*centre de santé communautaire*) and district referral health care centres (*centre de santé de référence*) where the first-level administration (district) is sited. Regional hospitals and regional health administrations represent the second health care level (region). The capital city hosts the third health care level, represented by teaching hospitals and the national health administration, where the national health policy is elaborated. In 2015, the country had 5 teaching hospitals, 8 regional hospitals covering 10 health regions, 63 district referral centres, and 1215 community health centres. The present study was focused on this last group, the primary health care centres that represent the entry point to the health system where health care is delivered by general physicians, nurses, and in a few cases, minimally trained health care workers (HCWs).

2.3. Study Design, Sites, and Duration

From July 2015 to February 2017, we carried out a pilot teledermatology programme based on the store-and-forward (SAF) model, focused on front-line health care delivery services. Of the 10 health regions in Mali, we selected three regions for the purpose (Koulikoro, Sikasso, and Mopti); the rest were excluded for either security reasons or the close presence of a dermatologist. In each health region, selected three health districts were also selected: the administrative centre of the health region plus two or three more health districts randomly selected thereafter, depending on the size of the region (Figure 1). Overall, 9 health districts were involved in the study planned to last for 18 months: 6 months for pre and post programme evaluation and training, and 12 months for utilization of the system.

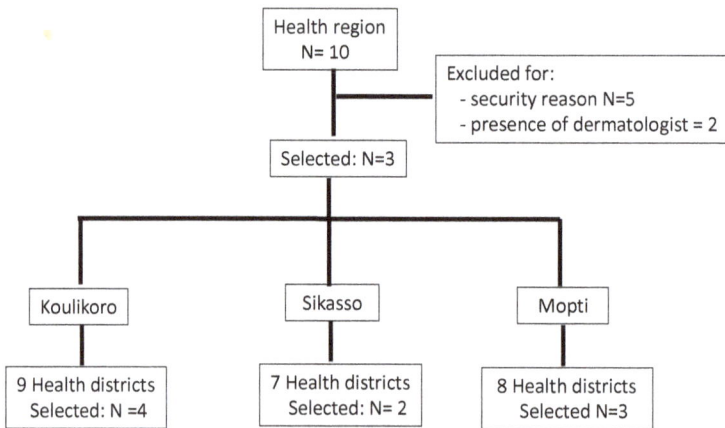

Figure 1. Flow chart of the selection of study sites: health region and districts.

2.4. Intervention—Equipment and Participants

The first step of our intervention was training. In each health centre, two health care workers were invited to participate in the training session which was held in the main dermatological ward, at the Marchoux Institute in the capital city Bamako where expert dermatologists were posted. During three consecutive days, the selected HCWs were respectively given information on the algorithmic approach for the management of common skin diseases identified in the pilot project [15], the use of a digital camera, and computer skills including type writing, the use of Internet (email), and the tele-expertise platform named 'Bogou' [22] (that means mutual assistance or help in all situations in the Djerma and Songhoï languages spoken in Mali, Niger, and Cameroon). This e-platform is a web-based application with secured access through a personal login and password [23]. It was developed with Java to run on several operating systems and work reliably with unstable and low-bandwidth connections. All data in *Bogou* are encrypted using a public and private key system [23]. Dermatological training was focused on common SDs, i.e pyoderma, superficial mycoses including tinea capitis, scabies, and conditions with pale patches inclusive of leprosy; attendees were encouraged to refer via the platform all skin disorders assessed as being beyond their competency and any case that did not fit with the algorithm. Theoretical training was also completed with clinical case studies and practical exercises. At the end of the training session, participants were issued with a booklet addressing the management of common SDs as cited above, a digital camera, and a kit for Internet connection including a 3G key USB.

2.5. Teledermatology Operating Procedures

In practice, when encountering a case that needed a consultation with a dermatologist, the health agent captures one or more pictures with a digital camera, logs on to a computer, uploads the images from the camera, connects to the platform, and uploads the pictures with a short medical history of the patient. The dermatologist (expert) immediately receives an email alert indicating an assignment for a case for diagnosis that has been sent. The expert also will log onto the platform, analyse the images, and send back concise details on the disorders and treatment recommendations. At any time, all participating HCWs could access pictures and responses. Importantly, the workload involved in responding to the HCWs relied mainly on one individual (OF) backed by a second in case the first one was not available; only one response to each request was given. The validity of all diagnoses and management strategies given was checked by another dermatologist based in France, who had expertise in tropical dermatology (AM). Clinical supervision was performed quarterly by a team (dermatologist and computer scientists) to confirm difficult diagnoses through skin biopsy and to solve technical issues.

2.6. Evaluation

We planned to evaluate the feasibility of the study and its impact on the management of common SD. While implementing and performing the programme, all relevant issues and challenges were recorded. The following indicators were also evaluated: total number of store-and-forward teledermatology consults via the *Bogou* platform, the number of cases that received a clear diagnosis and treatment, the turnaround time to receive the response from experts, the pattern of SDs referred to experts, the diagnosis concordance between experts, and the proportion and pattern of SDs as seen by HCWs before and after intervention. All SDs diagnosed via teledermatology were also compared to those seen in a dermatological setting where experts were working over the same period of time. Patient and care provider feedback was also assessed to measure the level of satisfaction and acceptance of the system.

2.7. Data Collection and Statistical Analysis

A standardized questionnaire was used to collect the data from patients who visited the targeted health centres for skin diseases and patients managed via the system. The opinions of both HCWs and the patients were also collected and then sorted by level of satisfaction. The software SPSS.16.0 (IBM Company, Chicago, IL, USA) was used for data capture and analysis. The chi-squared test was used to compare two proportions.

3. Results

3.1. Characteristics of the Study Sites and Trainees:

Overall, 20 HCW from 9 health centres were involved in the study: 9 nurses and 11 general physicians. Before the study, 6 out of 20 HCW had never touched a computer and had no email address (nurses only). Of the 9 health centres, only 4 had an Internet connection (Table 1). Not a single centre had a digital camera.

3.2. Skin Diseases Diagnosed by HCWs

Before the intervention, the proportion of dermatological consultation varied from 8% (Ngolobougou, 51/612) to 65% (Sikasso, 692/1067) with a mean of 20%. After the training session, these proportions were respectively 9% and 63% (Table 1). There was a slight increase in the dermatological activity of all centres, but the difference was not significant.

The pre-programme evaluation revealed that the five top diagnoses of SDs retrieved in the health centre logbook were: wounds (10.8%), allergies (8.8%), mycosis (5%), genital infection (7.3%), and pruritus (4.7%) (Table 2). At the post-programme evaluation, pyoderma (28.4%), eczema (13.5%), dermatophytosis (6.9%), tinea capitis (5.3%), and prurigo (4.4%) were the most common SDs. There was a huge decrease in the proportion of patients with unclear diagnosis, which decreased from 53.7%

(322/599) to 12.4% (84/679) before and after training, respectively ($p < 10^{-6}$). Clearer diagnoses were also observed during the post-programme period.

Table 1. Evaluation of health centres: proportion of skin diseases before and after training and distribution of trainees and cases posted via the platform.

Health Centre	Number of Trainees	Number of Cases Posted via the Platform	Before Training		After Training	
			Number of Skin Diseases (%)	Number of Consults	Number of Skin Diseases (%)	Number of Consults
Koulikoro [a]	2	9	82	900	76	756
Banamba [a]	3	32	185	1512	185	1426
Nara	2	3	95	542	85	501
Sikasso [a]	2	16	692 (65)	1067	706 (63)	1121
Ngolobougou	1	36	51 (8)	612	65 (9)	723
Kadiolo	2	6	60	415	79	608
Mopti [a]	4	35 [b]	108	902	166	1091
Douentza	2	17 [b]	45	480	60	461
Bankass	2	26	78	678	106	816
TOTAL	20	180	1396	7108	1528	7503

[a] Centres where the Internet connection was available before teledermatology intervention; [b] centre exclusively run by a nurse.

Table 2. Pattern of skin diseases observed in health centres before and after intervention: report on the six-month period.

Skin Diseases	Before Intervention	After Intervention
Dermatosis	322	84
Eczema	6	92
Dermatophytosis	-	47
Mycoses	30	7
Tinea capitis	3	36
Pyoderma	16	193
Wounds	65	-
Urticaria	-	11
Allergy	53	14
Follicular infection	8	-
Pruritus	28	-
Scabies	3	15
Onychodystrophy	-	13
Candidiasis	-	20
Measles	-	12
Herpes zoster	-	3
Herpes labialis	-	5
Genital infection	44	8
Prurigo		30
Erysipelas	7	11
Rash	4	8
Molluscum contagiosum	-	3
Aphthous ulcers	-	3
Patches	6	-
Intertrigo	-	6
Chickenpox	-	20
Vitiligo	-	4
Lipoma	-	1
Miliaria	-	22
Burn	4	-
Keloid	-	4
Ulceration	-	7
Total	**599**	**679**

3.3. Management of Skin Diseases via Teledermatology

This started immediately after training and continued over one year, from October 2015 to October 2016. Overall, 180 patients who consulted at the targeted health facilities were diagnosed and treated via our platform. The mean number of patients managed per month was 15, with a range of 5 (January) to 24 (August). Regarding the centre activity, the number of patients seen ranged from 3 patients (Nara) to 36 patients (Banamba) (Table 1). The number of images sent per patient varied from 0 to 13, with an average of 3.6. All patients except one accepted being photographed. The average turnaround time to receive the expert's response was 32 h (range from 13 min to 20 days). Except in two cases referred to the dermatological ward in the capital city (one case of bullous pemphigoid and one case of psoriasis) all patients were managed locally. Analysis of diseases diagnosed via the platform illustrated a wide range of conditions (Table 2) (Figures 2–5). The five top diagnoses were: eczema (25/180), dermatophytosis (22/180), pyoderma (10/180), prurigo (11/180), and psoriasis (7/180). However, other conditions such as keratoderma plantaris, vitiligo, small pox, pemghigus, drug-related eruption, and psoriasis were also seen. Miscellaneous diseases included lupus erythematosus (2 cases), leprosy (1 case), transient pustular melanosis (1 case), haemangioma (1 case), epidermal cyst (1 case), syringoma (1 case), and alopecia areata (1 case) (Table 3). The overall diagnosis concordance between dermatologists involved in the programme was 95% amongst the 40 cases randomly selected. Experts had divergent diagnoses in two cases in which the quality of the images was judged unsuitable for correct diagnosis. Importantly, clinical supervision of the health centres enabled the diagnosis of five patients through skin biopsy: two cases of psoriasis and one case each of pemphigus, lichen planus, and epidermal cyst, respectively. The quality of information and photographs given to experts was considered not good enough for diagnosis in six patients (3%). In addition, we failed to diagnose five more cases. Overall, 11 patients had no diagnosis.

Table 3. Miscellaneous skin conditions diagnosed via the platform in 22 cases out of 180 cases posted from health centres.

Skin Disorders	Frequency
Sun burn	2
Eczematised miliaria	2
Hemangioma	1
Alopecia areata	2
Epidermal cyst	1
Vulvovaginitis	1
Leprosy	1
Viral exanthema	1
Multiple keloid	2
Transient pustular melanosis	1
Onychodystrophy	1
Eruptive hidradenoma	1
Lichen simplex	1
Plantar ulcer	1
Congenital keratoderma	2
Varicose veins	2
Total	**22**

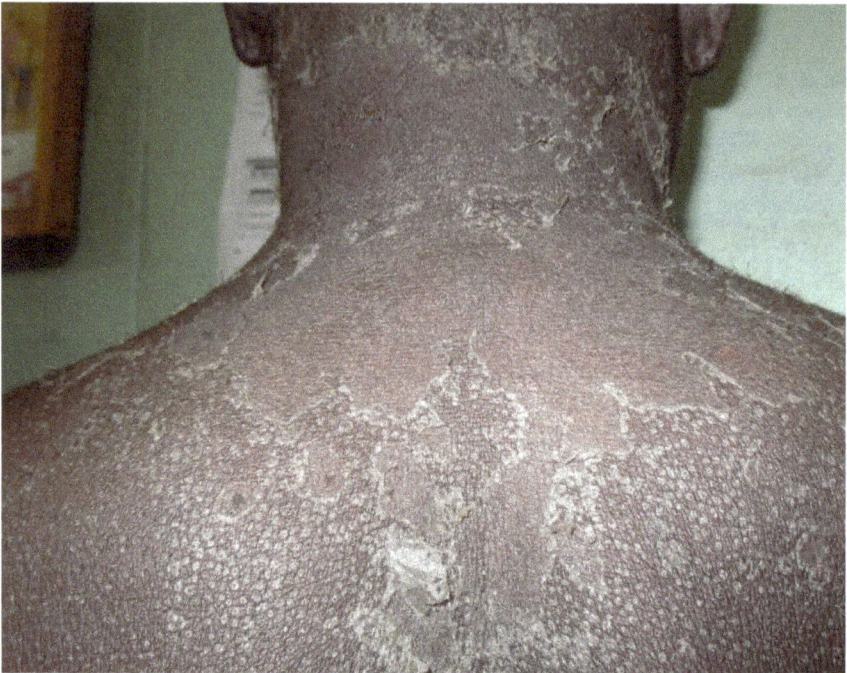

Figure 2. Drug eruption caused by amoxicillin intake following dental extraction.

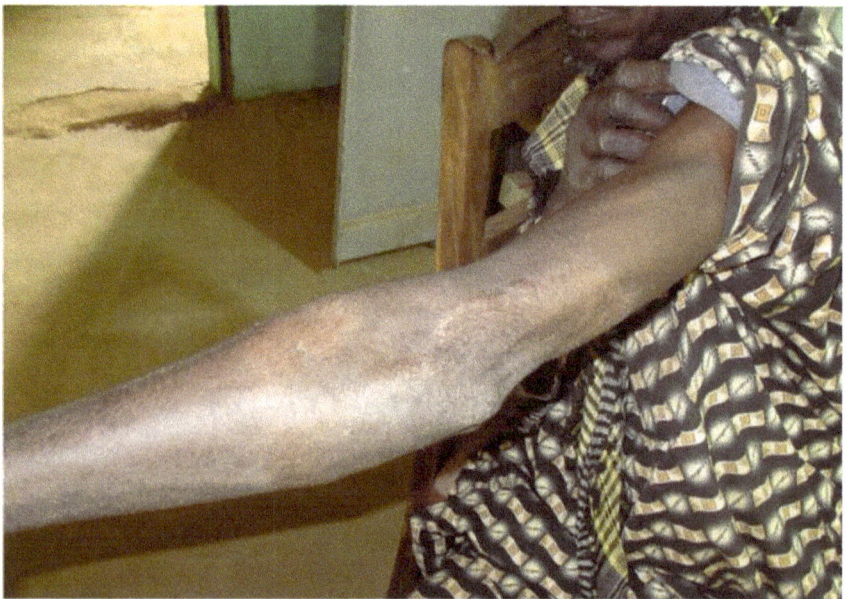

Figure 3. Paucibacillary leprosy: note the large hypochromic patch of the arm.

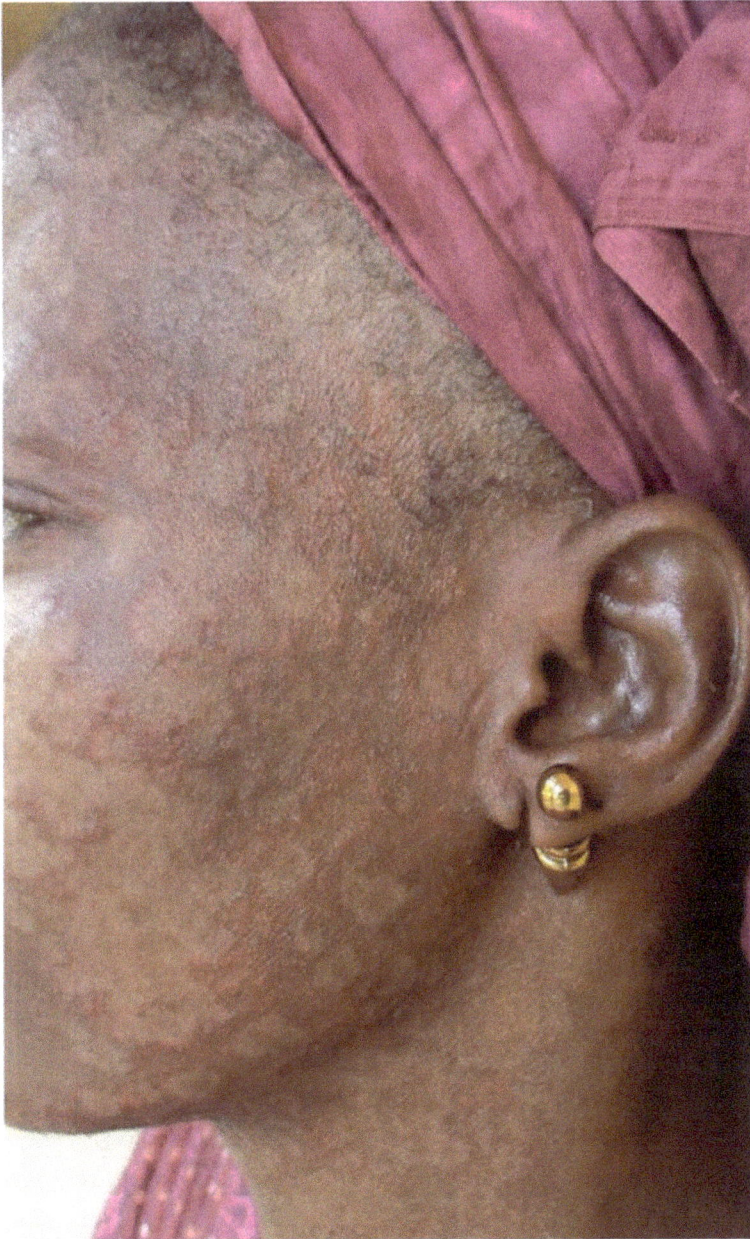

Figure 4. Tinea facei in women using skin bleaching creams (clobetasol and hydroquinone).

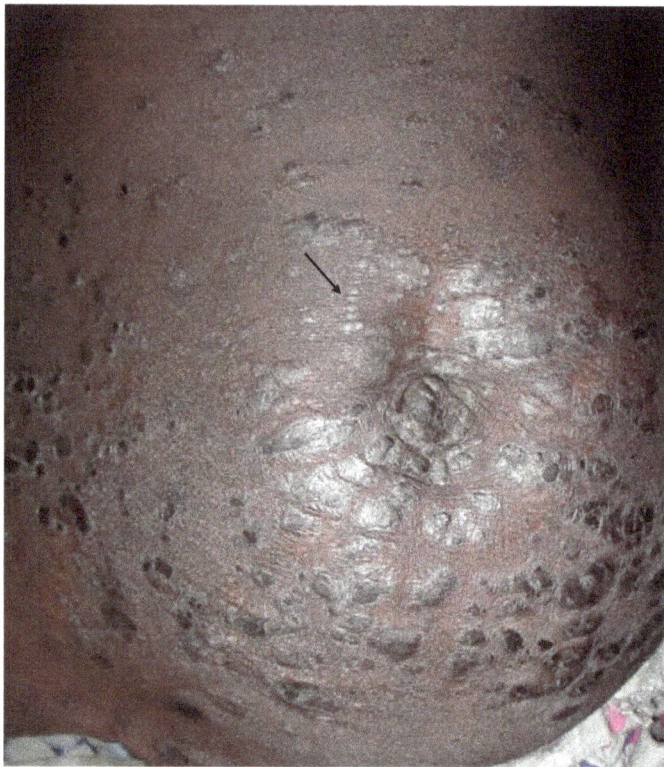

(A)

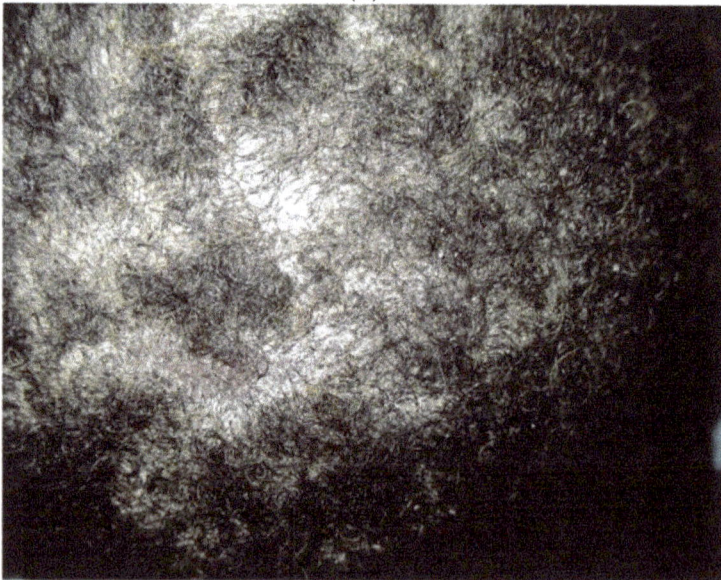

(B)

Figure 5. (**A**) Psoriasis in a 35-year-old woman: erythematous papules and plaque over the abdomen. Note the Köbner phenomenon; (**B**) Scalp involvement of the patient.

In the dermatology clinic of the capital city, 24,520 patients were consulted during the study period. The five top diagnoses observed in these patients were: eczema, dermatophytosis, bacterial infection and prurigo, or pruritus and plantar keratoderma. This pattern was similar to that of cases managed via teledermatology during the same period (Figures 6 and 7).

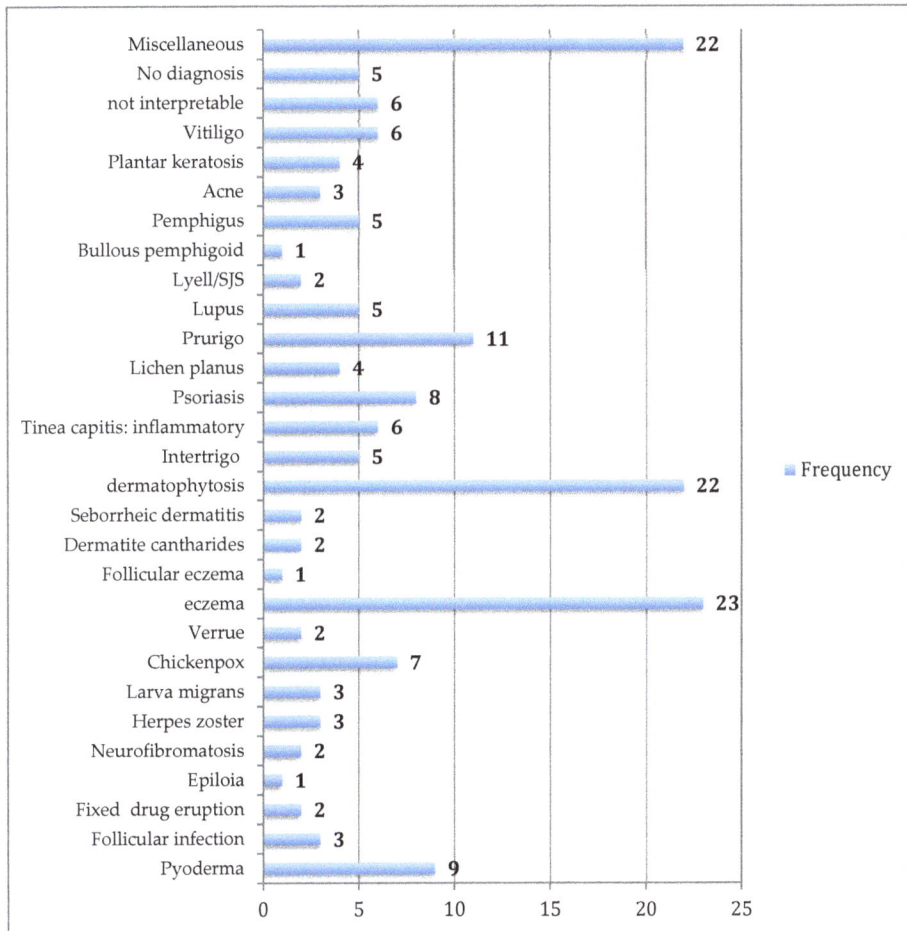

Figure 6. Pattern of skin diseases diagnosed via the platform in 180 cases posted by primary health care workers.

3.4. Satisfaction of HWCs and Patients

Interviews regarding the level of satisfaction involved 10 health providers and 37 patients managed via the system. Eight out of 10 HCWs declared that they were satisfied by the management of patients via the platform, this included four who were strongly satisfied. The time to receive the response from the expert was considered to be reasonable for seven out of 10 HCWs and response times for two were 'moderately' acceptable. According to some health care providers, our intervention enhanced both health centres and general health care practices. They stated: "I felt more confident when facing a patient with SD"; or: "presently, people look at me differently (with more attention) when compared to the time before the programme started". They also though that some programme aspects could be improved: the time to receive the response from the expert, and the platform. The concept of an android version for mobile phones and improved quality of the Internet connection in each region were considered relevant.

All the 37 patients interviewed stated that they were strongly satisfied and would recommend teledermatology to other patients. The fact that they were locally managed was very much appreciated. They also expressed the need to sustain this initiative.

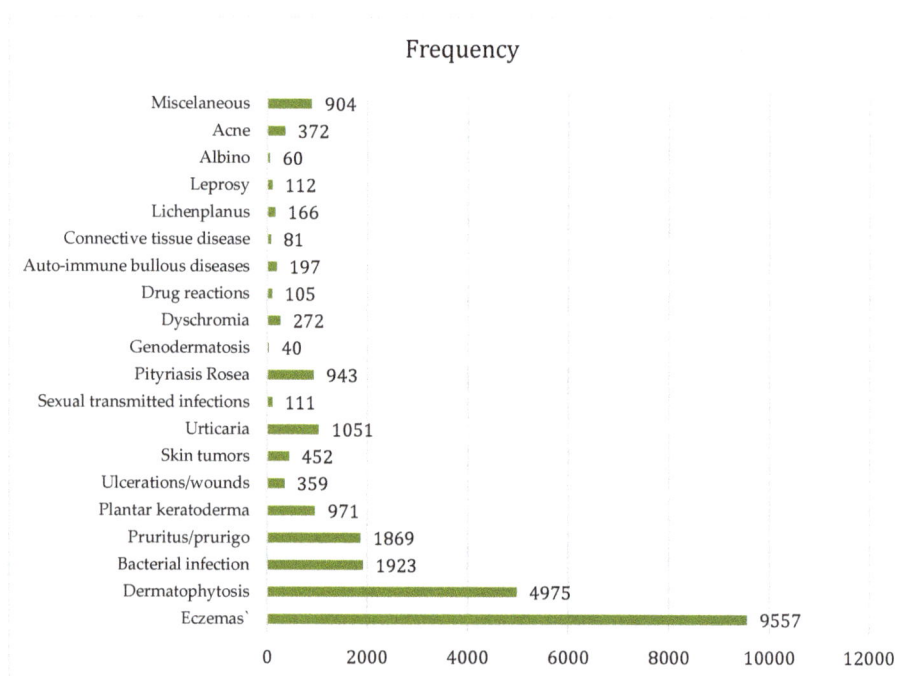

Frequency

Category	Frequency
Miscelaneous	904
Acne	372
Albino	60
Leprosy	112
Lichenplanus	166
Connective tissue disease	81
Auto-immune bullous diseases	197
Drug reactions	105
Dyschromia	272
Genodermatosis	40
Pityriasis Rosea	943
Sexual transmitted infections	111
Urticaria	1051
Skin tumors	452
Ulcerations/wounds	359
Plantar keratoderma	971
Pruritus/prurigo	1869
Bacterial infection	1923
Dermatophytosis	4975
Eczemas`	9557

Figure 7. Pattern of skin diseases seen in the Referral centre of Dermatology at the Marchoux Institute in 2015: 24,520 cases.

4. Discussion

This study was a teledermatology pilot programme based on a store-and-forward model and designed to work at a primary health care level in a developing country. Its implementation and evaluation definitely validated the feasibility of a teledermatology programme in a resource-limited area. The usefulness and challenges of such a programme has also been highlighted. There was a huge improvement in the management of all skin diseases in the targeted primary centres, for both common skin diseases and those beyond the expertise of the HCWs. A large number skin diseases were identified and managed locally by health care workers whose knowledge was also improved as long as the intervention continued. The equipment used for connection in this study was very simple, low-cost, and suitable when compared to a live interactive model that requires more equipment and greater technological expertise.

However, several limitations should be addressed. These include the selection of only three health regions, the small number of randomly selected health centres as compared to the total number of health centres in Mali, and the small number of teledermatology requests from one centre (Banamba) due to either the quality of the Internet connection or the lack of HCW commitment to ask for help.

Several papers have addressed the usefulness and effectiveness of teledermatology programmes [16,24]. The greatest number of published studies were performed in the United States, followed by the United Kingdom, Spain, the Netherlands, Italy, and Austria [25] Very few studies were conducted in Africa [26] or in sites such as prisons with greater health care needs [27]. As used in our study, store-and-forward continued to be the most common delivery modality [28]. The present study helps to bridge the gap of health care quality between front line health facilities and dermatologic wards. In rural areas where is a high prevalence of SDs and lack of specialists the needs of care for many people are also met.

The post-programme evaluation of health centres revealed that the management of common SDs was improved as shown by the decrease in the proportion of patients with either unclear diagnosis or 'dermatoses' (allergy, mycosis), and an increase in the number of clear diagnoses, i.e. pyoderma, dermatophytosis, scabies, and eczema. In the pre-programme evaluation, not a single case of very common disorders such as prurigo, urticaria, chickenpox, and miliaria was recorded in the centre logbook. After training, there was a huge improvement in the management of these disorders due to the dermatologic training. Along with this management shift, the skills of HCWs regarding computer science were also improved. One of our HCWs, who had never touched a computer, sent 17 requests for tele-expertise. In addition, two health centres were completely run by nurses, who were beginners in terms of computer science and the Internet. While no case of prurigo was mentioned in the pre-programme evaluation, many cases were noticed after intervention. This improvement could be in part related to the training module of common SDs to which participants have been exposed. It also confirmed the effectiveness of one-day training of primary HCWs in the management of common SDs with an algorithmic approach [15] that was likely to have helped to control the number of requests for teledermatology and avoided experts being swamped by HCW requests. We assume that the trained health staff managed many skin disorders themselves and e-referred only those for which dermatological expertise was required; this indicates that the programme expectations were met. The improvement in the diagnosis of SD in the targeted health centres as shown in the post-intervention evaluation might also have been a result of the continuing medical education created by the regularly-sent responses of experts via the e-platform that all HCW had the possibility to see and learn from. The clinical supervision by dermatologist confirmed cases in which the diagnosis was uncertain. The similarity of leading causes for visits in both primary and specialized health centres, as shown in this study, indicates that the pattern of SDs is not related to the level of health care facilities, but to the epidemiology of SDs. It also points out the necessity to set up and to sustain such initiatives, particularly in areas with poor geographic accessibility and weak coverage by dermatologists.

Despite the profound penetration of information and communication technology in Africa, the actual functioning of such tools has been repeatedly questioned given the frequent shortages of electric power, maintenance issues, and the low quality of connectivity. This prompted us to choose low-level technology with an adapted tool that comprised a 3G key connection and digital camera, as computers were available in all centres. This equipment worked well, and more than 90% of patients were properly managed. It should be underlined that the estimated cost of the teledermatology kit tool can be can easily covered by the cost of referral of one patient from Mopti to Bamako, the capital city. The mobile version of *Bogou*, which has been recently put into production, will lead in the future to a considerable drop in equipment costs. Indeed, almost every HWC has a smartphone in Mali.

Some issues not addressed in this study should be addressed further, in particular in developing countries when setting up a teledermatology programme. These include privacy issues as well as ethical and medicolegal responsibility in cases of injury and unsolved cases.

5. Conclusions

The implementation of a teledermatology programme based on a store-and-forward process in primary health care services is feasible and can positively impact the management of skin disorders. Development and testing of specific and secure applications for the e-management of skin disorders should be promoted. The expansion of such programmes is appealing in resource-limited countries where there are financial constraints and dermatologists are lacking.

Author Contributions: Conceptualization, O.F., C.O.B.; Methodology, O.F., C.O.B., S.K.; Software, C.O.B., M.N., A.G.; Training, Y.F., Y.K., M.G., B.G., A.K., K.T.; Validation, A.M.; Formal Analysis, O.F., L.C., B.T.; Investigation, A.D., L.C., S.B., B.T., B.K.; Resources, S.T.T.; Data Curation, S.T.T.; Writing—Original Draft Preparation, O.F., C.O.B., A.G.; Writing—Review and Editing, O.F., A.M.; Supervision, S.K.; Project Administration, O.F.; Funding Acquisition, O.F.

Funding: This research was funded by The Foundation Pierre Fabre (France).

Acknowledgments: We are grateful to Prof. Roderick J Hay (London) for advice concerning the manuscript and Dr. Florence Poli for her constant support to Malian dermatologists.

Conflicts of Interest: The funders had no role in the design of the study; in the collection, analyses, or interpretation of data; in the writing of the manuscript, and in the decision to publish the results.

References

1. Anonymous. Skin disease and public health medicine. *Lancet* **1991**, *337*, 1008–1009. [CrossRef]
2. Figueroa, J.I.; Fuller, L.C.; Abraha, A.; Hay, R.J. Dermatology in southwestern Ethiopia: Rationale for a community approach. *Int. J. Dermatol.* **1998**, *37*, 752–758. [CrossRef] [PubMed]
3. Mahé, A.; Prual, A.; Konaté, M.; Bobin, P. Skin diseases of children in Mali: A public health problem. *Trans. R. Soc. Trop. Med. Hyg.* **1995**, *89*, 467–470. [CrossRef]
4. Walker, S.L.; Shah, M.; Hubbard, V.G.; Pradhan, H.M.; Ghimire, M. Skin disease is common in rural Nepal: Results of a point prevalence study. *Br. J. Dermatol.* **2008**, *158*, 334–338. [CrossRef] [PubMed]
5. Saw, S.M.; Koh, D.; Adjani, M.R.; Wong, M.L.; Hong, C.Y.; Lee, J.; Chia, S.E.; Munoz, C.P.; Ong, C.N. A population-based prevalence survey of skin diseases in adolescents and adults in rural Sumatra, Indonesia, 1999. *Trans. R. Soc. Trop. Med. Hyg.* **2001**, *95*, 384–388. [CrossRef]
6. Abdel-Hafez, K.; Abdel-Aty, M.A.; Hofny, E.R. Prevalence of skin diseases in rural areas of Assiut Governorate, Upper Egypt. *Int. J. Dermatol.* **2003**, *42*, 887–892. [CrossRef] [PubMed]
7. Leekassa, R.; Bizuneh, E.; Alem, A.; Fekadu, A.; Shibre, T. Community diagnosis of common skin diseases in the Zay community of the Zeway Islands, Ethiopia. *Ethiop. Med. J.* **2005**, *43*, 189–195. [PubMed]
8. Dogra, S.; Kumar, B. Epidemiology of skin diseases in school children: A study from northern India. *Pediatr. Dermatol.* **2003**, *20*, 470–473. [CrossRef] [PubMed]
9. Bechelli, L.M.; Haddad, N.; Pimenta, W.P.; Pagnano, P.M.; Melchior, J.E.; Fregnan, R.C.; Zanin, L.C.; Arenas, A. Epidemiological survey of skin diseases in schoolchildren living in the Purus Valley (Acre State, Amazonia, Brazil). *Dermatologica* **1981**, *163*, 78–93. [CrossRef] [PubMed]
10. Gibbs, S.A.M. Skin disease and socioeconomic conditions in rural Africa: Tanzania. *Int. J. Dermatol.* **1996**, *35*, 633–639. [CrossRef] [PubMed]
11. National Health Administration of the Minister of Health. *Direction Nationale de la Santé. Données du Système d'Information Sanitaire National: Annuaire Statistique 2007*; Ministère de la Santé: Bamako, Mali, 2007; p. 145. (In French).
12. Karimkhani, C.; Dellavalle, R.P.; Coffeng, L.E.; Flohr, C.; Hay, R.J.; Langan, S.M.; Nsoesie, E.O.; Ferrari, A.J.; Erskine, H.E.; Silverberg, J.I.; et al. Global skin disease morbidity and mortality: an update from the global burden of disease study 2013. *JAMA Dermatol.* **2017**, *153*, 406–412. [CrossRef] [PubMed]
13. Faye, O.; Keita, S.; N'diaye, H.; Konare, H.; Coulibaly, I. Evaluation du niveau de connaissance des agents de santé sur le diagnostic de la lèpre à Bamako (MALI): Proposition pour l'avenir de la lutte anti-lépreuse. *Mali. Méd.* **2003**, *18*, 32–34. (In French)
14. Mahé, A.; Cissé, I.A.; Faye, O.; N' Diaye, H.T.; Niamba, P. Skin diseases in Bamako (Mali). *Int. J. Dermatol.* **1998**, *37*, 673–676. [CrossRef] [PubMed]
15. Mahé, A.; Faye, O.; N'Diaye, H.T.; Konaré, H.D.; Coulibaly, I.; Kéita, S.; Traoré, A.K.; Hay, R.J. Integration of basic dermatological care into primary health care services in Mali. *Bull World Health Organ.* **2005**, *83*, 935–943. [PubMed]
16. Warshaw, E.M.; Hillman, Y.J.; Greer, N.L.; Hagel, E.M.; MacDonald, R.; Rutks, I.R.; Wilt, T.J. Teledermatology for diagnosis and management of skin conditions: A systematic review. *J. Am. Acad. Dermatol.* **2011**, *64*, 759–772. [CrossRef] [PubMed]

17. Heffner, V.A.; Lyon, V.B.; Brousseau, D.C.; Holland, K.E.; Yen, K. Store-and-forward teledermatology versus in-person visits: A comparison in pediatric teledermatology clinic. *J. Am. Acad. Dermatol.* **2009**, *60*, 956–961. [CrossRef] [PubMed]
18. Edison, K.E.; Ward, D.S.; Dyer, J.A.; Lane, W.; Chance, L.; Hicks, L.L. Diagnosis, diagnostic confidence, and management concordance in live-interactive and store-and-forward teledermatology compared to in-person examination. *Telemed. E-Health,* **2008**, *14*, 889–895. [CrossRef] [PubMed]
19. Moreno-Ramirez, D.; Ferrandiz, L.; Nieto-Garcia, A.; Carrasco, R.; Moreno-Alvarez, P.; Galdeano, R.; Bidegain, E.; Rios-Martin, J.J.; Camacho, F.M. Store-and-forward teledermatology in skin cancer triage: Experience and evaluation of 2009 teleconsultations. *Arch. Dermatol.* **2007**, *143*, 479–483. [CrossRef] [PubMed]
20. Moreno-Ramirez, D.; Ferrandiz, L.; Bernal, A.P.; Duran, R.C.; Martin, J.J.; Camacho, F. Teledermatology as a filtering system in pigmented lesion clinics. *J. Telemed. Telecare* **2005**, *11*, 298–303. [CrossRef] [PubMed]
21. Oliveira, M.R.; Wen, C.L.; Neto, C.F.; Silveira, P.S.; Rivitti, E.A.; Böhm, G.M. Web site for training nonmedical health-care workers to identify potentially malignant skin lesions and for teledermatology. *Telemed. J. E-Health* **2002**, *8*, 323–332. [CrossRef] [PubMed]
22. Bogou. Available online: http://raft.unige.ch/bogou/ (accessed on 18 July 2018).
23. Bediang, G.; Perrin, C.; Ruiz de Castañeda, R.; Kamga, Y.; Sawadogo, A.; Bagayoko, C.O.; Geissbuhler, A. The RAFT telemedicine network: Lessons learnt and perspectives from a decade of educational and clinical services in low-and middle-incomes countries. *Front. Public Health* **2014**, *2*, 180. [CrossRef] [PubMed]
24. Tran, K.; Ayad, M.; Weinberg, J.; Cherng, A.; Chowdhury, M.; Monir, S.; Hariri, M.; Kovarik, C. Mobile teledermatology in the developing world: Implications of a feasibility study on 30 Egyptian patients with common skin diseases. *J. Am. Acad. Dermatol.* **2011**, *64*, 302–309. [CrossRef] [PubMed]
25. Trettel, A.; Eissing, L.; Augustin, M. Telemedicine in dermatology: Findings and experiences worldwide—A systematic literature review. *J. Eur. Acad. Dermatol. Venereol.* **2018**, *32*, 215–224. [CrossRef] [PubMed]
26. Delaigue, S.; Bonnardot, L.; Olson, D.; Morand, J.J. Overview of teledermatology in low-resource settings. *Med. Sante Trop.* **2015**, *25*, 365–372. [PubMed]
27. Khatibi, B.; Bambe, A.; Chantalat, C.; Resche-Rigon, M.; Sanna, A.; Fac, C.; Bagot, M.; Guibal, F. Teledermatology in a prison setting: A retrospective study of 500 expert opinions. *Ann. Dermatol. Venereol.* **2016**, *143*, 418–422. [CrossRef] [PubMed]
28. Yim, K.M.; Florek, A.G.; Oh, D.H.; McKoy, K.; Armstrong, A.W. Teledermatology in the United States: An Update in a Dynamic Era. *Telemed. J. E-Health* **2018**, in press. [CrossRef] [PubMed]

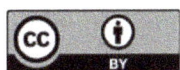

Tropical Medicine and
Infectious Disease

MDPI

Review

Advances in the Treatment of Yaws

Michael Marks [ID]

Clinical Research Department, London School of Hygiene & Tropical Medicine, Keppel Street,
London WC1E 7HT, UK; michael.marks@lshtm.ac.uk; Tel.: +44-20-7636-8635

Received: 31 July 2018; Accepted: 27 August 2018; Published: 29 August 2018

Abstract: Yaws is one of the three endemic treponematoses and is recognised by the World Health Organization as a neglected tropical disease. Yaws is currently reported in 15 countries in the Pacific, South-East Asia, West and Central Africa, predominantly affects children, and results in destructive lesions of the skin and soft tissues. For most of the twentieth century penicillin-based treatment was the standard of care and resistance to penicillin has still not been described. Recently, oral azithromycin has been shown to be an effective treatment for yaws, facilitating renewed yaws eradication efforts. Resistance to azithromycin is an emerging threat and close surveillance will be required as yaws eradication efforts are scaled up globally.

Keywords: yaws; *Treponema pallidum*

1. Introduction

Yaws, caused by *Treponema pallidum* subsp. *pertenue*, is one of the three endemic treponematoses (along with *T.p.* subsp. *endemicum*, the causative agent of bejel, and *T. carateum*, the causative agent of pinta) and is recognised by the World Health Organization as a neglected tropical disease (NTD) [1,2]. The disease predominantly affects children and results in destructive lesions of the skin and soft tissues. Yaws is still found in Africa, South-East Asia and the Pacific. *T.p.* subsp. *pertenue* is closely related to *T.p.* subsp. *pallidum*, the causative agent of syphilis [3] but neither sexual nor mother-to-child transmission of yaws is believed to occur [2].

2. Epidemiology

Yaws is currently reported in 15 countries in the Pacific, South-East Asia, West and Central Africa [4–9]. Currently the most cases are reported in Papua New Guinea, the Solomon Islands and Ghana and all have reported in excess of 15,000 cases in recent years. In the mid-twentieth century, yaws was endemic in South America and the Caribbean, but control programmes in the mid-twentieth century (see below) are believed to have eliminated yaws from the majority of countries in the region [10,11]. India interrupted transmission in 2004 and declared elimination in 2006 [12] following a sustained programme that began in 1996.

Yaws is restricted to warm and humid environments [13]. Transmission is skin to skin contact from active infectious lesions [14]. Early studies had suggested that flies may play a role in transmission but there is no definitive proof that this occurs [14–16]. The majority of active infections cases occur in children aged under 15 years. Closely-related treponemal infections have been identified in primate populations, but zoonotic transmission to humans has not been established [17,18].

3. Clinical Features

As with other treponemal infections, yaws is characterized by a multi-stage disease process predominantly involving skin, bones and cartilage.

The initial stage of primary yaws is the development of an erythematous lesion that occurs at the site of inoculation after an incubation period of 9–90 days [14,19]. These lesions may break down forming an ulcerated plaque over a period of 1–2 weeks. Primary lesions occur most frequently on the lower limbs or buttocks [13,20], whilst genital lesions are extremely uncommon. If patients are left untreated then primary lesions will heal spontaneously, with scarring, over a period of 3–6 months [21].

Without treatment individuals will progress to secondary yaws. Secondary yaws predominantly involves the skin and bones [20,22]. As with secondary syphilis, both generalised lymphadenopathy and constitutional symptoms, including fever and malaise, are frequently reported in patients with secondary yaws [19]. A wide-range of skin manifestations occur in secondary yaws including macular lesions and hyperkeratotic lesions on the palms and soles ('crab yaws') [14,19,20]. Osteoperiostitis, affecting the fingers (resulting in dactylitis) or long bones (forearm, fibula, tibula) is the most common bony manifestation of secondary yaws. Following treatment of early yaws (primary or secondary) skin lesions usually resolve within 2–4 weeks and bone pain may start to resolve in as little as 48 h [23].

In the absence of treatment of early yaws, patients go on to develop latent infection. During this clinical stage of disease patients have reactive serology but no clinical evidence of infection. Relapse from latent to active disease can occur for a period of up to 5–10 years and serve as a source of onward transmission. Previously up to 10% of patients were reported to develop the late-stage manifestations of tertiary yaws, but this is now much less commonly reported [19]. Tertiary disease may manifest as gummatous nodules resulting in tissue necrosis, a destructive osteitis which can cause destruction of the maxilla (gangosa), or bowing of the shins (sabre shin), or a hypertrophic periostitis causing exostosis of the paranasal maxilla (gondou).

Clinical diagnosis is supported by serological testing. Diagnostic testing combines a treponemal assay (such as the *Treponema pallidum* particle agglutination assay) and a non-treponemal assay (such as the rapid plasma regain assay). Treponemal tests are more specific but remain positive for life. The titre of non-treponemal assays rises following infection and falls following treatment. A four-fold fall in titre (e.g., from 1:16 to 1:4) is considered consistent with serological cure. Newer point-of-care treponemal and non-treponemal assays have increasingly taken on the role of traditional lab-based assays [24,25].

An important recent discovery has been the finding that *Haemophilus ducreyi* may cause ulcerative skin lesions similar to those seen in patients with early yaws [26,27]. *H. ducreyi* may cause lesions in both patients who have non-reactive and reactive serological tests for yaws, which complicates assessment of patients with suspected active yaws as serological point of care tests cannot be used to accurately provide a definitive diagnosis. When molecular tests are used, a large proportion of patients suspected to have active early yaws are found in fact to have latent yaws (reactive serological tests) and a different cause for the current skin lesion.

4. Penicillin-Based Treatment

Early studies conducted in Haiti demonstrated that penicillin-based treatments were highly efficacious in the treatment of yaws [23] and penicillin-based therapy was subsequently adopted as the standard of care worldwide for all endemic treponematoses [14]. Different penicillin-based regimes are effective for the treatment of yaws, but long-acting intramuscular benzathine benzylpenicillin was the most commonly used regimen. Lower doses were used than those recommended for the treatment of venereal syphilis (1.2 million units for the treatment of adults and 0.6 million units for the treatment of children) [14]. Although there have been rare reports of 'treatment failure' with penicillin-based therapy, the inability to distinguish treatment failure from reinfection makes these data extremely difficult to interpret, especially in highly endemic settings [28]. As with syphilis, no evidence of penicillin resistance has developed in yaws despite it being the first-line treatment for more than 50 years.

During the mid-twentieth century, successful treatment campaigns were conducted targeting yaws and the other endemic treponematoses [29]. In 1949, the World Health Assembly passed a resolution supporting efforts for the control and elimination of the endemic treponematoses, including yaws. WHO and UNICEF led a global effort between 1952 and 1964, based on penicillin treatment. At the time, the recommended strategy varied, based on the prevalence of active yaws in the community (Table 1). Although not ultimately successful in achieving eradication, the programme did significantly reduce the global prevalence of yaws by as much as 98% [30]. Following these efforts, the incidence of the disease rebounded in a number of countries in the 1970s, ultimately leading to a further World Health Assembly resolution in 1978, which resulted in some countries renewing control efforts [29].

Table 1. Historical strategy for the eradication of yaws: 1952–1964.

Prevalence of Clinically Active Yaws	Treatment Strategy
Hyperendemic: above 10%	Benzathine benzylpenicillin to the whole community (total mass treatment)
Mesoendemic: 5–10%	Treat all active cases, all children under 15 and all contacts of infectious cases (juvenile mass treatment)
Hypoendemic: under 5%	Treat all active cases and all household and other contacts (selective mass treatment)

5. Azithromycin-Based Treatment

Despite its efficacy, treatment with penicillin remains challenging in many settings. Injectable penicillin requires access to a secure cold chain and trained staff to administer therapy, both of which are not always available in the remote locations where yaws is found. Treatment also carried a small but important risk of anaphylaxis. Supplies of benzathine benzylpenicillin have also been insecure in recent years [31], with implications for reliable access to treatment.

Azithromycin, an oral macrolide antibiotic, had previously been demonstrated to be effective in the treatment of syphilis [32] with cure rates equivalent to those of benzathine benzylpenicillin. Given the high degree of genetic homology between syphilis and yaws, azithromycin was an attractive option for study as an alternative treatment for yaws. In a landmark study conducted in Papua New Guinea, patients with early (primary and secondary) yaws were randomised to receive treatment with either a single dose of intramuscular benzathine benzylpenicillin or a single, oral dose of azithromycin. Azithromycin was shown to be non-inferior to benzathine benzylpenicillin with a cure rate greater than 95% in both arms [33]. Subsequently, a study conducted in Ghana also confirmed the non-inferiority of azithromycin compared to benzathine benzylpenicillin [34].

These initial studies all enrolled patients with early active yaws and used a dose of 30 mg/kg (max. 2 g). Two outstanding questions were whether azithromycin was effective for the treatment of latent infection and whether the lower dose of azithromycin used for the treatment of trachoma (20 mg/kg—max. 1 g) was also efficacious in the treatment of yaws. In a longitudinal cohort study in Papua New Guinea, treatment with azithromycin was demonstrated to have a cure rate for patients with latent yaws equivalent to the cure rate of patients with active yaws [35]. The efficacy of the low versus standard dose azithromycin was compared in a randomised control trial in patients with both early active and latent yaws, conducted in Papua New Guinea and Ghana. The clinical cure rate was equivalent in both low and standard dose arms. The serological cure rate in patients with active yaws was slightly lower in the low-dose arm. In patients with latent yaws the serological cure rate was equivalent with both doses of azithromycin [36]. Taken together with observational data, this suggests that low-dose azithromycin is also effective in the treatment of yaws, although the 30 mg/kg dose remains the standard of care.

Unlike with penicillin, resistance to azithromycin is well described in *T. pallidum*. Resistance is mediated by one of two mutations in the 23s rDNA and can be detected by specific molecular tests [37–41]. In the context of large scale azithromycin-based treatment programmes (see below), treatment failure and genotypic resistance to azithromycin has now also been described in yaws [42].

6. Community Treatment with Azithromycin

Azithromycin has been widely distributed at the community level for the treatment of trachoma [43] and the WHO recommends mass drug administration (MDA) of azithromycin for the elimination of trachoma as a public health problem as part of the SAFE (Surgery, Antibiotics, Facial cleanliness and Environmental improvement) strategy [44]. MDA of azithromycin has been shown to be safe and indeed there is considerable evidence that MDA may result in significant off-target benefits including reductions in child mortality [45].

Taken together, the evidence of the safety of MDA with azithromycin and the efficacy of azithromycin for the treatment of yaws provide the rationale behind the revised WHO strategy for the eradication of yaws (the Morges strategy). This strategy emphasises MDA of azithromycin in communities where yaws is endemic. Following an initial round of MDA (referred to as total community treatment—TCT) it may be appropriate to conduct further MDA or to switch to a strategy of treating active cases and their contacts (total targeted treatment—TTT) [46]. No clear evidence currently exists to guide the decision regarding when to switch between TCT and TTT, but modelling studies suggest that TCT is a preferable strategy because it ensures a higher coverage of latent yaws cases [47,48].

Initial assessments of the efficacy of azithromycin MDA were conducted in both the Pacific and West Africa. In a study in the Solomon Islands, communities received a single round of MDA of azithromycin (conducted for the elimination of trachoma as a public health problem) at a dose of 20 mg/kg (max. 1g) and were followed up at 6 and 18 months following MDA [49–51]. A significant reduction in the prevalence of both active and latent yaws was seen at both 6 and 18 months following MDA. In Ghana, MDA with azithromycin (30 mg/kg, max. 2 g) was conducted in a single district and follow-up conducted at 12 months. As in the Solomon Islands, a significant reduction in both active and latent yaws was documented [52].

The most comprehensive evaluation of the WHO Morges strategy was conducted in Lihir, Papua New Guinea [53]. In this study of more than 15,000 individuals, an initial round of mass treatment was undertaken, followed by six-monthly rounds of surveillance and treatment of new cases and their contacts. In keeping with the studies discussed above, this study demonstrated a marked reduction in the prevalence of both active and latent yaws. Despite this initial success, interruption of transmission was not achieved [42]. Ongoing transmission was driven both by cases imported from outside the study site and cases arising in individuals missed during the initial mass treatment phase of the study. Thirty-six months into the study, a single case of treatment failure was detected. The patient had been treated at 30 months with azithromycin but at month 36 had clinical evidence of progression and serological evidence of treatment failure. Subsequent molecular testing confirmed genotypic azithromycin resistance in this case. Alongside the index case, several contacts were detected at month 36 and month 42 of the study with azithromycin-resistant yaws. Although subsequent treatment with benzathine benzylpenicillin was used to successfully ring-fence the outbreak, these data highlight the risk of emerging azithromycin resistance threatening yaws eradication efforts [42].

Trop. Med. Infect. Dis. **2018**, 3, 92

7. Conclusions

There has been considerable progress in the treatment of yaws in the last decade. Azithromycin has emerged as an effective and easily deliverable oral treatment option that can be used to treat both individual cases and during community MDA. The emergence of azithromycin resistance highlights the need for ongoing surveillance to support yaws eradication efforts globally. Further studies are needed to better define the optimum MDA strategy including the number of rounds and population coverage required to interrupt the transmission of yaws.

Funding: This research received no external funding.

Conflicts of Interest: The authors declare no conflict of interest.

References

1. Marks, M.; Solomon, A.W.; Mabey, D.C. Endemic treponemal diseases. *Trans. R. Soc. Trop. Med. Hyg.* **2014**, *108*, 601–607. [CrossRef] [PubMed]
2. Mitjà, O.; Asiedu, K.; Mabey, D. Yaws. *Lancet* **2013**, *381*, 763–773. [CrossRef]
3. Cejková, D.; Zobaníková, M.; Chen, L.; Pospíšilová, P.; Strouhal, M.; Qin, M.; Mikalová, L.; Norris, S.J.; Muzny, D.M.; Gibbs, R.A.; et al. Whole genome sequences of three *Treponema pallidum* ssp. *pertenue* strains: Yaws and syphilis treponemes differ in less than 0.2% of the genome sequence. *PLoS Negl. Trop. Dis.* **2012**, *6*, e1471.
4. Agadzi, V.K.; Aboagye-Atta, Y.; Nelson, J.W.; Perine, P.L.; Hopkins, D.R. Resurgence of yaws in Ghana. *Lancet* **1983**, *2*, 389–390. [CrossRef]
5. Asiedu, K. The return of yaws. *Bull. World Health Organ.* **2008**, *86*, 507–508. [PubMed]
6. Tharmaphornpilas, P.; Srivanichakorn, S.; Phraesrisakul, N. Recurrence of yaws outbreak in Thailand, 1990. *Southeast Asian J. Trop. Med. Public Health* **1994**, *25*, 152–156. [PubMed]
7. Fegan, D.; Glennon, M.; Macbride-Stewart, G.; Moore, T. Yaws in the Solomon Islands. *J. Trop. Med. Hyg.* **1990**, *93*, 52–57. [PubMed]
8. Fegan, D.; Glennon, M.J.; Thami, Y.; Pakoa, G. Resurgence of yaws in Tanna, Vanuatu: Time for a new approach? *Trop. Doct.* **2010**, *40*, 68–69. [CrossRef] [PubMed]
9. Manning, L.A.; Ogle, G.D. Yaws in the periurban settlements of Port Moresby, Papua New Guinea. *Papua New Guinea Med. J.* **2002**, *45*, 206–212.
10. John, R.K.S. Yaws in the Americas. *Rev. Infect. Dis.* **1985**, *7*, S266–S272. [CrossRef]
11. Scolnik, D.; Aronson, L.; Lovinsky, R.; Toledano, K.; Glazier, R.; Eisenstadt, J.; Eisenberg, P.; Wilcox, L.; Rowsell, R.; Sliverman, M. Efficacy of a targeted, oral penicillin-based yaws control program among children living in rural South America. *Clin. Infect. Dis.* **2003**, *36*, 1232–1238. [CrossRef] [PubMed]
12. Bora, D.; Dhariwal, A.C.; Lal, S. Yaws and its eradication in India—A brief review. *J. Commun. Dis.* **2005**, *37*, 1–11. [PubMed]
13. Hackett, C.J. Extent and nature of the yaws problem in Africa. *Bull. World Health Organ.* **1953**, *8*, 127–182.
14. Perine, P.L.; Hopkins, D.R.; Niemel, P.L.A.; St.-John, R.; Causse, G.; Antal, G.M. *Handbook of Endemic Treponematoses: Yaws, Endemic Syphilis and Pinta*; World Health Organization: Geneva, Switzerland, 1984; Available online: http://apps.who.int/iris/handle/10665/37178?locale=en (accessed on 2 May 2013).
15. Houinei, W.; Godornes, C.; Kapa, A.; Knauf, S.; Mooring, E.Q.; González-Beiras, C.; Watup, R.; Paru, R.; Advent, P.; Bieb, S.; et al. *Haemophilus ducreyi* DNA is detectable on the skin of asymptomatic children, flies and fomites in villages of Papua New Guinea. *PLoS Negl. Trop. Dis.* **2017**, *11*, e0004958. [CrossRef] [PubMed]
16. Knauf, S.; Raphael, J.; Mitjà, O.; Lejora, I.A.V.; Chuma, I.S.; Batamuzi, E.K.; Keyyu, J.D.; Fyumagwa, R.; Lüert, S.; Godornes, C.; et al. Isolation of *Treponema* DNA from necrophagous flies in a natural ecosystem. *EBioMedicine* **2016**, *11*, 85–90. [CrossRef] [PubMed]
17. Harper, K.N.; Fyumagwa, R.D.; Hoare, R.; Wambura, P.N.; Coppenhaver, D.H.; Sapolsky, R.M.; Alberts, S.C.; Tung, J.; Rogers, J.; Kilewo, M.; et al. *Treponema pallidum* infection in the wild baboons of East Africa: Distribution and genetic characterization of the strains responsible. *PLoS ONE* **2012**, *7*, e50882. [CrossRef] [PubMed]

18. Knauf, S.; Liu, H.; Harper, K.N. Treponemal infection in nonhuman primates as possible reservoir for human yaws. *Emerg. Infect. Dis.* **2013**, *19*, 2058–2060. [CrossRef] [PubMed]
19. Koff, A.B.; Rosen, T. Nonvenereal treponematoses: Yaws, endemic syphilis, and pinta. *J. Am. Acad. Dermatol.* **1993**, *29*, 519–535. [CrossRef]
20. Mitjà, O.; Hays, R.; Lelngei, F.; Laban, N.; Ipai, A.; Pakarui, S.; Bassat, Q. Challenges in recognition and diagnosis of yaws in children in Papua New Guinea. *Am. J. Trop. Med. Hyg.* **2011**, *85*, 113–116. [CrossRef] [PubMed]
21. Sehgal, V.N. Leg ulcers caused by yaws and endemic syphilis. *Clin. Dermatol.* **1990**, *8*, 166–174. [CrossRef]
22. Mitjà, O.; Hays, R.; Ipai, A.; Wau, B.; Bassat, Q. Osteoperiostitis in early yaws: Case series and literature review. *Clin. Infect. Dis.* **2011**, *52*, 771–774. [CrossRef] [PubMed]
23. Rein, C.R. Treatment of yaws in the Haitian peasant. *J. Natl. Med. Assoc.* **1949**, *41*, 60–65. [PubMed]
24. Marks, M.; Goncalves, A.; Vahi, V.; Sakana, O.; Puiahi, E.; Zhang, Z.; Dalipanda, T.; Bottomley, C.; Mabey, D.; Solomin, A.W. Evaluation of a rapid diagnostic test for yaws infection in a community surveillance setting. *PLoS Negl. Trop. Dis.* **2014**, *8*, e3156. [CrossRef] [PubMed]
25. Ayove, T.; Houniei, W.; Wangnapi, R.; Bieb, S.V.; Kazadi, W.; Luke, L.N.; Manineng, C.; Moses, P.; Paru, R.; Esfandiari, J.; et al. Sensitivity and specificity of a rapid point-of-care test for active yaws: A comparative study. *Lancet Glob. Health* **2014**, *2*, e415–e421. [CrossRef]
26. Marks, M.; Chi, K.H.; Vahi, V.; Pillay, N.; Sokana, O.; Pavluck, A.; Mabey, D.C.; Chen, C.Y.; Solomon, A.W. *Haemophilus ducreyi* associated with skin ulcers among children, Solomon Islands. *Emerg. Infect. Dis.* **2014**, *20*, 1705–1707. [CrossRef] [PubMed]
27. Mitjà, O.; Lukehart, S.A.; Pokowas, G.; Moses, P.; Kapa, A.; Godones, C.; Robson, J.; Cherian, S.; Houniei, W.; Kazadi, W.; et al. *Haemophilus ducreyi* as a cause of skin ulcers in children from a yaws-endemic area of Papua New Guinea: A prospective cohort study. *Lancet Glob. Health* **2014**, *2*, e235–e241. [CrossRef]
28. Backhouse, J.L.; Hudson, B.J.; Hamilton, P.A.; Nesteroff, S.I. Failure of penicillin treatment of yaws on Karkar Island, Papua New Guinea. *Am. J. Trop. Med. Hyg.* **1998**, *59*, 388–392. [CrossRef] [PubMed]
29. Asiedu, K.; Amouzou, B.; Dhariwal, A.; Karam, M.; Lobo, D.; Patnaik, S.; Meheus, A. Yaws eradication: Past efforts and future perspectives. *Bull. World Health Organ.* **2008**, *86*, 499. [CrossRef] [PubMed]
30. Antal, G.M.; Causse, G. The control of endemic treponematoses. *Rev. Infect. Dis.* **1985**, *7*, S220–S226. [CrossRef] [PubMed]
31. Nurse-Findlay, S.; Taylor, M.M.; Savage, M.; Mello, M.B.; Saliyou, S.; Lavayen, S.; Seghers, F.; Campbell, M.L.; Birgirimana, F.; Ouedraogo, L.; et al. Shortages of benzathine penicillin for prevention of mother-to-child transmission of syphilis: An evaluation from multi-country surveys and stakeholder interviews. *PLoS Med.* **2017**, *14*, e1002473. [CrossRef] [PubMed]
32. Riedner, G.; Rusizoka, M.; Todd, J.; Maboko, L.; Hoelscher, M.; Mmbando, D.; Samky, E.; Lyamuya, E.; Mabey, D.; Grosskurth, H.; et al. Single-dose azithromycin versus penicillin G benzathine for the treatment of early syphilis. *N. Engl. J. Med.* **2005**, *353*, 1236–1244. [CrossRef] [PubMed]
33. Mitjà, O.; Hays, R.; Ipai, A.; Penias, M.; Paru, R.; Fagaho, D.; Lazzari, E.; Bassat, Q. Single-dose azithromycin versus benzathine benzylpenicillin for treatment of yaws in children in Papua New Guinea: An open-label, non-inferiority, randomised trial. *Lancet* **2012**, *379*, 342–347.
34. Kwakye-Maclean, C.; Agana, N.; Gyapong, J.; Nortey, P.; Adu-Sarkodie, Y.; Aryee, E.; Asiedu, K.; Ballard, R.; Binka, F. A single dose oral azithromycin versus intramuscular benzathine penicillin for the treatment of yaws—A randomized non-inferiority trial in Ghana. *PLoS Negl. Trop. Dis.* **2017**, *11*, e0005154. [CrossRef] [PubMed]
35. Mitjà, O.; González-Beiras, C.; Godornes, C.; Kolmau, R.; Houniei, W.; Abel, H.; Kapa, A.; Paru, A.; Bieb, S.V.; Wangi, J.; et al. Effectiveness of single-dose azithromycin to treat latent yaws: A longitudinal comparative cohort study. *Lancet Glob. Health* **2017**, *5*, e1268–e1274.
36. Marks, M.; Mitjà, O.; Bottomley, C.; Kwakye, C.; Houniei, W.; Bauri, M.; Adwere, P.; Abdulai, A.A.; Dua, F.; Boateng, L.; et al. Comparative efficacy of low-dose versus standard-dose azithromycin for patients with yaws: A randomised non-inferiority trial in Ghana and Papua New Guinea. *Lancet Glob. Health* **2018**, *6*, e401–e410. [CrossRef]
37. Grimes, M.; Sahi, S.K.; Godornes, B.C.; Tantalo, L.C.; Roberts, N.; Bostick, D.; Marra, C.M.; Lukehart, S.A. Two mutations associated with macrolide resistance in *Treponema pallidum*: Increasing prevalence and correlation with molecular strain type in Seattle, Washington. *Sex Transm. Dis.* **2012**, *39*, 954–958. [CrossRef] [PubMed]

38. Lukehart, S.A.; Godornes, C.; Molini, B.J.; Sonnett, P.; Hopkins, S.; Mulcahy, F.; Engelman, J.; Mitchell, S.J.; Rompalo, A.M.; Marra, C.M.; et al. Macrolide resistance in *Treponema pallidum* in the United States and Ireland. *N. Engl. J. Med.* **2004**, *351*, 154–158. [CrossRef] [PubMed]

39. Chen, C.Y.; Chi, K.H.; Pillay, A.; Nachamkin, E.; Su, J.R.; Ballard, R.C. Detection of the A2058G and A2059G 23S rRNA gene point mutations associated with azithromycin resistance in *Treponema pallidum* by use of a TaqMan real-time multiplex PCR assay. *J. Clin. Microbiol.* **2013**, *51*, 908–913. [CrossRef] [PubMed]

40. Šmajs, D.; Paštěková, L.; Grillová, L. Macrolide resistance in the syphilis spirochete, *Treponema pallidum* ssp. *pallidum*: Can we also expect macrolide-resistant yaws strains? *Am. J. Trop. Med. Hyg.* **2015**, *93*, 678–683.

41. Šmajs, D.; Pospíšilová, P. Macrolide resistance in yaws. *Lancet* **2018**, *391*, 1555–1556. [CrossRef]

42. Mitjà, O.; Godornes, C.; Houinei, W.; Kapa, A.; Paru, R.; Abel, H.; González-Beiras, C.; Bieb, S.V.; Wangi, J.; Barry, A.E.; et al. Re-emergence of yaws after single mass azithromycin treatment followed by targeted treatment: A longitudinal study. *Lancet Lond. Engl.* **2018**, *391*, 1599–1607. [CrossRef]

43. Solomon, A.W.; Holland, M.J.; Alexander, N.D.E.; Massae, P.A.; Aguirre, A.; Natividad-Sancho, A.; Molina, S.; Safari, S.; Shao, J.F.; Courtright, P.; et al. Mass treatment with single-dose azithromycin for trachoma. *N. Engl. J. Med.* **2004**, *351*, 1962–1971. [CrossRef] [PubMed]

44. Emerson, P.M.; Burton, M.J.; Solomon, A.W.; Bailey, R.; Mabey, D.C. The SAFE strategy for trachoma control: Using operational research for policy, and implementation. *Bull. World Health Organ.* **2006**, *84*, 613–619. [CrossRef] [PubMed]

45. Keenan, J.D.; Bailey, R.L.; West, S.K.; Arzika, A.M.; Hart, J.; Weaver, J.; Kalua, K.; Mrango, Z.; Ray, K.J.; Cook, C.; et al. Azithromycin to reduce childhood mortality in sub-Saharan Africa. *N. Engl. J. Med.* **2018**, *378*, 1583–1592. [CrossRef] [PubMed]

46. The World Health Organization. Eradication of yaws—The Morges Strategy. *Wkly. Epidemiol. Rec.* **2012**, *87*, 189–194.

47. Marks, M.; Mitjà, O.; Fitzpatrick, C.; Asiedu, K.; Solomon, A.W.; Mabey, D.C.; Funk, S. Mathematical modeling of programmatic requirements for yaws eradication. *Emerg. Infect. Dis.* **2017**, *23*, 22–28. [CrossRef] [PubMed]

48. Dyson, L.; Marks, M.; Crook, O.M.; Sokana, O.; Solomon, A.W.; Bishop, A.; Mabey, D.C.W.; Hollingsworth, T.D. Targeted treatment of yaws with household contact tracing: How much do we miss? *Am. J. Epidemiol.* **2018**, *187*, 837–844. [CrossRef] [PubMed]

49. Marks, M.; Vahi, V.; Sokana, O.; Puiahi, E.; Pavluck, A.; Zhang, Z.; Dalipanda, T.; Bottomley, C.; Mabey, D.C.; Solomon, A.W. Mapping the epidemiology of yaws in the Solomon Islands: A cluster randomized survey. *Am. J. Trop. Med. Hyg.* **2015**, *92*, 129–133. [CrossRef] [PubMed]

50. Marks, M.; Vahi, V.; Sokana, O.; Chi, K.H.; Puiahi, E.; Kilua, G.; Pillay, A.; Dalipanda, T.; Bottomley, C.; Solomon, A.W.; et al. Impact of community mass treatment with azithromycin for trachoma elimination on the prevalence of yaws. *PLoS Negl. Trop. Dis.* **2015**, *9*, e0003988. [CrossRef] [PubMed]

51. Marks, M.; Sokanam, O.; Nachamkin, E.; Puiahi, E.; Kilua, G.; Pillay, A.; Bottomley, C.; Solomon, A.W.; Mabey, D.C. Prevalence of active and latent yaws in the Solomon Islands 18 months after azithromycin mass drug administration for trachoma. *PLoS Negl. Trop. Dis.* **2016**, *10*, e0004927. [CrossRef] [PubMed]

52. Abdulai, A.A.; Agana-Nsiire, P.; Biney, F.; Kwakye-Maclea, C.; Kyei-Faried, S.; Amponsa-Achiano, K.; Simpson, S.V.; Bonsu, G.; Ohene, S.A.; Ampofo, W.K.; et al. Community-based mass treatment with azithromycin for the elimination of yaws in Ghana—Results of a pilot study. *PLoS Negl. Trop. Dis.* **2018**, *12*, e0006303. [CrossRef] [PubMed]

53. Mitjà, O.; Houinei, W.; Moses, P.; Kapa, A.; Paru, R.; Hays, R.; Lukehart, S.; Godornes, C.; Bieb, S.V.; Grice, T.; Siba, P.; et al. Mass treatment with single-dose azithromycin for yaws. *N. Engl. J. Med.* **2015**, *372*, 703–710. [CrossRef] [PubMed]

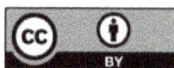

*Tropical Medicine and
Infectious Disease*

MDPI

Review

Onchodermatitis: Where Are We Now?

Michele E. Murdoch

Department of Dermatology, West Herts Hospitals NHS Trust, Vicarage Road, Watford,
Hertfordshire WD18 0HB, UK; michele.murdoch@nhs.net; Tel.: +44-1923-217139

Received: 30 July 2018; Accepted: 28 August 2018; Published: 1 September 2018

Abstract: Onchocerciasis causes debilitating pruritus and rashes as well as visual impairment and blindness. Prior to control measures, eye disease was particularly prominent in savanna areas of sub-Saharan Africa whilst skin disease was more common across rainforest regions of tropical Africa. Mass drug distribution with ivermectin is changing the global scene of onchocerciasis. There has been successful progressive elimination in Central and Southern American countries and the World Health Organization has set a target for elimination in Africa of 2025. This literature review was conducted to examine progress regarding onchocercal skin disease. PubMed searches were performed using keywords 'onchocerciasis', 'onchodermatitis' and 'onchocercal skin disease' over the past eight years. Articles in English, or with an English abstract, were assessed for relevance, including any pertinent references within the articles. Recent progress in awareness of, understanding and treatment of onchocercal skin disease is reviewed with particular emphasis on publications within the past five years. The global burden of onchodermatitis is progressively reducing and is no longer seen in children in many formerly endemic foci.

Keywords: onchodermatitis; onchocercal skin disease; onchocerciasis; ivermectin

---

1. Introduction

Onchocerciasis, caused by infection with the filarial worm *Onchocerca volvulus*, is one of the eleven neglected tropical diseases (NTDs) recently targeted for elimination by the World Health Organization (WHO) [1]. More than 99% of all cases are concentrated in 28 countries in sub-Saharan Africa. Small foci also occurred in the Americas, but there has been successful progressive elimination in this region and infection is currently found in a single large transmission zone (the 'Yanomani area') which straddles the border of Venezuela and Brazil [2]. Small foci of infection also persist in Yemen [3].

Historically onchocerciasis was better known for its clinical effects of visual impairment and blindness, prompting its alternative name of 'river blindness'. Over recent years, however, there has been significantly increased awareness of the skin manifestations associated with this disease and indeed the main clinical manifestations of onchocerciasis in the twenty countries formerly covered by the African Program for Onchocerciasis Control (APOC) were related to skin disease [4].

Currently the WHO estimates that 198 million people are at risk of infection, though this number may increase as the mapping of areas of low transmission is finalized [5]. The Global Burden of Disease (GBD) Study 2013 estimated a global prevalence of 17 million infected cases [6]. The Democratic Republic of Congo (DRC) had the highest number of onchocerciasis cases at 8.3 million [7]. In its 2015 iteration, the GBD collaborators estimated an overall prevalence of 15.53 million, comprising 12.22 million with skin disease and 1.03 million cases with vision loss due to onchocerciasis [8]. The most recent available data in GBD Study 2016 estimates a global prevalence of 14.65 million [9].

When ivermectin was first licensed for human use in 1987 Merck, Sharp and Dome (MSD), now known as Merck and MSD, made the unprecedented decision to donate the drug (Mectizan®) to the world to treat onchocerciasis for as long as needed and it has remained the mainstay of treatment to date. In 2015 Dr. William Campbell, MSD and Prof. Satosh Ōmura of the Kitasato Institute shared the Nobel Prize in Physiology or Medicine for their development and use of ivermectin for onchocerciasis [10].

APOC was launched in 1995 with the objective of removing onchocerciasis as a public health and socio-economic problem in Africa [11]. The countries included in the program were: Angola, Burundi, Cameroon, Central African Republic, Chad, Congo, Democratic Republic of Congo (DRC), Equatorial Guinea, Ethiopia, Gabon, Kenya, Liberia, Malawi, Mozambique, Nigeria, Rwanda, South Sudan, Sudan, Uganda, and Tanzania. In 1997, APOC adopted community-directed treatment with ivermectin (CDTi) as its core strategy and the coverage and compliance with ivermectin steadily increased. In 2009 APOC changed its strategy to a target of elimination of the disease in Africa [12]. APOC closed at the end of 2015 and WHO established a new structure, the Expanded Special Project for Elimination of Neglected Tropical Diseases (ESPEN), to co-ordinate technical support for activities focused on five neglected tropical diseases in Africa, including onchocerciasis elimination [13].

Onchocerciasis control and elimination efforts are among the most sustained, successful, and cost-effective public health campaigns ever launched. By improving the general health of individuals, they contribute to improvements in worker productivity, gender equality and education and hence they actively contribute towards achieving several of the Millennium Development Goals [14].

2. Cutaneous Features

In 1989 Hay et al. reported an association between infection and skin changes associated with onchocerciasis in Ecuador [15]. The development of a formal clinical classification and grading system describing the cutaneous changes in onchocerciasis [16] facilitated more formal and extensive mapping of the true global burden of onchocercal skin disease (OSD). The categories of onchocercal skin disease delineated were (i) acute papular onchodermatitis (APOD) (ii) chronic papular onchodermatitis (CPOD) (iii) lichenified onchodermatitis (LOD) (iv) atrophy (v) depigmentation and (vi) hanging groin. The system was designed for easy use in the field by nurses or primary healthcare attendants, had good inter-observer variation *kappa* results and could be adapted for computer coding for large scale surveys.

A pre-control population survey of 6790 residents in savanna mesoendemic villages in Kaduna State, northern Nigeria [17] where onchocercal blindness was common, revealed that 38.6% of the residents aged five and above complained of itching with normal skin or had one or more forms of onchocercal skin disease including nodules. The presence of nodules was the most common finding (21.2%), followed by atrophy (6.1% of those <50 years), APOD (3.4%), depigmentation (3.2%), and CPOD (2.3%). A further 9.5% of residents complained of itching but had clinically normal skin. Atrophy, hanging groin and nodules were more common in females, whereas APOD was more common in males. After controlling for age and sex, microfilarial positivity was a risk factor for CPOD, depigmentation, hanging groin and nodules (OR 1.54, $p = 0.046$; OR 2.29, $p = 0.002$; OR 2.18, $p = 0.002$, and OR 3.80, $p \leq 0.001$ respectively). Similar though weaker odds ratios were found with microfilarial load *per se*.

The first multi-country study to explore OSD across Africa comprised seven rainforest or savanna-forest mosaic areas where onchocercal blindness was not common [18]. Following a census, individuals were randomly selected for examination in five of the study sites, though protocol deviation in the other two sites meant that individuals were asked to come to a central point for examination. Overall, onchocercal skin lesions (excluding nodules) affected 28% of the population aged five years and above. The commonest type of OSD was CPOD (13%), followed by depigmentation (10%) and APOD (7%). The prevalence of itching increased with age until 20 years and then plateaued, affecting 42% of the population aged 20 years and above. The prevalence of any onchocercal skin lesion and/or itching combined showed a very high correlation with the level of endemicity (as determined by the prevalence of nodules) of $r = 0.8$, $p < 0.001$.

In Yemen and Abu Hamid in Sudan, an atypical and severe form of onchodermatitis known as *sowda* (or lichenified onchodermatitis) is prominent. *Sowda* is common in older children, teenagers, and young adults but current expertise now suggests that all ages, including the elderly can be affected [19]. Typically, *sowda* presents as an extremely itchy hyperpigmented plaque or plaques on one leg; less commonly both legs or an arm or shoulder can be involved. There is also often marked rubbery enlargement of the draining lymph nodes. Eye disease and palpable subcutaneous nodules are uncommon in Yemen and use of ivermectin has concentrated on treating skin disease in this country. A general concept is that onchocerciasis has a spectrum of skin changes, with *sowda* representing one end of a clinico-parasitological spectrum with low parasite loads and high levels of immune response.

A pre-control study in Edo State, Nigeria examined 2020 individuals who had visited primary health centers in each community and were recruited using simple random sampling. The area was hyperendemic for onchocerciasis with a skin snip positivity rate of 83%. The prevalence of depigmentation was very high at 87.5%, itching was 84.16% and nodules 75.42% [20]. Another pre-control study in Anfilo District of West Wellega, Ethiopia used a multistage sampling technique and a total of 1114 individuals ≥15 years were examined [21]. The prevalence of positive skin snips was 74.8% and nodules 12.1%. The prevalence of pruritus was 64.3%, leopard skin (19.1%), 'skin lesions' 11.3%, lymphadenopathy 16.4%, and hanging groin the least prevalent at 5.2%. The overall prevalence of pruritus and/or these clinical signs was 26.4%, being more prevalent in males (32.4%) than in females (20.8%, $p < 0.05$). A study in Enugu State, Nigeria revealed lichenified onchodermatitis was the most common clinical manifestation of onchocerciasis, occurring in 42/119 (35.29%) of infected persons (as denoted by the presence of palpable onchocercal nodules) [22].

There is a paucity of literature exploring concurrence of skin and eye morbidities. In a hyperendemic area of Cameroon, with a 63% nodule prevalence among males aged ≥ 20, individuals aged five years and older were invited to present themselves at a central point and 765 people were examined [23]. Onchocercal visual impairment (which included low vision and blindness) and depigmentation were found to concur significantly (OR 9.0, 95% CI 3.9–20.8), which was partly explained by age and exposure to infection (OR 3.0, 95% CI 1.2–7.7). Host immune characteristics such as the HLA-DQ alleles associated with depigmentation [24] might play a role in the pathogenesis of both depigmentation and visual impairment.

3. Imported Onchodermatitis

Growth in international travel and immigration means patients with onchocerciasis may be diagnosed in countries in the western world but it is probably under-reported because of its relatively non-specific presentations and limited awareness among physicians practicing outside endemic countries.

A retrospective study of 6168 patients diagnosed with one or more NTDs at a Tropical Medicine Referral Unit in Madrid, Spain between 1989–2007 found that onchocerciasis was the most common NTD in immigrants [25]. A diagnosis of definite onchocerciasis was based on positive skin snips or pruritus +/− skin lesions suggestive of onchocerciasis and a positive Mazzotti test (performed in patients with negative skin snips and no evidence of ocular onchocerciasis). Probable onchocerciasis was diagnosed in immigrants in the presence of pruritus +/− suggestive skin lesions and response to treatment with ivermectin. Onchocerciasis was present in 240 (9.1%) of immigrants (169 definite and 71 probable cases). All but two cases in immigrants occurred in African patients, with the majority coming from Equatorial Guinea (213/240, 88.8%), a reflection of the historical links between that country and Spain. The other countries of origin were Cameroon, Nigeria, Angola, and Zaire and one each from Republic of Guinea, Mali, Togo, D.R. Congo, Ghana, Sierra Leone, Sao Tome, Ivory Coast, Colombia, and Ecuador. (N.B. Zaire's name was changed back to D.R. Congo in 1997). The number of new cases of onchocerciasis per new African immigrants significantly decreased each year over the period of the study. In a further group of immigrants who had travelled back to endemic countries to visit family and friends, there were 14 more cases of onchocerciasis.

With respect to the group of travelers who had visited endemic areas in this study, definite onchocerciasis was diagnosed in those with positive skin snips or positive serology in the presence of pruritus +/− suggestive skin lesions. In contrast to immigrants, who presumably had had long periods of exposure to infection prior to immigration, the number of travelers with onchocerciasis was much smaller at only 17. Of these, 16 had had a trip duration >3 months, range 3–336 months, and 1 patient had travelled for 1 month). All had travelled to sub-Saharan Africa and some patients had visited more than one country during their trip.

A literature search for English and French articles between 1994 and 2014 identified 29 cases of onchocerciasis in migrants from endemic countries and in expatriates and travelers from non-endemic areas [26]. The most frequent clinical manifestations in these cases plus the authors' index case were pruritus (76.7%), unilateral leg or forearm swelling (43.3%) and rash (40%), whereas only two (6.9%) complained of eye symptoms. Eosinophilia was very common (92%). Eye symptoms, lymphadenopathy and chronic dermatitis were seen more frequently in migrants, whereas rash and arm swelling were more frequent in returned travelers and expatriates.

A review of 31 filarial cases in a French University Centre between 2002 and 2011 revealed 4 cases due to onchocerciasis comprising 3 immigrants from Cameroon, Sierra Leone, and Senegal with onchodermatitis and one traveler from Central Africa with arm swelling [27]. Another review of 289 NTD cases from 2000 and 2015 at the Infectious and Tropical Diseases Unit, Florence, Italy revealed just two cases of onchocerciasis from sub-Saharan Africa with typical cutaneous manifestations and they both presented within the first five years of the review [28].

In a group of 27 migrants who came to Israel from an onchocerciasis-endemic area in Ethiopia and who were referred for an atopic eczema-like rash, 14 had positive skin snips or positive IgG$_4$ antifilarial serology [29]. The migrants who did not have laboratory proof of infection had similar clinical findings. Considering the group as a whole, patients' main complaint was relentless pruritus, which began with an average of 2.2 years after immigration, which a range of 1 year prior to immigration to 11 years after immigration. The most common finding was LOD in combination with atrophy and depigmentation 8/27 (30%), followed by CPOD 7/27 (26%).

The largest case series of imported onchocerciasis to date reviewed 400 cases attending a reference clinical unit in Madrid, Spain [30]. All the migrants came from sub-Saharan countries and the most frequently occurring dermatological symptom was pruritus.

4. Burden of Disease

Onchocerciasis is mainly a non-fatal disease and its public health impact is therefore best understood in terms of DALYs (DALYs = Years of Lives Lost (YLL) + Years Lived with Disability (YLD)). Both skin and eye disease caused by onchocerciasis result in a decrease in productivity [31]. Initially only the burden from onchocercal eye disease was considered in global estimates, but the burden from 'itch' was first included in the GBD Study 1990, based on data from the multicountry prevalence study in Africa [18]. Physical onchocercal skin disease manifestations have also been included since the GDB Study 2010. There is now evidence that *O. volvulus* infection is causing onchocerciasis-associated epilepsy including nodding syndrome, and this condition is associated with high mortality, because in remote onchocerciasis-endemic regions a large number of individuals are not treated or treated too late with anti-epileptic drugs. Such sequelae have not been included in GBD estimates to date.

The GBD study 2013 estimated that onchocerciasis was the sixth highest cause of NTD-related YLDs globally and it was ranked highly in the top 10 leading causes of YLDs in Liberia, Cameroon and South Sudan. In all these countries, the burden from onchocerciasis is predominantly due to onchocercal skin disease [7]. In its 2015 iteration the GBD Study provided an overall global estimate of 1,135,700 (YLDs) due to onchocercal infection [8]. In the GBD Study 2016, onchocerciasis was ranked as the first leading cause of YLDs for Liberia, as the second leading cause for DRC and South Sudan, the fifth for Cameroon and the sixth cause for both Central African Republic and Sierra Leone [9].

5. Immunopathogenesis

Filarial parasites are known to induce a large range of immunoregulatory mechanisms to evade and down-modulate the host's immune system in order to ensure the parasite's survival [32]. Such mechanisms include induction of regulatory T cells, which promote high levels of non-complement binding IgG$_4$ [33]. Survival of *O. volvulus* within the human host is thus the result of a complex interplay with the host's immune system, which itself may be dependent on genetic factors, and pathology ensues when pro-inflammatory processes override any immunomodulatory effects.

Wolbachia are endosymbiotic bacteria found in most human filariae, (except *Loa loa*), and appear to be essential for the filarial worm's fertility and survival. In an experimental murine model *Wolbachia* were found to be an essential component in the development of anterior segment onchocercal eye disease and mediated corneal pathology by activating Toll-like receptors on mammalian cells, which in turn stimulated recruitment and activation of neutrophils and macrophages [34].

Recruitment of neutrophils by *Wolbachia* around adult female worms in *O. ochengi* infection in cattle has been shown to confound eosinophil degranulation and may act to protect the adult worms from the host immune system [35]. Furthermore, the major inflammatory motif of *Wolbachia* lipoproteins are able to directly activate human neutrophils in vitro [36].

The formation of neutrophil extracellular traps (NETS), a process referred to as NETosis, is now regarded as a novel effector mechanism, consisting of the extrusion of nuclear contents with neutrophil-derived granular and cytoplasmic proteins, which may limit microbial spread by entrapment and limit collateral inflammatory tissue damage by entrapping and degrading soluble cytokines and chemokines. Tamarozzi et al. visualized extracellular NETS and neutrophils around adult *O. volvulus* in nodules excised from untreated patients but not in nodules from patients treated with doxycycline, which kills *Wolbachia*. [37]. In addition, whole *Wolbachia* or latex microspheres coated with a synthetic *Wolbachia* lioprotein of the major nematode *Wolbachia* TLR2/6 ligand, peptidoglycan associated lipoprotein, induced NETosis in human neutrophils in vitro and TLR6-deficient mice were used to demonstrate that TLR6 was essential for this process. It is possible that NETosis triggered by *Wolbachia* is an anti-parasite response to limit the density of tens of thousands of uterine-released microfilariae (mf) produced daily by each adult female worm and that *Wolbachia*-induced NETs may directly modify inflammatory processes in the skin.

TGF-β was preferentially observed in the skin of infected individuals with 'generalized' or hyporeactive onchocerciasis and was reduced in patients with the hyperreactive form of onchocercal skin disease (LOD or *sowda*) [38]. In a similar vein, 'hyperreactive onchocerciasis' has been found to be characterized by a combination of accentuated Th17 and Th2 immune responses and reduced regulatory T cells [39].

Secretory extracellular superoxide dismutase (*OvES-SOD*) from *O. volvulus*, which is found in the excretory/secretory products of adult worms, was able to trigger responses in sera from onchocerciasis patients, with IgG titers significantly higher in sera from individuals with the 'hyperreactive' form compared with sera from those with the generalized form of onchocerciasis [40]. The authors proposed that, in addition to its role in superoxide anion reduction in the extracellular space, the *OvEC-SOD* may help regulate inflammatory responses.

In patients who became mf-negative after repeated ivermectin treatments, parasite-specific cellular immune responsiveness and Th1 and Th2-type cytokine production becomes reactivated. Similarly, mf-negative patients after repeated ivermectin treatments have enhanced pro-inflammatory chemokines and reduced regulatory chemokines and cytokines [41].

Immunocytochemical examination of nodules using immuno-markers for blood and lymphatic vessels has suggested an intimate relationship between adult *O. volvulus* worms and lymphatic vessels, including the likely proliferation of lymphatic endothelial cells [42]. This has raised the possibility that the lymphatic system may be more involved in the migration of adult *O. volvulus* worms than was previously believed and may explain the lymphoedema that is sometimes seen in onchocerciasis [16]. Microfilariae, which have been documented in the blood in heavily-infected onchocerciasis patients and after treatment, might also migrate via the lymphatic system. Angiogenesis and lymphangiogenesis within nodules is characterized by the expression of CXCL 12, CXCR4, VEGF-C, angiopoietin-1 and angiopoietin-2. A proportion of macrophages in the inflammatory infiltrate in nodules were positive for the lymphatic endothelial cell marker Lyve-1 and some were integrated into the endothelium of the lymphatic vessels [43] and angiogenesis and lymphangiogenesis within nodules may provide new targets for drug treatment.

Imported Skin Disease Pathogenesis

Baum et al. [29] noted a long interval for some Ethiopian immigrants in Israel before they developed any symptoms and hypothesized that environmental factors resulting from immigration from a developing to an industrialized country triggered an immunological shift to strong T-helper (Th) 2 responses, in a similar manner that an increased prevalence in asthma had been noted in Ethiopian migrants several years after migrating to Israel.

6. Immunogenetics

HLA class II variants may influence susceptibility to infection by *O. volvulus* and subsequent host immune responses causing pathology. Correlation between allelic variants of HLA-DQA1 and HLA-DQB1 and various forms of onchocercal skin disease have previously been documented in a Nigerian population [24], and recently a protective role of DQA1*0401 against *O. volvulus* infection has been demonstrated in both Cayapas Amerindians and Afro-Ecuadorians. Furthermore HLA-DQA1*0102 and *0103 seemed to represent risk factors for infection in Afro-Ecuadorians and HLA-DQA1*0301 was a possible susceptibility allele in the Cayapas population [44].

7. New Diagnostics

The quest for elimination of onchocerciasis requires newer, more sensitive diagnostic tests to verify that transmission of infection has been suppressed or interrupted. Such tests differ from previously used tests to diagnose infection in individuals.

7.1. Detection of Parasite in Humans

The sensitivity of the skin snip assay has been increased by replacing microscopic examination of the snip with detection of amplified parasite DNA. Most assays target the tandemly repeated sequence in the *O. volvulus* genome called the 0–150 repeat. Real-time PCR and isothermal loop amplification (LAMP) assays have also been developed [45,46]. On comparison of three PCR methods for evaluating onchocerciasis elimination efforts in areas co-endemic with other filarial nemaodes, the qPCR-O150 assay was deemed to be more appropriate for evaluating skin snips of OV-16 positive children when deciding when to stop MDA [47]. A novel O-5S qPCR assay targeting the *O. volvulus* O-5S rRNA gene, had 100% specificity and proved more sensitive than O-150 qPCR assay (66.5% vs 39% positivity rate) [48].

7.2. Serological Tests to Detect Exposure to O. volvulus

The Ov16 ELISA is now recommended by WHO guidelines for demonstrating the interruption of transmission of *O. volvulus* [49]. According to these guidelines, the serological threshold for stopping MDA is an Ov16 antibody prevalence of <0.1% among children under 10 years of age who act as sentinels for recent infection, but the current tools are not reliably specific enough and an Ov16 threshold of <2% may ultimately prove to be the most reliable serological threshold for stopping MDA [50]. Current assays have focused on IgG_4 detection, but the IgG_4 response takes time to develop and thus will not immediately reflect recent exposure. Two commercially available rapid diagnostic tests (RDTs) are a single Ov16 test and a combination test using Ov16 and the *W. bancrofti* antigen Wb123 [51]. The SD BIOLONE Ov16 rapid test was successfully field-tested in Senegal [52].

7.3. Detection of Parasite in Vector Blackflies

The O-150 PCR DNA amplification assay is the most widely used assay to screen pools of flies to verify elimination of transmission. Instead of using human bait to catch the vector blackflies, as has been done in the past, the Esperanza window trap has been used in Mexico with success [53,54] and such traps are being evaluated for use in Africa [55].

7.4. Detection of Biomarkers

Recent research has also produced assays to detect potentially viable adult worms such as specific metabolites produced by female worms [56,57] and detection of parasite microRNA in the blood [58,59] though the latter may not be present in sufficient concentration to act as a biomarker for infection [60].

8. Treatment

8.1. Effect of Ivermectin on Cutaneous Disease

Ivermectin, a macrocyclic lactone, interacts with post-synaptic glutamate-gated chloride channels resulting in paralysis of mf, which are therefore transported to regional lymph nodes and killed by effector cells. Release of uterine mf is also temporarily inhibited.

The first multi-country study on the short-term effect of ivermectin on onchocercal skin disease in Africa was performed by Brieger and colleagues in four study sites in Nigeria, Ghana and Uganda [61]. They followed up rural villagers for 18 months and found that from 6 months onwards, the prevalence of severe itching was reduced by 40–50% among those receiving ivermectin compared to the trend in the placebo group. The prevalence of APOD, CPOD, and LOD combined was significantly reduced in the ivermectin group at 9 months and the severity at 3 months. Furthermore, there was no difference between ivermectin given at 3, 6, or 12 monthly intervals.

The first assessment of the effect of mass treatment with ivermectin in the Onchocerciasis Elimination Program for the Americas was Banic et al.'s report [62] in the hyperendemic Yanomani communities of Roraima State, Brazil. Pre-treatment, 18/103 individuals (17.5%) had atrophy +/or 'scaling' of the skin. After three years of twice-yearly ivermectin therapy, there was a very significant reduction in the prevalence and intensity of infection by skin snips but there was no reduction in the prevalence of nodules or onchodermatitis.

The first multi-country study on the longer term impact of ivermectin on onchocercal skin disease involved seven study sites in Cameroon, Sudan, Nigeria and Uganda [63]. Two cross-sectional surveys were performed at baseline and after five or six years of CDTi. In phase I, 5193 individuals were examined and 5180 people participated in phase II. Within each study site, 10 villages underwent a census to cover approximately 1500 persons. Individuals aged five years and above were asked to present themselves for examination at a central point until a sample size of approximately 750 was obtained. The effect of five or six rounds of annual CDTi was profound with significant ($p < 0.001$) reductions in the odds of itching (OR 0.32), APOD (OR 0.28), CPOD (OR 0.34), depigmentation (OR 0.31) and nodules (OR 0.37). Reduction in the odds of LOD was also significant (OR 0.54, $p < 0.03$).

In Anfilo district, Western Ethiopia, 971 participants aged 15 years and above were examined after 6 years of annual CDTi and the prevalence of microfilaridermia, pruritus, leopard skin, nodules, and hanging groin were reduced by 45.6%, 54.4%, 61.3%, 77.7%, and 88.5% respectively [64].

In a previously hyperendemic rainforest area with a nodular rate of ≥40% in Anambra State, Nigeria, a cross-sectional survey of 894 subjects after a decade of CDTi identified nodules in 86 (9.62%) persons and 186 (20.81%) had one or more forms of onchocercal skin disease. There was a total absence of OSD in children < 10 years old and only 5 (5.43%) with OSD in the second decade of life, indicative of some encouraging success of the CDTi program. The rate of APOD however increased with age up to the third decade and decreased thereafter suggesting on-going transmission, either due to poor compliance or low coverage of treatment. All the individuals with APOD had missed the annual ivermectin treatment more than once during the program. CPOD, LOD, ATR, and DPM all increased with age for both sexes [65].

In 2015 after more than 15 years of CDTi in the West Region of Cameroon, a cross-sectional survey of 2058 individuals aged 5 years and above was performed to assess progress towards elimination. The weighted prevalence of positive skin snip results was 5.5% and that of nodules 2.1%. The weighted prevalence of skin disease excluding nodules was 1.7% and varied from 1.1% in men to 2.2% in women. Of note, treatment compliance was again found to be poor with only 39.3% of participants declaring they had taken five treatments during the last five years [66].

Prior to control measures on the island of Bioko, Equatorial Guinea, a survey in the mid 1980s reported that 28.8% of the study population suffered from dermatitis, pigmentation changes and cutaneous atrophy. After vector elimination in 2005 and more than 16 years of CDTi on Bioko Island, a community-based cross-sectional survey was performed in 2014, including a full cutaneous examination [67]. Although these workers found that 50.4% individuals reported never having taken ivermectin and only 28% had taken it more than twice within the past five years, there was a reduction in pruritus and skin lesions (14.9% complained of pruritus, 3% had nodules, 1.3% had 'onchodermatitis' and a further 1.8% had leopard skin. Nodules were more common in subjects older than 10 years and pruritus was more frequently found in adults (17.6%) than children (5.9%, $p = 0.002$).

With standard annual dosing, ivermectin was initially thought to have minimal macrofilarical activity, but recent mathematical modelling suggests that multiple doses of ivermectin, even at standard (150 μg/kg) doses and annual frequency, can have a modest permanent sterilizing effect after four or more consecutive treatments. The life expectancy of adult *O. volvulus* was reduced by 50% and 70% respectively after three years of annual or 3-monthly treatment with ivermectin [68]. There have been reports of suboptimal responses in some patients in Ghana after repeated treatment. In a Ghanian study of 42 patients treated with ivermectin and 204 randomly selected individuals, a significantly higher *MDR1* variant allele frequency was noted in suboptimal responders (21%) than in patients who responded to treatment (12%) or the random population sample (11%). *CYP3A5*1/CYP3A5*1 and CYP3A5*1/CYP3A5*3* genotypes were also significantly different for responders and suboptimal responders, suggesting a possible role of these haplotypes in an individual's response to ivermectin [69].

In Yemen, ivermectin was initially distributed only to *sowda*, (or lichenified onchodermatitis), cases four times a year, but a mass drug distribution program to treat the entire community has now begun. In the northern endemic valleys, there has been a marked reduction in the number of *sowda* cases from more than 50% pre-drug treatment to approximately 6% and in most areas it is uncommon to find new cases of *sowda* [19].

8.2. Effect on Imported Skin Disease

In Baum et al.'s study of Ethiopian immigrants to Israel [29], both patients with confirmed, and those with suspected, onchocerciasis, responded equally to ivermectin with reduction in itching and lichenification. Overall 9/17 (52%) had remission of more than 12 months, 5/17 (30%) had temporary relief lasting 3–12 months and required repeat treatment and 3/17 (18%) did not respond to treatment.

Puente's case series [30] reported that ivermectin was used as first-line therapy and adverse events were described in 11 (3.2%) cases.

8.3. Effect of Ivermectin on Psychosocial and Socio-Economic Aspects of Onchodermatits

In the past sufferers with OSD were considered unclean and were stigmatized because of fear of transmission of OSD, resulting in social ostracism. OSD has also been associated with reduced productivity [31], difficulties breastfeeding, poor school attendance and reduced marriage prospects for affected teenage girls. Vlassof et al.'s pre-control multicountry study in Africa had identified that one third of residents with OSD reported low self-esteem, about half of those affected perceived onchocercal skin disease as a very serious health issue and 1–2% had even considered suicide [70]. Higher levels of stigma were noted in individuals with APOD, CPOD or LOD than persons with depigmentation.

After a decade of CDTi, a questionnaire presented to subjects in Anambra State, Nigeria identified that itching and onchocercal skin manifestations remained the most troublesome symptom and sign of onchocerciasis and social seclusion (or stigmatization) the most worrisome consequence. A preponderance of onchodermatitis on the limbs (visible area of the body to others), plus involvement of the buttocks (an area considered 'private') were deemed contributory factors for the psychological impact of the skin disease [71]. In a random sample exit interview of 594/40,914 persons treated with ivermectin in Ezinihitte, Nigeria, (an area with predominantly onchocercal skin disease) the most common reason cited for seeking treatment was 'to gain treatment and prevention of skin problems' [72]. The fifth and sixth rank-order reasons were 'to prevent hanging groin' and 'to prevent/relieve enlargement of the scrotum or clitoris'. Genital lymphoedema is caused by filarial blockage of lymphatics in the pelvic region. Although both hanging groin and genital lymphoedema have low prevalence, they have important implications for married life and sexuality.

A multicountry study in Africa in Cameroon, DRC, Nigeria, and Uganda after at least four years of CDTi used random sampling of household treatment records to capture factors that reflected individuals' perception of benefits of CDTi. In this study, overall 84.7% of respondents indicated that ivermectin treatment had many benefits: social benefits included improved ability to work, peer acceptance and improved school attendance; individual benefits included self-respect/esteem, election to political office and improved domestic relationships and health benefits included improved skin texture and less ill health. Improvement in skin was perceived for the individual by 40.4% and for the household by 39.5% of respondents. Reduction in itching was perceived for the individual by 54.5% of respondents and for the household by 52.2% of respondents [73].

A subsequent multicountry study using multi-stage sampling after 7–10 years of CDTi revealed that although people with OSD were still stigmatized and people still feared sexual intimacy with affected persons, avoidance of people with OSD had decreased from 32.7% before CDTi activities to 4.3% [74]. People who had lived in the community for less than 5 years tended to stigmatize those with OSD more than those who had lived in the community for longer and the youth stigmatized the most. Reasons given for avoiding people with OSD included 'considered infectious', 'looked ugly', 'were irritating', 'were dirty', 'were scary' and 'were embarrassing'. An example of the changes in perception towards OSD is this quote from a young Nigerian man in a focus group discussion: *"Although we know better now, there is still the fear that something like hanging groin is hereditary. Really, people no longer avoid sufferers so much but I know that here we think that if it gets to the stage where one's groin is hanging, then it will be hereditary. Before no-one would go into marriage with a girl whose mother had leopard skin because it was believed that she would develop it and no female would ordinarily marry a man whose father had hanging groin. But these things are changing now because we know better".*

An interesting study asked schoolchildren aged 6–16 years to draw their perceptions of onchocerciasis and CDTi in their communities. Out of a total of 50 drawings generated, 30 pictures were categorized as showing symptoms of the disease, which included rashes and swellings (nodules), and a further 5 represented multiple perceptions on symptoms, benefits, and effects of treatment [75]. The results highlighted that children were cognizant of the external signs of onchocerciasis and the authors recommended that children be included in health promotion activities to maintain successful compliance with CDTi.

9. Update on Onchocerciasis Control Programs and Elimination

9.1. Onchocerciasis Elimination Program for the Americas (OEPA)

Right from its outset in 1993, this program used six-monthly mass ivermectin distribution with a target coverage of 85% with the goal of elimination of onchocerciasis from the region. Ivermectin distribution four times/year was also used in some areas. WHO has recently produced guidelines to help countries know when they can safely stop MDA and transition to a period of post-treatment surveillance (PTS) based on entomological evaluation to detect infection in the blackfly vector and serological evaluation in humans to detect the presence of antibodies to *O. volvulus* Ov16 antigen [49]. When all foci in a country have satisfactorily completed the PTS, the country may request a visit by a WHO verification team to assess elimination of transmission. By the end of 2012, transmission had been eliminated in 11 of the 13 foci in the Americas [6]. Elimination was first demonstrated by Colombia in 2103 [76], followed by Ecuador in 2014, Mexico in 2015 and Guatemala in 2016 [77]. Elimination of transmission in Ecuador was particularly gratifying as the main vector here, *Simulium exiguum*, was a very effective transmitter of infection and the skin and eye disease in this focus was probably the most severe in the Americas [78].

The remaining two onchocerciasis foci in the Americas form a single epidemiological transmission unit (the Yanomani Area) along the border between Brazil and Venezuela. There are challenges to treating the Yanomani Area, which is a remote area and difficult to reach. Furthermore, the Yanomani people can freely move across the country borders whereas program officials cannot, so increased political co-operation between the countries is needed.

9.2. African Program for Onchocerciasis Control (APOC)

The African Program for Onchocerciasis Control (APOC) initially focused on control of the disease as a public health problem. It was uncertain whether ivermectin could actually interrupt transmission and eliminate the parasite in Africa, as here the vectors are very efficient and the epidemiology very different, with large endemic areas that were often not well defined. The first evidence that elimination of onchocerciasis with ivermectin treatment was feasible in Africa came from studies in Senegal and Mali published in 2009 [79] and 2012 [80], which led to a paradigm shift from one of control of the disease to a target of elimination.

A further encouragement came from Tekle et al.'s report of a skin snip survey in 3703 individuals above the age of one year performed after 15–17 years of CDTi in Kaduna State, Nigeria. (These were the same villages where the onchocerciasis skin classification had originally been field-tested). These workers found that all examined individuals were skin snip negative, which was the first evidence from an APOC country that elimination of onchocerciasis infection with ivermectin might be feasible in Africa [81]. Unfortunately, Boko Haram activities interrupted fieldwork and entomological evaluations are still awaited.

From its outset APOC included a small number of projects where it was judged that local eradication of the vector would be possible and cost-effective and could be combined with CDTi. The island of Bioko, Equatorial Guinea [82], and the Itwara focus in Uganda [83] both achieved vector elimination. Bioko Island had no subsequent reported cases of infection and a recent study on 5–9-year-old school children revealed no evidence of infection by skin snipping and blood spot for Ov16 and Wb123 IgG$_4$ [84]. Current WHO serological criteria for stopping MDA were therefore met and 3 years of post-treatment surveillance are currently underway to identify any new cases of infection.

The Abu Hamed focus in Sudan, which had predominantly the severe form of skin disease *sowda* or lichenified onchodermatitis, was the first focus in Africa to have successfully completed the entire WHO-recommended process to confirm elimination [85].

In 2007 Uganda launched a national elimination policy based on twice-yearly ivermectin treatment and vector control/elimination. By 2017, 1,157,303 people in six foci were living free of onchocerciasis, which is the largest population to date declared free under WHO elimination guidelines, providing further evidence that elimination of onchocerciasis in Africa is possible [86]. Ethiopia, Mali, Niger, and Senegal also have eliminated onchocerciasis in subnational areas. Although APOC faced certain challenges it achieved overall major success as a control program [11]. All areas where *O. volvulus* might be transmitted and where ivermectin has not been distributed in the past, now require careful

Trop. Med. Infect. Dis. **2018**, *3*, 94

'elimination mapping' to determine whether they are onchocerciasis endemic or not so that appropriate treatment plans can be made [87].

9.3. Yemen

Since February 2016 Yemen has been using MDA with ivermectin in *sowda*-endemic areas with the goal of eliminating onchocerciasis in that country [88].

9.4. Challenges Faced by APOC

APOC faced several challenges, especially in conflict and post-conflict situations and in areas co-endemic with *Loa loa*. In DRC for example, the country had been devastated by political unrest and two civil wars and even after the signing of peace in 2003, fighting continued in the eastern provinces. Although the annual therapeutic and geographical coverage of CDTi projects slowly increased from 2001–2012, targets could not be met [89]. In Sierra Leone, civil conflict also resulted in limited onchocerciasis control activities from 1991–2002, but after the war, good CDTi was achieved between 2005 and 2009. In 2010, after 5 rounds of ivermectin, 10 out of 12 endemic districts had a >50% reduction in mf prevalence and 11 of 12 districts had ≥50% reduction in mean mf density among the positives, suggesting that Sierra Leone will now be on course to achieve elimination by the year 2025 [90].

Co-endemicity with *L. loa* has been another significant challenge for APOC. In areas co-endemic with loaisis, ivermectin treatment in people with high loads of *L. loa* mf can cause severe and occasionally fatal encephalopathy reactions. Little was known about the geographical distribution of loiasis in DRC at the start of CDTi projects and in 2004 adverse events in CDTi areas co-infected with loiasis resulted in 14 deaths [89]. Mass treatment was temporally halted whilst the situation was re-evaluated. A rapid assessment procedure for *L. loa* which assesses an individual's history of eye worm (RAPLOA) was subsequently introduced in co-endemic areas. If ≥40% of the population report eye worm, this is deemed to pose an unacceptable risk of encephalopathy and MDA is withheld from that area. Recently the LoaScope, a mobile phone-based imaging device that can rapidly determine the mf density of *L. loa* infections, has proven useful in determining more accurately whether or not MDA can safely proceed. In the Okola health district of Cameroon, persons with very high *L. loa* microfilarial counts (>20,000 mf/mL) were thus able to be excluded from ivermectin therapy and no serious adverse events occurred [91]. Individuals at risk of ivermectin-related side-effects in loiasis- co-endemic areas may safely be treated with doxycycline but a course of treatment (4–6 weeks) is required.

Additional challenges to APOC included cross-border transmission of infection. Although Uganda has some areas clear of disease, conflict in the north of the country meant that maximum control activities have only been carried out over the past 3–4 years and cross-borders areas continue to cause difficulties because of delay in programs in the DRC and South Sudan. A strategy meeting between Uganda and DRC, initially triggered by the Ebola outbreak, led to improved cross-border co-operation for onchocerciasis control and elimination [92] and lessons learnt from the Sierra Leone, Liberia, and Guinea (Conakry) Mano River Union collaboration on onchocerciasis should help with other neglected tropical disease programs in the future [93]. Although international borders that intersect endemic regions present the biggest challenge, intra-country borders (e.g., administrative districts, or loiasis-endemic and non-endemic areas) can also pose problems [94]. Migrant populations are also part of cross-border challenges. Non-compliance with treatment has been another issue is some areas [95] but can be improved using traditional kinship structures [96]. Hostility towards health workers occurred during the Ebola outbreak as some people feared they were responsible for spreading Ebola [97].

9.5. Health and Economic Impacts of MDA with Ivermectin

Using updated disability weights for visual impairment, blindness, and troublesome itching (0.033, 0.195 and 0.108 respectively), Coffeng et al. estimated that APOC had cumulatively averted an impressive 19 million DALYs from 1995 up until 2015 [98]. This represented some 80% reduction in loss of DALYs for APOC countries, though in reality the true burden averted by APOC is even larger still as these updated estimates did not include disfiguring skin disease and onchocerciasis-associated epilepsy, including nodding and Nakalanga syndrome [99–101].

Redekop et al., considered mild and moderate skin disease and moderate and severe vision loss and blindness and estimated that the global economic benefit (productivity loss prevented) for the period 2011–2030 for onchocerciasis was 7.1 billion I$ (International dollars) if a target of elimination by 2020 was achieved [102].

GBD 2010 data has been used to estimate the global health impact of meeting the London Declaration 2012 targets on NTDs [103]. Regarding onchocerciasis, for the period 2011–2020, 7 million DALYs were averted and for 2021–2030, 12.6 million DALYS, giving a total of 19.6 million DALYS averted over the entire period, compared to a counterfactual scenario of no control/elimination program. The projected health benefits were thus deemed to justify the enormous effort involved. With respect to Ethiopia, the GBD study 2015 data, estimated that the age-standardized DALY rates for onchocerciasis have encouragingly decreased by a dramatic 66.2% between 1990 and 2015 [104].

Using a mathematical dynamical transmission model called ONCHOSIM, Kim et al. simulated trends for the prevalence of severe itching, low vision, and blindness in two scenarios of elimination of onchocerciasis in Africa versus a control scenario of continuing measures simply aimed at keeping the disease at a locally acceptable level [105]. Using the same vision disability weights as above but a disability weight for severe itching of 0.187 [106,107] Kim and colleagues estimated that elimination of the disease in Africa would avert 4.3 million–5.6 million (DALYs) over 2013–2045 compared with staying in the control mode. The decrease in the prevalence of severe itching was faster than those of low vision and blindness and the majority of DALYs averted were associated with the reduction in severe itching cases.

As ivermectin is a broad-spectrum anti-parasitic agent, it also has an effect on so-called off-target diseases, including soil-transmitted helminthiasis, lymphatic filariasis and scabies. Krotneva et al. [108] have estimated that between 1995 and 2010 annual MDA with ivermectin cumulatively averted about an extra 500 thousand DALYs from these co-endemic infections. This represents approximately an additional 5.5% relative to the total burden of 8.9 million DALYs averted from onchocerciasis, thus indicating that the overall cost-effectiveness of APOC is even higher than previously thought.

9.6. Effect on HIV

As HIV and helminth co-infection may be associated with a higher viral load and lower CD4+ cell counts, treatment with ivermectin could potentially benefit people living with HIV beyond simply treating the worm infection. Specific evidence for this to date is limited but there is no suggestion that anti-helminthic drugs are harmful for HIV-positive individuals [109]. NTDs may also lead to a worse prognosis in TB and malaria sufferers and further research on these interactions is needed [110].

9.7. ESPEN

Successful integrated chemotherapy for both onchocerciasis (with ivermectin) and lymphatic filariasis (ivermectin + albendazole) has been underway in some co-endemic areas [111]. APOC has now closed and a new programme has been established called the Expanded Special Project for Elimination of Neglected Tropical Diseases (ESPEN). This new program has different funding and governance and aims to co-implement control activities of onchocerciasis alongside other neglected tropical diseases and WHO currently recommends the use of preventive chemotherapy (PC) for lymphatic filariasis, onchocerciasis, schistosomiasis, soil-transmitted helminthiasis (hookworm, ascariasis and trichuriasis) and trachoma.

10. Newer Treatments

Alternative (or complementary) strategies (ATSs) are needed in some African settings in order to achieve elimination of onchocerciasis by 2025. Examples of ATSs include additional vector control [112,113] biannual or pluriannual CDTi, community-directed treatment with combinations of antihelminthics or new drugs and 'test and treat' strategies. As itching can reappear several months after an annual dose of ivermectin there should be more advocacy for bi-annual ivermectin distribution, but this is logistically difficult in remote areas.

10.1. Anti-Wolbachia Treatments

In loiasis co-endemic areas, treatment with ivermectin carries the risk of serious and sometimes fatal reactions due to the associated rapid killing of *L. loa mf*. As *L. loa* does not contain *Wolbachia*, anti-*Wolbachia* antibiotics such as doxycycline can be safely used to treat onchocerciasis in co-endemic areas. Antibiotics that are already registered for human use are undergoing evaluation for anti-*Wolbachia* activity to try to identify drugs that could have shorter treatment regimes, than the current six-week course of doxycycline. High-dose rifampicin has had promising results in animal studies [114]. A Cochrane review performed in 2015 [115] identified three randomized controlled trials that compared the effectiveness of doxyciline plus ivermectin versus ivermectin alone. The authors concluded that there was only limited evidence of very low quality from two of the studies that a six-week course of doxyciline followed by ivermectin may result in more frequent macrofilaricidal and microfilaricidal acitivity and sterilization of female adult worms compared with ivermectin alone. Only one study measured clinical outcomes, which were visual outcomes at six months but the results were graded as very low quality and hence the vision-related outcomes were uncertain. Similar RCTs assessing skin-related outcomes have not been reported to date.

In loiasis co-endemic areas, community-directed delivery of a six-week course of doxycycline proved feasible and doxycycline was a safe and effective macrofilaricidal agent [116]. A meta-analytical model using field trial data estimated that the efficacy of doxycycline (the maximum proportional reduction of adult female *O. volvulus* worms positive for *Wolbachia*) was 91–94%, irrespective of a variety of treatment regimes of four, five or six weeks. The life span of adult worms was reduced by 70–80%, from approximately 10 years to 2–3 years [117]. A pilot trial in Ghana confirmed that a four-week course of doxycycline was sufficient for *Wolbachia* depletion and that minocycline 200 mg/day for three weeks was more potent than a three-week course of doxycycline [118]. An Anti-*Wolbachia* Consortium (A-WOL) has been established to look for new drugs with macrofilaricidal activity by targeting *Wolbachia* and the capacity of this screening program has been significantly enhanced via the development of a high-throughput assay [119].

10.2. Moxidectin

Moxidectin is a more effective microfilaridial agent than ivermectin and 12 months after moxidectin treatment, dermal mf were still lower or comparable to the nadir seen one month after ivermectin treatment [120]. A double-blind, parallel group superiority trial in four study sites in Ghana, Liberia and DRC confirmed that at 12 months post-dosing, the skin microfilarial density was lower in the moxidectin group than the ivermectin group (adjusted geometric mean difference 3.9 [3.2–4.9], $p < 0.0001$) [121]. EpiOncho modelling suggests that the number of years to reach thresholds for onchoerciasis elimination with annual moxidectin is similar to that with biannual CDTi [122]. A not-for-profit organization, Medicines Development for Global Health, is planning for affordable access to moxidectin for countries to incorporate moxidectin into their control and elimination programmes. Moxidectin now has FDA approval for onchocerciasis in adults but further research is needed to clarify where and when it will be possible to use it on a community-wide basis.

10.3. Ivermectin-Diethylcarbamazine-Albendazole

Triple therapy is being considered, but a lot more work is still needed to identify whether or not it has a role in treatment of onchocerciasis. A strategy is needed to ensure that *O. volvulus*-infected patients with high microfilarial loads are excluded from treatment, as diethylcarbamazine can cause general and irreversible ocular side effects [123].

10.4. Emodepside

Emodepside, which has known efficacy in animal models, paralyses adult filarial worms by facilitating a nematode Ca^{2+}-activated K^+ channel called SLO-1 in a sustained way, but does not affect human channels [124]. It is therefore hoped it may prove to be a useful macrofilaricidal agent for human use and is undergoing a phase 1 study to determine its safety, tolerability, and pharmacokinetics in healthy volunteers by the Drugs for Neglected Diseases Initiative (DNDi) (NCT02661178).

10.5. Genome Assemblies

Recently genome assemblies for *O. volvulus* and *Wolbachia* have been generated, allowing identification of enzymes that are likely to be essential for *O. volvulus* survival. This will hopefully provide a rich resource of potential new targets for drug development [125].

10.6. Vaccine

In 2015 an international consortium launched a new global initiative, known as TOVA ('The Onchocerciasis Vaccine for Africa'), with the goal of evaluating and pursuing vaccine development as a complementary control tool to eliminate onchocerciasis. Two recombinant proteins, *Ov*-103 and *Ov*-RAL-2, have been identified that individually or in combination induced significant protection against infection in animal models [126], and it is hoped that initial vaccine candidates could be in human safety trials by 2022 [127].

11. Concept of Skin NTDs and Integrated Control and Management of Neglected Tropical Skin Diseases

In addition to onchocerciasis, several other neglected tropical diseases (NTDs) have cutaneous manifestations and a new proposal is for an integrated strategy for the management of skin NTDs using preventive chemotherapy, or intensified disease management, or both, depending on the overall health needs of an area [128]. Such an approach will require (i) assessment of which diseases are present within an area (ii) roll-out of training packages to help workers screen for several conditions and (iii) care pathways for diagnosis and treatment in the local community and onward referral to health centers and district hospitals as needed, with appropriate strengthening of health infrastructure. Targeting skin NTDs should also help treat other common skin conditions and hopefully lead to wider public health benefits. WHO has recently produced a training guide to help front-line health workers recognize NTDs through examination of the skin [129], and the key pointers identified for onchodermatitis were (i) itchy skin, (ii) subcutaneous lumps (large lumps suggest onchocercal nodules; small itchy lumps suggest acute or chronic onchodermatitis) and (iii) patches (raised dark scaly patches on one leg suggests lichenified onchodermatitis, and non-itchy speckled loss of pigment on shins suggests onchocercal depigmentation).

Hofstraat and Brakel reviewed social stigma towards NTDs in general and proposed that further research was needed to study the efficacy of joint approaches to reduce stigmatization in society and that lessons learnt from leprosy should be incorporated [130].

12. Mathematical Modelling of Onchodermatitis

The mathematical model ONCHOSIM has been extended to include predicted trends for various forms of onchocercal skin disease up to 2025 [131]. The prevalence of reversible skin disease (e.g., troublesome itching, acute and chronic papular and lichenified onchodermatitis) was shown to decline rapidly with waning infection prevalence, with the rate of the decline depending on achieved therapeutic coverage. In contrast, irreversible manifestations such as cutaneous atrophy, depigmentation and hanging groin declined much more slowly. ONCHOSIM has its drawbacks as it was not set up initially for chemotherapy. Other elimination simulation models exist, including SIMONA which has been used in the Americas.

13. Conclusions

In 2016, more than 131 million people were treated with ivermectin for onchocerciasis and 85.9% of all districts globally had achieved effective coverage of $\geq$65% [132]. As a result of MDA with ivermectin, onchocerciasis has been significantly reduced in many countries, transmission has been eliminated in four Central and South American countries and in foci in several African countries, and onchodermatitis is no longer seen in children in many formerly endemic foci. Continued vigilance is needed to check for the development of resistance to ivermectin, a single-dose macrofilaricidal agent remains the 'Holy Grail' for drug developers, and alternative strategies need to be implemented in some areas. Much concerted effort needs to continue to hope to achieve WHO's target for elimination of onchocerciasis by 2025. Even after transmission has been interrupted, certain individuals will have irreversible deforming hanging groin, visible depigmentation and onchocerciasis-associated epilepsy but hopefully the incessant and debilitating pruritus due to onchocerciasis will become a thing of the past.

Funding: This research received no external funding.

Conflicts of Interest: The author declares no conflict of interest.

References

1. World Health Organization. *Accelerating work to overcome the global impact of neglected tropical diseases: A roadmap for implementation*; World Health Organization: Geneva, Switzerland, 2012; pp. 1–42.
2. World Health Organization. Elimination of onchocerciasis in the WHO region of the Americas: Ecuador's progress towards verification of elimination. *Wkly. Epid. Rec.* **2014**, *89*, 401–405.
3. Mahdy, M.A.K.; Abdul-Ghani, R.; Abdulrahman, T.A.A.; Al-Eryani, S.M.A.; Al-Mekhlafi, A.M.; Alhaidari, S.A.A.; Azazy, A.A. Onchocerca volvulus infection in Tihama region-west of Yemen: Continuing transmission in ivermectin-targeted endemic foci and unveiled endemicity in districts with previously unknown status. *PLoS Negl. Trop.Dis.* **2018**, *12*, 1–16. [CrossRef] [PubMed]
4. Murdoch, M.E. Onchodermatitis. *Curr. Opin. Infect. Dis.* **2010**, *23*, 124–131. [CrossRef] [PubMed]
5. World Health Organization. Progress report on the elimination of human onchocerciasis, 2016–2017. *Wkly. Epidemiol. Rec.* **2017**, *92*, 681–694.
6. Vos, T.; Barber, R.M.; Bell, B.; Bertozzi-Villa, A.; Biryukov, S.; Bolliger, I.; Charlson, F.; Davis, A.; Degenhardt, L.; Dicker, D.; et al. Global, regional, and national incidence, prevalence, and years lived with disability for 301 acute and chronic diseases and injuries in 188 countries, 1990–2013: A systemic analysis for the Global Burden of Disease Study 2013. *Lancet* **2015**, *386*, 743–800. [CrossRef]
7. Herricks, J.R.; Hotez, P.J.; Wanga, V.; Coffeng, L.E.; Haagsma, J.A.; Basáñez, M.G.; Buckle, G.; Budke, C.M.; Carabin, H.; Fèvre, E.M.; et al. The global burden of disease study 2013: What does it mean for the NTDs? *PLoS Negl. Trop. Dis.* **2017**, *11*, e0005424. [CrossRef] [PubMed]
8. Vos, T.; Allen, C.; Arora, M.; Barber, R.M.; Bhutta, Z.A.; Brown, A.; Carter, A.; Casey, D.C.; Charlson, F.J.; Chen, A.Z.; et al. Global, regional, and national incidence, prevalence, and years lived with disability for 310 diseases and injuries, 1990–2015: A systematic analysis for the Global Burden of Disease Study 2015. *Lancet* **2016**, *388*, 1545–1602. [CrossRef]
9. Vos, T.; Abajobir, A.A.; Abbafati, C.; Abbas, K.M.; Abate, K.H.; Abd-Allah, F.; Abdulle, A.M.; Abebo, T.A.; Abera, S.F.; Aboyans, V.; et al. Global, regional, and national incidence, prevalence, and years lived with disability for 328 diseases and injuries for 195 countries, 1990–2016: A systematic analysis for the Global Burden of Disease Study 2016. *Lancet* **2017**, *390*, 1211–1259. [CrossRef]

10. Stokstad, E.; Vogel, G. Neglected tropical diseases get the limelight in Stockholm. *Science* **2015**, *350*, 144–145. [CrossRef] [PubMed]

11. Fobi, G.; Yameogo, L.; Noma, M.; Aholou, Y.; Koroma, J.B.; Zouré, H.M.; Ukety, T.; Lusamba-Dikassa, P.S.; Mwikisa, C.; Boakye, D.A.; et al. Managing the fight against onchocerciasis in Africa: APOC Experience. *PLoS Negl. Trop. Dis.* **2015**, *9*, e0003542. [CrossRef] [PubMed]

12. Hopkins, A.D. From 'control to elimination': A strategic change to win the end game. *Int. Health* **2015**, *7*, 304–305. [CrossRef] [PubMed]

13. Hopkins, A.D. Neglected tropical diseases in Africa: A new paradigm. *Int. Health* **2016**, *8*, i28–i33. [CrossRef] [PubMed]

14. Dunn, C.; Callahan, K.; Katabarwa, M.; Richards, F.; Hopkins, D.; Withers, P.C.; Buyon, L.E.; McFarland, D. The contributions of onchocerciasis control and elimination programs toward the achievement of the Millennium Development Goals. *PLoS Negl. Trop. Dis.* **2015**, *9*, e0003703. [CrossRef] [PubMed]

15. Hay, R.J.; Mackenzie, C.D.; Guderian, R.; Noble, W.C.; Proano, J.R.; Williams, J.F. Onchodermatitis-correlation between skin disease and parasitic load in an endemic focus in Ecuador. *Br. J. Dermatol.* **1989**, *121*, 187–198. [CrossRef] [PubMed]

16. Murdoch, M.E.; Hay, R.J.; Mackenzie, C.D.; Williams, J.F.; Ghalib, H.W.; Cousens, S.; Abiose, A.; Jones, B.R. A clinical classification and grading system of the cutaneous changes in onchocerciasis. *Br. J. Dermatol.* **1993**, *129*, 260–269. [CrossRef] [PubMed]

17. Murdoch, M.E.; Murdoch, I.E.; Evans, J.; Yahaya, H.; Njepuome, N.; Cousens, S.; Jones, B.R.; Abiose, A. Pre-control relationship of onchocercal skin disease with onchocercal infection in Guinea Savanna, Northern Nigeria. *PLoS Negl. Trop. Dis.* **2017**, *11*, e0005489. [CrossRef] [PubMed]

18. Murdoch, M.E.; Asuzu, M.C.; Hagan, M.; Makunde, W.H.; Ngoumou, P.; Ogbuagu, K.F.; Okello, D.; Ozoh, G.; Remme, J. Onchocerciasis: The clinical and epidemiological burden of skin disease in Africa. *Ann. Trop. Med. Parasitol.* **2002**, *96*, 283–296. [CrossRef] [PubMed]

19. Al-Kubati, A.S.; Mackenzie, C.D.; Boakye, D.; Al-Qubati, Y.; Al-Samie, A.R.; Awad, I.E.; Thylefors, B.; Hopkins, A. Onchocerciasis in Yemen: Moving forward towards an elimination program. *Int. Health* **2018**, *10*, i89–i96. [CrossRef] [PubMed]

20. Olusegun, A.F.; Ehis, O.C. Hyperendemicity of onchocerciasis in Ovia Northeast Local Government Area, Edo State, Nigeria. *Malays. J. Med. Sci.* **2010**, *17*, 20–24.

21. Dori, G.U.; Belay, T.; Belete, H.; Panicker, K.N.; Hailu, A. Parasitological and clinico-epidemiological features of onchocerciasis in West Wellega, Ethiopia. *J. Parasit. Dis.* **2012**, *36*, 10–18. [CrossRef] [PubMed]

22. Eyo, J.E.; Onyishi, G.C.; Ugokwe, C.U. Rapid epidemiological assessment of onchocerciasis in a tropical semi-urban community, Enugu State, Nigeria. *Iran. J. Parasitol.* **2013**, *8*, 145–151. [PubMed]

23. Coffeng, L.E.; Fobi, G.; Ozoh, G.; Bissek, A.C.; Nlatté, B.O.; Enyong, P.; Olinga, J.M.; Zouré, H.G.M.; Habbema, J.D.F.; Stolk, W.A.; et al. Concurrence of dermatological and ophthalmological morbidity in onchocerciasis. *Trans. R. Soc. Trop. Med. Hyg.* **2012**, *106*, 243–251. [CrossRef] [PubMed]

24. Murdoch, M.E.; Payton, A.; Abiose, A.; Thomson, W.; Panicker, V.K.; Dyer, P.A.; Jones, B.R.; Maizels, R.M.; Oilier, W.E.R. HLA-DQ alleles associate with cutaneous features of onchocerciasis. *Hum. Immunol.* **1997**, *55*, 46–52. [CrossRef]

25. Norman, F.F.; de Ayala, A.P.; Pérez-Molina, J.A.; Monge-Maillo, B.; Zamarrón, P.; López-Vélez, R. Neglected tropical diseases outside the tropics. *PLoS Negl. Trop. Dis.* **2010**, *4*, e762. [CrossRef] [PubMed]

26. Antinori, S.; Parravicini, C.; Galimberti, L.; Tosoni, A.; Giunta, P.; Galli, M.; Corbellino, M.; Ridolfo, A.L. Is imported onchocerciasis a truly rare entity? Case report and review of the literature. *Travel Med. Infect. Dis.* **2017**, *16*, 11–17. [CrossRef] [PubMed]

27. Develoux, M.; Hennequin, C.; Le Loup, G.; Paris, L.; Magne, D.; Belkadi, G.; Pialoux, G. Imported filariasis in Europe: A series of 31 cases from Metropolitan France. *Eur. J. Intern. Med.* **2017**, *37*, e37–e39. [CrossRef] [PubMed]

28. Zammarchi, L.; Vellere, I.; Stella, L.; Bartalesi, F.; Strohmeyer, M.; Bartoloni, A. Spectrum and burden of neglected tropical diseases observed in an infectious and tropical diseases unit in Florence, Italy (2000–2015). *Intern. Emerg. Med.* **2017**, *12*, 467–477. [CrossRef] [PubMed]

29. Baum, S.; Greenberger, S.; Pavlotsky, F.; Solomon, M.; Enk, C.D.; Schwartz, E.; Barzilai, A. Late-onset onchocercal skin disease among Ethiopian immigrants. *Br. J. Dermatol.* **2014**, *171*, 1078–1083. [CrossRef] [PubMed]

30. Puente, S.; Ramirez-Olivencia, G.; Lago, M.; Subirats, M.; Perez-Blazquez, E.; Bru, F.; Garate, T.; Vicente, B.; Belhassen-Garcia, M.; Muro, A. Dermatological manifestations in onchocerciasis: A retrospective study of 400 imported cases. *Enferm. Infect. Microbiol. Clin.* **2017**. [CrossRef] [PubMed]

31. Lenk, E.J.; Redekop, W.K.; Luyendijk, M.; Rijnsburger, A.J.; Severens, J.L. Productivity loss related to neglected tropical diseases eligible for preventive chemotherapy: A systematic literature review. *PLoS Negl. Trop. Dis.* **2016**, *10*, e0004397. [CrossRef] [PubMed]

32. Tamarozzi, F.; Halliday, A.; Gentil, K.; Hoerauf, A.; Pearlman, E.; Taylor, M.J. Onchocerciasis: The role of *Wolbachia* bacterial endosymbionts in parasite biology, disease pathogenesis, and treatment. *Clin. Microbiol. Rev.* **2011**, *24*, 459–469. [CrossRef] [PubMed]

33. Adjobimey, T.; Hoerauf, A. Induction of immunoglobulin G4 in human filariasis: An indicator of immunoregulation. *Ann. Trop. Med. Parasitol.* **2010**, *104*, 455–464. [CrossRef] [PubMed]

34. Kwarteng, A.; Ahuno, S.T.; Akoto, F.O. Killing filarial nematode parasites: Role of treatment options and host immune response. *Infect. Dis. Poverty* **2016**, *5*, 86. [CrossRef] [PubMed]

35. Hansen, R.D.E.; Trees, A.J.; Bah, G.S.; Hetzel, U.; Martin, C.; Bain, O.; Tanya, V.N.; Makepeace, B.L. A worm's best friend: Recruitment of neutrophils by *Wolbachia* confounds eosinophil degranulation against the filarial nematode *Onchocerca ochengi*. *Proc. R. Soc. B Biol. Sci.* **2011**, *278*, 2293–2302. [CrossRef] [PubMed]

36. Tamarozzi, F.; Wright, H.L.; Johnston, K.L.; Edwards, S.W.; Turner, J.D.; Taylor, M.J. Human filarial *Wolbachia* lipopeptide directly activates human neutrophils in vitro. *Parasite Immunol.* **2014**, *36*, 494–502. [CrossRef] [PubMed]

37. Tamarozzi, F.; Turner, J.D.; Pionnier, N.; Midgley, A.; Guimaraes, A.F.; Johnston, K.L.; Edwards, S.W.; Taylor, M.J. *Wolbachia* endosymbionts induce neutrophil extracellular trap formation in human onchocerciasis. *Sci. Rep.* **2016**, *6*, 35559. [CrossRef] [PubMed]

38. Korten, S.; Hoerauf, A.; Kaifi, J.T.; Büttner, D.W. Low levels of transforming growth factor-beta (TGF-beta) and reduced suppression of Th2-mediated inflammation in hyperreactive human onchocerciasis. *Parasitology* **2011**, *138*, 35–45. [CrossRef] [PubMed]

39. Katawa, G.; Layland, L.E.; Debrah, A.Y.; von Horn, C.; Batsa, L.; Kwarteng, A.; Arriens, S.; Taylor, D.W.; Specht, S.; Hoerauf, A.; et al. Hyperreactive onchocerciasis is characterized by a combination of Th17-Th2 immune responses and reduced regulatory T cells. *PLoS Negl. Trop. Dis.* **2015**, *9*, e3414. [CrossRef] [PubMed]

40. Ajonina-Ekoti, I.; Ndjonka, D.; Tanyi, M.K.; Wilbertz, M.; Younis, A.E.; Boursou, D.; Kurosinski, M.A.; Eberle, R.; Lüersen, K.; Perbandt, M.; et al. Functional characterization and immune recognition of the extracellular superoxide dismutase from the human pathogenic parasite *Onchocerca volvulus* (OvEC-SOD). *Acta Trop.* **2012**, *124*, 15–26. [CrossRef] [PubMed]

41. Lechner, C.J.; Gantin, R.G.; Seeger, T.; Sarnecka, A.; Portillo, J.; Schulz-Key, H.; Karabou, P.K.; Helling-Giese, G.; Heuschkel, C.; Banla, M.; et al. Chemokines and cytokines in patients with an occult *Onchocerca volvulus* infection. *Microbes Infect.* **2012**, *14*, 438–446. [CrossRef] [PubMed]

42. Mackenzie, C.D.; Huntington, M.K.; Wanji, S.; Lovato, R.V.; Eversole, R.R.; Geary, T.G. The association of adult *Onchocerca volvulus* with lymphatic vessels. *J. Parasitol.* **2010**, *96*, 219–221. [CrossRef] [PubMed]

43. Attout, T.; Hoerauf, A.; Dénécé, G.; Debrah, A.Y.; Marfo-Debrekyei, Y.; Boussinesq, M.; Wanji, S.; Martinez, V.; Mand, S.; Adjei, O.; et al. Lymphatic vascularisation and involvement of Lyve-1+ macrophages in the human *Onchocerca* nodule. *PLoS ONE* **2009**, *4*, e0008234. [CrossRef] [PubMed]

44. de Angelis, F.; Garzoli, A.; Battistini, A.; Iorio, A.; de Stefano, G.F. Genetic response to an environmental pathogenic agent: HLA-DQ and onchocerciasis in northwestern Ecuador. *Tissue Antigens* **2011**, *79*, 123–129. [CrossRef] [PubMed]

45. Unnasch, T.R.; Golden, A.; Cama, V.; Cantey, P.T. Diagnostics for onchocerciasis in the era of elimination. *Int. Health* **2018**, *10*, i20–i26. [CrossRef] [PubMed]

46. Thiele, E.A.; Cama, V.A.; Lakwo, T.; Mekasha, S.; Abanyie, F.; Sleshi, M.; Kebede, A.; Cantey, P.T. Detection of onchocerca volvulus in skin snips by microscopy and real-time polymerase chain reaction: Implications for monitoring and evaluation activities. *Am. J. Trop. Med. Hyg.* **2016**, *94*, 906–911. [CrossRef] [PubMed]

47. Prince-Guerra, J.L.; Cama, V.A.; Wilson, N.; Thiele, E.A.; Likwela, J.; Ndakala, N.; wa Muzinga, J.M.; Ayebazibwe, N.; Ndjakani, Y.D.; Pitchouna, N.A.; et al. Comparison of PCR methods for *Onchocerca volvulus* detection in skin snip biopsies from the Tshopo Province, Democratic Republic of the Congo. *Am. J. Trop. Med. Hyg.* **2018**, *98*, 1427–1434. [CrossRef] [PubMed]

48. Mekonnen, S.A.; Beissner, M.; Saar, M.; Ali, S.; Zeynudin, A.; Tesfaye, K.; Adbaru, M.G.; Battke, F.; Poppert, S.; Hoelscher, M.; et al. O-5S quantitative real-time PCR: A new diagnostic tool for laboratory confirmation of human onchocerciasis. *Parasites Vectors* **2017**, *10*, 451. [CrossRef] [PubMed]

49. World Health Organization. *Guidelines for Stopping Mass Drug Administration and Verifying Elimination of Human Onchocerciasis: Criteria and Procedures*; WHO Press: Geneva, Switzerland, 2016.

50. Gass, K.M. Rethinking the serological threshold for onchocerciasis elimination. *PLoS Negl. Trop. Dis.* **2018**, *12*, e0006249. [CrossRef] [PubMed]

51. Steel, C.; Golden, A.; Stevens, E.; Yokobe, L.; Domingo, G.J.; De los Santos, T.; Nutman, T.B. Rapid point-of-contact tool for mapping and integrated surveillance of *Wuchereria bancrofti* and *Onchocerca volvulus* infection. *Clin. Vaccine Immunol.* **2015**, *22*, 896–901. [CrossRef] [PubMed]

52. Dieye, Y.; Storey, H.L.; Barrett, K.L.; Gerth-Guyette, E.; Di Giorgio, L.; Golden, A.; Faulx, D.; Kalnoky, M.; Ndiaye, M.K.N.; Sy, N.; et al. Feasibility of utilizing the SD BIOLINE Onchocerciasis IgG4 rapid test in onchocerciasis surveillance in Senegal. *PLoS Negl. Trop. Dis.* **2017**, *11*, e0005884. [CrossRef] [PubMed]

53. Rodríguez-Pérez, M.A.; Adeleke, M.A.; Burkett-Cadena, N.D.; Garza-Hernández, J.A.; Reyes-Villanueva, F.; Cupp, E.W.; Toé, L.; Salinas-Carmona, M.C.; Rodríguez-Ramírez, A.D.; Katholi, C.R.; et al. Development of a novel trap for the collection of blackflies of the *Simulium ochraceum* complex. *PLoS ONE* **2013**, *8*, e76814. [CrossRef] [PubMed]

54. Rodríguez-Pérez, M.A.; Adeleke, M.A.; Rodríguez-Luna, I.C.; Cupp, E.W.; Unnasch, T.R. Evaluation of a community-based trapping program to collect *Simulium ochraceum* sensu lato for verification of onchocerciasis elimination. *PLoS Negl. Trop. Dis.* **2014**, *8*, e3249. [CrossRef] [PubMed]

55. Toé, L.D.; Koala, L.; Burkett-Cadena, N.D.; Traoré, B.M.; Sanfo, M.; Kambiré, S.R.; Cupp, E.W.; Traoré, S.; Yameogo, L.; Boakye, D.; et al. Optimization of the Esperanza window trap for the collection of the African onchocerciasis vector *Simulium damnosum* sensu lato. *Acta Trop.* **2014**, *137*, 39–43. [CrossRef] [PubMed]

56. Denery, J.R.; Nunes, A.A.K.; Hixon, M.S.; Dickerson, T.J.; Janda, K.D. Metabolomics-based discovery of diagnostic biomarkers for onchocerciasis. *PLoS Negl. Trop. Dis.* **2010**, *4*, e834. [CrossRef] [PubMed]

57. Globisch, D.; Moreno, A.Y.; Hixon, M.S.; Nunes, A.A.K.; Denery, J.R.; Specht, S.; Hoerauf, A.; Janda, K.D. *Onchocerca volvulus*-neurotransmitter tyramine is a biomarker for river blindness. *Proc. Natl. Acad. Sci. USA* **2013**, *110*, 4218–4223. [CrossRef] [PubMed]

58. Tritten, L.; Burkman, E.; Moorhead, A.; Satti, M.; Geary, J.; Mackenzie, C.; Geary, T. Detection of circulating parasite-derived microRNAs in filarial infections. *PLoS Negl. Trop. Dis.* **2014**, *8*, e2971. [CrossRef] [PubMed]

59. Quintana, J.F.; Makepeace, B.L.; Babayan, S.A.; Ivens, A.; Pfarr, K.M.; Blaxter, M.; Debrah, A.; Wanji, S.; Ngangyung, H.F.; Bah, G.S.; et al. Extracellular *Onchocerca*-derived small RNAs in host nodules and blood. *Parasites Vectors* **2015**, *8*, 1–11. [CrossRef] [PubMed]

60. Lagatie, O.; Batsa-Debrah, L.; Debrah, A.; Stuyver, L.J. Plasma-derived parasitic microRNAs have insufficient concentrations to be used as diagnostic biomarker for detection of *Onchocerca volvulus* infection or treatment monitoring using LNA-based RT-qPCR. *Parasitol. Res.* **2017**, *116*, 1013–1022. [CrossRef] [PubMed]

61. Brieger, W.R.; Awedoba, A.K.; Eneanya, C.I.; Hagan, M.; Ogbuagu, K.F.; Okello, D.O.; Ososanya, O.O.; Ovuga, E.B.L.; Noma, M.; Kale, O.O.; et al. The effects of ivermectin on onchocercal skin disease and severe itching: Results of a multicentre trial. *Trop. Med. Int. Heal.* **1998**, *3*, 951–961. [CrossRef]

62. Banic, D.M.; Calvão-Brito, R.H.S.; Marchon-Silva, V.; Schuertez, J.C.; de Lima Pinheiro, L.R.; da Costa-Alves, M.; Têva, A.; Maia-Herzog, M. Impact of 3 years ivermectin treatment on onchocerciasis in Yanomami communities in the Brazilian Amazon. *Acta Trop.* **2009**, *112*, 125–130. [CrossRef] [PubMed]

63. Ozoh, G.A.; Murdoch, M.E.; Bissek, A.C.; Hagan, M.; Ogbuagu, K.; Shamad, M.; Braide, E.I.; Boussinesq, M.; Noma, M.M.; Murdoch, I.E.; et al. The African Programme for Onchocerciasis Control: Impact on onchocercal skin disease. *Trop. Med. Int. Heal.* **2011**, *16*, 875–883. [CrossRef] [PubMed]

64. Samuel, A.; Belay, T.; Yehalaw, D.; Taha, M.; Zemene, E.; Zeynudin, A. Impact of six years community directed treatment with ivermectin in the control of onchocerciasis, western Ethiopia. *PLoS ONE* **2016**, *11*, e0141029. [CrossRef] [PubMed]

65. Mbanefo, E.C.; Eneanya, C.I.; Nwaorgu, O.C.; Otiji, M.O.; Oguoma, V.M.; Ogolo, B.A. Onchocerciasis in Anambra State, Southeast Nigeria: Endemicity and clinical manifestations. *Postgrad. Med. J.* **2010**, *86*, 578–583. [CrossRef] [PubMed]

66. Kamga, G.R.; Dissak-Delon, F.N.; Nana-Djeunga, H.C.; Biholong, B.D.; Ghogomu, S.M.; Souopgui, J.; Kamgno, J.; Robert, A. Important progress towards elimination of onchocerciasis in the West Region of Cameroon. *Parasites Vectors* **2017**, *10*, 373. [CrossRef] [PubMed]
67. Moya, L.; Herrador, Z.; Ta-Tang, T.H.; Rubio, J.M.; Perteguer, M.J.; Hernandez-González, A.; García, B.; Nguema, R.; Nguema, J.; Ncogo, P.; et al. Evidence for suppression of onchocerciasis transmission in Bioko Island, Equatorial Guinea. *PLoS Negl. Trop. Dis.* **2016**, *10*, e0004829. [CrossRef] [PubMed]
68. Walker, M.; Pion, S.D.S.; Fang, H.; Gardon, J.; Kamgno, J.; Basáñez, M.G.; Boussinesq, M. Macrofilaricidal efficacy of repeated doses of ivermectin for the treatment of river blindness. *Clin. Infect. Dis.* **2017**, *65*, 2026–2034. [CrossRef] [PubMed]
69. Kudzi, W.; Dodoo, A.N.O.; Mills, J.J. Genetic polymorphisms in MDR1, CYP3A4 and CYP3A5 genes in a Ghanaian population: A plausible explanation for altered metabolism of ivermectin in humans? *BMC Med. Genet.* **2010**, *11*, 111. [CrossRef] [PubMed]
70. Vlassoff, C.; Weiss, M.; Ovuga, E.B.L.; Eneanya, C.; Nwel, P.T.; Babalola, S.S.; Awedoba, A.K.; Theophilus, B.; Cofie, P.; Shetabi, P. Gender and the stigma of onchocercal skin disease in Africa. *Soc. Sci. Med.* **2000**, *50*, 1353–1368. [CrossRef]
71. Mbanefo, E.C.; Eneanya, C.I.; Nwaorgu, O.C.; Oguoma, V.M.; Otiji, M.O.; Ogolo, B.A. Onchocerciasis in Anambra State, Southeast Nigeria: Clinical and psychological aspects and sustainability of community directed treatment with ivermectin (CDTI). *Postgrad. Med. J.* **2010**, *86*, 573–577. [CrossRef] [PubMed]
72. Abanobi, O.; Chukwuocha, U.; Onwuliri, C.; Opara, K. Primary motives for demand of ivermectin drug in mass distribution programmes to control onchocerciasis. *N. Am. J. Med. Sci.* **2011**, *3*, 89–94. [CrossRef] [PubMed]
73. Okeibunor, J.C.; Amuyunzu-Nyamongo, M.; Onyeneho, N.G.; Tchounkeu, Y.F.L.; Manianga, C.; Kabali, A.T.; Leak, S. Where would I be without ivermectin? Capturing the benefits of community-directed treatment with ivermectin in Africa. *Trop. Med. Int. Heal.* **2011**, *16*, 608–621. [CrossRef] [PubMed]
74. Tchounkeu, Y.F.L.; Onyeneho, N.G.; Wanji, S.; Kabali, A.T.; Manianga, C.; Amazigo, U.V.; Amuyunzu-Nyamongo, M. Changes in stigma and discrimination of onchocerciasis in Africa. *Trans. R. Soc. Trop. Med. Hyg.* **2012**, *106*, 340–347. [CrossRef] [PubMed]
75. Amuyunzu-Nyamongo, M.; Tchounkeu, Y.F.L.; Oyugi, R.A.; Kabali, A.T.; Okeibunor, J.C.; Manianga, C.; Amazigo, U.V. Drawing and interpreting data: Children's impressions of onchocerciasis and community-directed treatment with ivermectin (CDTI) in four onchocerciasis endemic countries in Africa. *Int. J. Qual. Stud. Health Well-Being* **2011**, *6*, 5918. [CrossRef] [PubMed]
76. Nicholls, R.S.; Duque, S.; Olaya, L.A.; López, M.C.; Sánchez, S.B.; Morales, A.L.; Palma, G.I. Elimination of onchocerciasis from Colombia: First proof of concept of river blindness elimination in the world. *Parasites Vectors* **2018**, *11*, 237. [CrossRef] [PubMed]
77. World Health Organization. Progress towards eliminating onchocerciasis in the WHO Region of the Americas: verification of elimination of transmission in Guatemala. *Wkly. Epid. Rec.* **2016**, *91*, 501–505.
78. Guevara, Á.; Lovato, R.; Proaño, R.; Rodriguez-Perez, M.A.; Unnasch, T.; Cooper, P.J.; Guderian, R.H. Elimination of onchocerciasis in Ecuador: Findings of post-treatment surveillance. *Parasites Vectors* **2018**, *11*, 265. [CrossRef] [PubMed]
79. Diawara, L.; Traore, M.O.; Badji, A.; Bissan, Y.; Doumbia, K.; Goita, S.F.; Konate, L.; Mounkoro, K.; Sarr, M.D.; Seck, A.F.; et al. Feasibility of onchocerciasis elimination with ivermectin treatment in endemic foci in Africa: First evidence from studies in Mali and Senegal. *PLoS Negl. Trop. Dis.* **2009**, *3*, e497. [CrossRef] [PubMed]
80. Traore, M.O.; Sarr, M.D.; Badji, A.; Bissan, Y.; Diawara, L.; Doumbia, K.; Goita, S.F.; Konate, L.; Mounkoro, K.; Seck, A.F.; et al. Proof-of-principle of onchocerciasis elimination with ivermectin treatment in endemic foci in Africa: Final results of a study in Mali and Senegal. *PLoS Negl. Trop. Dis.* **2012**, *6*, e1825. [CrossRef] [PubMed]
81. Tekle, A.H.; Elhassan, E.; Isiyaku, S.; Amazigo, U.V.; Bush, S.; Noma, M.; Cousens, S.; Abiose, A.; Remme, J.H. Impact of long-term treatment of onchocerciasis with ivermectin in Kaduna State, Nigeria: First evidence of the potential for elimination in the operational area of the African Programme for Onchocerciasis Control. *Parasites Vectors* **2012**, *5*, 28. [CrossRef] [PubMed]
82. Traoré, S.; Wilson, M.D.; Sima, A.; Barro, T.; Diallo, A.; Aké, A.; Coulibaly, S.; Cheke, R.A.; Meyer, R.R.F.; Mas, J.; et al. The elimination of the onchocerciasis vector from the island of Bioko as a result of larviciding by the WHO African Programme for Onchocerciasis Control. *Acta Trop.* **2009**, *111*, 211–218. [CrossRef] [PubMed]

83. Garms, R.; Lakwo, T.L.; Ndyomugyenyi, R.; Kipp, W.; Rubaale, T.; Tukesiga, E.; Katamanywa, J.; Post, R.J.; Amazigo, U.V. The elimination of the vector *Simulium neavei* from the Itwara onchocerciasis focus in Uganda by ground larviciding. *Acta Trop.* **2009**, *111*, 203–210. [CrossRef] [PubMed]

84. Herrador, Z.; Garcia, B.; Ncogo, P.; Perteguer, M.J.; Rubio, J.M.; Rivas, E.; Cimas, M.; Ordoñez, G.; de Pablos, S.; Hernández-González, A.; et al. Interruption of onchocerciasis transmission in Bioko Island: Accelerating the movement from control to elimination in Equatorial Guinea. *PLoS Negl. Trop. Dis.* **2018**, *12*, e0006471. [CrossRef] [PubMed]

85. Zarroug, I.M.A.; Hashim, K.; ElMubark, W.A.; Shumo, Z.A.I.; Salih, K.A.M.; ElNojomi, N.A.A.; Awad, H.A.; Aziz, N.; Katabarwa, M.; Hassan, H.K.; et al. The first confirmed elimination of an onchocerciasis focus in Africa: Abu Hamed, Sudan. *Am. J. Trop. Med. Hyg.* **2016**, *95*, 1037–1040. [CrossRef] [PubMed]

86. Katabarwa, M.N.; Lakwo, T.; Habomugisha, P.; Unnasch, T.R.; Garms, R.; Hudson-Davis, L.; Byamukama, E.; Khainza, A.; Ngorok, J.; Tukahebwa, E.; et al. After 70 years of fighting an age-old scourge, onchocerciasis in Uganda, the end is in sight. *Int. Health* **2018**, *10*, i79–i88. [CrossRef] [PubMed]

87. Rebollo, M.P.; Zoure, H.; Ogoussan, K.; Sodahlon, Y.; Ottesen, E.A.; Cantey, P.T. Onchocerciasis: Shifting the target from control to elimination requires a new first-step-elimination mapping. *Int. Health* **2018**, *10*, i14–i19. [CrossRef] [PubMed]

88. World Health Organization. Progress report on the elimination of human onchocerciasis, 2015–2016. *Wkly. Epid. Rec.* **2016**, *43*, 505–514.

89. Makenga-Bof, J.C.; Maketa, V.; Bakajika, D.K.; Ntumba, F.; Mpunga, D.; Murdoch, M.E.; Hopkins, A.; Noma, M.M.; Zouré, H.; Tekle, A.H.; et al. Onchocerciasis control in the Democratic Republic of Congo (DRC): Challenges in a post-war environment. *Trop. Med. Int. Heal.* **2015**, *20*, 48–62. [CrossRef] [PubMed]

90. Koroma, J.B.; Sesay, S.; Conteh, A.; Koudou, B.; Paye, J.; Bah, M.; Sonnie, M.; Hodges, M.H.; Zhang, Y.; Bockarie, M.J. Impact of five annual rounds of mass drug administration with ivermectin on onchocerciasis in Sierra Leone. *Infect. Dis. Poverty* **2018**, *7*, 30. [CrossRef] [PubMed]

91. Kamgno, J.; Pion, S.D.; Chesnais, C.B.; Bakalar, M.H.; D'Ambrosio, M.V.; Mackenzie, C.D.; Nana-Djeunga, H.C.; Gounoue-Kamkumo, R.; Njitchouang, G.R.; Nwane, P.; et al. A test-and-not-treat strategy for onchocerciasis in *Loa loa* endemic areas. *N. Engl. J. Med.* **2017**, *377*, 2044–2052. [CrossRef] [PubMed]

92. Lakwo, T.; Ukety, T.; Bakajika, D.; Tukahebwa, E.; Awaca, P.; Amazigo, U. Cross-border collaboration in onchocerciasis elimination in Uganda: Progress, challenges and opportunities from 2008 to 2013. *Glob. Health* **2018**, *14*, 16. [CrossRef] [PubMed]

93. Gustavsen, K.; Sodahlon, Y.; Bush, S. Cross-border collaboration for neglected tropical disease efforts-Lessons learned from onchocerciasis control and elimination in the Mano River Union (West Africa). *Glob. Health* **2016**, *12*, 44. [CrossRef] [PubMed]

94. Bush, S.; Sodahlon, Y.; Downs, P.; Mackenzie, C.D. Cross-border issues: An important component of onchocerciasis elimination programmes. *Int. Health* **2018**, *10*, i54–i59. [CrossRef] [PubMed]

95. Senyonjo, L.; Oye, J.; Bakajika, D.; Biholong, B.; Tekle, A.; Boakye, D.; Schmidt, E.; Elhassan, E. Factors associated with ivermectin non-compliance and its potential role in sustaining *Onchocerca volvulus* transmission in the west region of Cameroon. *PLoS Negl. Trop. Dis.* **2016**, *10*, e0004905. [CrossRef] [PubMed]

96. Katabarwa, M.N.; Habomugisha, P.; Agunyo, S.; McKelvey, A.C.; Ogweng, N.; Kwebiiha, S.; Byenume, F.; Male, B.; McFarland, D. Traditional kinship system enhanced classic community-directed treatment with ivermectin (CDTI) for onchocerciasis control in Uganda. *Trans. R. Soc. Trop. Med. Hyg.* **2010**, *104*, 265–272. [CrossRef] [PubMed]

97. Bogus, J.; Gankpala, L.; Fischer, K.; Krentel, A.; Weil, G.J.; Fischer, P.U.; Kollie, K.; Bolay, F.K. Community attitudes toward mass drug administration for control and elimination of neglected tropical diseases after the 2014 outbreak of Ebola virus disease in Lofa County, Liberia. *Am. J. Trop. Med. Hyg.* **2016**, *94*, 497–503. [CrossRef] [PubMed]

98. Coffeng, L.E.; Stolk, W.A.; Zouré, H.G.M.; Veerman, J.L.; Agblewonu, K.B.; Murdoch, M.E.; Noma, M.; Fobi, G.; Richardus, J.H.; Bundy, D.A.P.; et al. African Programme for Onchocerciasis Control 1995-2015: Updated health impact estimates based on new disability weights. *PLoS Negl. Trop. Dis.* **2014**, *8*, e2759. [CrossRef] [PubMed]

99. Colebunders, R.; Mandro, M.; Njamnshi, A.K.; Boussinesq, M.; Hotterbeekx, A.; Kamgno, J.; O'Neill, S.; Hopkins, A.; Suykerbuyk, P.; Basáñez, M.G.; et al. Report of the first international workshop on onchocerciasis-associated epilepsy. *Inf. Dis. Poverty* **2018**, *7*, 23. [CrossRef] [PubMed]

100. Colebunders, R.; Nelson Siewe, F.J.; Hotterbeekx, A. Onchocerciasis-associated epilepsy, an additional reason for strengthening onchocerciasis elimination programs. *Trends. Parasitol.* **2018**, *34*, 208–216. [CrossRef] [PubMed]

101. Chesnais, C.B.N.A.; Zoung-Bissek, A.C.; Tatah, G.Y.; Nana-Djeunga, H.C.; Kamgno, J.; Colebunders, R.; Boussinesq, M. First evidence by a cohort study in Cameroon that onchocerciasis does induce epilepsy. In Proceedings of the 1st international workshop on onchocerciasis- associated epilepsy, Antwerp, Belgium, 12–14 October 2017. *Lancet Infect. Dis.* **2018**, in press.

102. Redekop, W.K.; Lenk, E.J.; Luyendijk, M.; Fitzpatrick, C.; Niessen, L.; Stolk, W.A.; Tediosi, F.; Rijnsburger, A.J.; Bakker, R.; Hontelez, J.A.C.; et al. The socioeconomic benefit to individuals of achieving the 2020 targets for five preventive chemotherapy neglected tropical diseases. *PLoS Negl. Trop. Dis.* **2017**, *11*, e0005289. [CrossRef] [PubMed]

103. de Vlas, S.J.; Stolk, W.A.; le Rutte, E.A.; Hontelez, J.A.C.; Bakker, R.; Blok, D.J.; Cai, R.; Houweling, T.A.J.; Kulik, M.C.; Lenk, E.J.; et al. Concerted efforts to control or eliminate neglected tropical diseases: How much health will be gained? *PLoS Negl. Trop. Dis.* **2016**, *10*, e0004386. [CrossRef] [PubMed]

104. Deribew, A.; Kebede, B.; Tessema, G.A.; Adama, Y.A.; Misganaw, A.; Gebre, T.; Hailu, A.; Biadgilign, S.; Amberbir, A.; Desalegn, B.; et al. Mortality and disability-adjusted life-years (Dalys) for common neglected tropical diseases in Ethiopia, 1990–2015: Evidence from the Global Burden of Disease Study 2015. *Ethiop. Med. J.* **2017**, *55*, 3–14. [PubMed]

105. Kim, Y.E.; Stolk, W.A.; Tanner, M.; Tediosi, F. Modelling the health and economic impacts of the elimination of river blindness (onchocerciasis) in Africa. *BMJ Glob. Heal.* **2017**, *2*, e000158. [CrossRef] [PubMed]

106. Salomon, J.A.; Vos, T.; Hogan, D.R.; Gagnon, M.; Naghavi, M.; Mokdad, A.; Begum, N.; Shah, R.; Karyana, M.; Kosen, S.; et al. Common values in assessing health outcomes from disease and injury: Disability weights measurement study for the Global Burden of Disease Study 2010. *Lancet* **2012**, *380*, 2129–2143. [CrossRef]

107. Salomon, J.A.; Vos, T.; Murra, C.J.L. Disability weights for vision disorders in Global Burden of Disease study-Authors' reply. *Lancet* **2013**, *381*, 23–24. [CrossRef]

108. Krotneva, S.P.; Coffeng, L.E.; Noma, M.; Zouré, H.G.M.; Bakoné, L.; Amazigo, U.V.; de Vlas, S.J.; Stolk, W.A. African Program for Onchocerciasis Control 1995–2010: Impact of annual ivermectin mass treatment on off-target infectious diseases. *PLoS Negl. Trop. Dis.* **2015**, *9*, e0004051. [CrossRef] [PubMed]

109. Means, A.R.; Burns, P.; Sinclair, D.; JL, W. Antihelminthics in helminth-endemic areas: Effects on HIV disease progression (Review). *Cochrane Database Syst. Rev.* **2016**. [CrossRef] [PubMed]

110. Simon, G.G. Impacts of neglected tropical disease on incidence and progression of HIV/AIDS, tuberculosis, and malaria: Scientific links. *Int. J. Infect. Dis.* **2016**, *42*, 54–57. [CrossRef] [PubMed]

111. Luroni, L.T.; Gabriel, M.; Tukahebwa, E.; Onapa, A.W.; Tinkitina, B.; Tukesiga, E.; Nyaraga, M.; Auma, A.M.; Habomugisha, P.; Byamukama, E.; et al. The interruption of *Onchocerca volvulus* and *Wuchereria bancrofti* transmission by integrated chemotherapy in the Obongi focus, North Western Uganda. *PLoS ONE* **2017**, *12*, e0189306. [CrossRef] [PubMed]

112. Lakwo, T.; Garms, R.; Wamani, J.; Tukahebwa, E.M.; Byamukama, E.; Onapa, A.W.; Tukesiga, E.; Katamanywa, J.; Begumisa, S.; Habomugisha, P.; et al. Interruption of the transmission of *Onchocerca volvulus* in the Kashoya-Kitomi focus, western Uganda by long-term ivermectin treatment and elimination of the vector *Simulium neavei* by larviciding. *Acta Trop.* **2017**, *167*, 128–136. [CrossRef] [PubMed]

113. Boakye, D.; Tallant, J.; Adjami, A.; Moussa, S.; Tekle, A.; Robalo, M.; Rebollo, M.; Mwinza, P.; Sitima, L.; Cantey, P.; et al. Refocusing vector assessment towards the elimination of onchocerciasis from Africa: A review of the current status in selected countries. *Int. Health* **2018**, *10*, i27–i32. [CrossRef] [PubMed]

114. Aljayyoussi, G.; Tyrer, H.E.; Ford, L.; Sjoberg, H.; Pionnier, N.; Waterhouse, D.; Davies, J.; Gamble, J.; Metugene, H.; Cook, D.A.N.; et al. Short-course, high-dose rifampicin achieves *Wolbachia* depletion predictive of curative outcomes in preclinical models of lymphatic filariasis and onchocerciasis. *Sci. Rep.* **2017**, *7*, 210. [CrossRef] [PubMed]

115. Abegunde, A.T.; Ahuja, R.M.; Okafor, N.J. Doxycycline Plus Ivermectin Versus Ivermectin Alone for Treatment of Patients with Onchocerciasis (Review). Available online: https://www.cochranelibrary.com/cdsr/doi/10.1002/14651858.CD011146/epdf/full (accessed on 11 June 2014).

116. Tamarozzi, F.; Tendongfor, N.; Enyong, P.A.; Esum, M.; Faragher, B.; Wanji, S.; Taylor, M.J. Long term impact of large scale community-directed delivery of doxycycline for the treatment of onchocerciasis. *Parasites Vectors* **2012**, *5*, 53. [CrossRef] [PubMed]

117. Walker, M.; Specht, S.; Churcher, T.S.; Hoerauf, A.; Taylor, M.J.; Basáñez, M.G. Therapeutic efficacy and macrofilaricidal activity of doxycycline for the treatment of river blindness. *Clin. Infect. Dis.* **2015**, *60*, 1199–1207. [CrossRef] [PubMed]

118. Klarmann-Schulz, U.; Specht, S.; Debrah, A.Y.; Batsa, L.; Ayisi-Boateng, N.K.; Osei-Mensah, J.; Mubarik, Y.; Konadu, P.; Ricchiuto, A.; Fimmers, R.; et al. Comparison of doxycycline, minocycline, doxycycline plus albendazole and albendazole alone in their efficacy against onchocerciasis in a randomized, open-label, pilot trial. *PLoS Negl. Trop. Dis.* **2017**, *11*, e0005156. [CrossRef] [PubMed]

119. Clare, R.H.; Cook, D.A.N.; Johnston, K.L.; Ford, L.; Ward, S.A.; Taylor, M.J. Development and validation of a high-throughput anti-*Wolbachia* whole-cell screen: A route to macrofilaricidal drugs against onchocerciasis and lymphatic filariasis. *J. Biomol. Screen.* **2015**, *20*, 64–69. [CrossRef] [PubMed]

120. Awadzi, K.; Opoku, N.O.; Attah, S.K.; Lazdins-Helds, J.; Kuesel, A.C. A randomized, single-ascending-dose, ivermectin-controlled, double-blind study of moxidectin in *Onchocerca volvulus* infection. *PLoS Negl. Trop. Dis.* **2014**, *8*, e2953. [CrossRef] [PubMed]

121. Opoku, N.O.; Bakajika, D.K.; Kanza, E.M.; Howard, H.; Mambandu, G.L.; Nyathirombo, A.; Nigo, M.M.; Kasonia, K.; Masembe, S.L.; Mumbere, M.; et al. Single dose moxidectin versus ivermectin for *Onchocerca volvulus* infection in Ghana, Liberia, and the Democratic Republic of the Congo: A randomised, controlled, double-blind phase 3 trial. *Lancet* **2018**. [CrossRef]

122. Turner, H.C.; Walker, M.; Attah, S.K.; Opoku, N.O.; Awadzi, K.; Kuesel, A.C.; Basáñez, M.G. The potential impact of moxidectin on onchocerciasis elimination in Africa: an economic evaluation based on the phase II clinical trial data. *Parasites Vectors* **2015**, *8*, 167. [CrossRef] [PubMed]

123. Fischer, P.U.; King, C.L.; Jacobson, J.A.; Weil, G.J. Potential value of triple drug therapy with ivermectin, diethylcarbamazine, and albendazole (ida) to accelerate elimination of lymphatic filariasis and onchocerciasis in Africa. *PLoS Negl. Trop. Dis.* **2017**, *11*, e0005163. [CrossRef] [PubMed]

124. Crisford, A.; Ebbinghaus-Kintscher, U.; Schoenhense, E.; Harder, A.; Raming, K.; O'Kelly, I.; Ndukwe, K.; O'Connor, V.; Walker, R.J.; Holden-Dye, L. The cyclooctadepsipeptide anthelmintic emodepside differentially modulates nematode, insect and human calcium-activated potassium (SLO) channel alpha subunits. *PLoS Negl. Trop. Dis.* **2015**, *9*, e0004062. [CrossRef] [PubMed]

125. Cotton, J.A.; Bennuru, S.; Grote, A.; Harsha, B.; Tracey, A.; Beech, R.; Doyle, S.R.; Dunn, M.; Hotopp, J.C.D.; Holroyd, N.; et al. The genome of *Onchocerca volvulus*, agent of river blindness. *Nat. Microbiol.* **2016**, *2*, 16216. [CrossRef] [PubMed]

126. Lustigman, S.; Makepeace, B.L.; Klei, T.R.; Babayan, S.A.; Hotez, P.; Abraham, D.; Bottazzi, M.E. *Onchocerca volvulus*: The road from basic biology to a vaccine. *Trends Parasitol.* **2018**, *34*, 64–79. [CrossRef] [PubMed]

127. Lustigman, S. Sara Lustigman: Developing a vaccine to accelerate onchocerciasis elimination. *Trends Parasitol.* **2018**, *34*, 1–3.

128. Mitjà, O.; Marks, M.; Bertran, L.; Kollie, K.; Argaw, D.; Fahal, A.H.; Fitzpatrick, C.; Fuller, L.C.; Garcia Izquierdo, B.; Hay, R.; et al. Integrated control and management of neglected tropical skin diseases. *PLoS Negl. Trop. Dis.* **2017**, *11*, e0005136. [CrossRef] [PubMed]

129. World Health Organization. Recognizing Neglected Tropical Diseases Through Changes on the Skin. A Training Guide for Front-line Health Workers. 2018. Available online: http://apps.who.int/iris/bitstream/handle/10665/272723/9789241513531-eng.pdf (accessed on 3 March 2018).

130. Hofstraat, K.; van Brakel, A.H. Social stigma towards neglected tropical diseases: A systematic review. *Int. Health* **2016**, *8*, i53–i70. [CrossRef] [PubMed]

131. Vinkeles Melchers, N.V.S.; Coffeng, L.E.; Murdoch, M.E.; Pedrique, B.; Bakker, R.; Ozoh, G.A.; de Vlas, S.J.; Stolk, W.A. Impact of ivermectin mass treatment on the burden of onchocercal skin and eye disease: detailed model predictions up to 2025. *Am. J. Trop. Med. Hyg.* **2016**, *95*, 345.

132. World Health Organization. Summary of global update on preventive chemotherapy implementation in 2016: crossing the billion. *Wkly. Epid. Rec.* **2017**, *92*, 589–593.

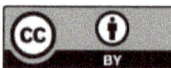

Tropical Medicine and
Infectious Disease

MDPI

Review

Mycetoma: The Spectrum of Clinical Presentation

Ahmed Hassan Fahal [1,*], Suliman Hussein Suliman [2] and Roderick Hay [3]

[1]   The Mycetoma Research Centre, University of Khartoum, Khartoum 11111, Sudan
[2]   Department of Surgery, Faculty of Medicine, University of Khartoum, Khartoum 11111, Sudan;
       sul.hus.sul@gmail.com
[3]   The International Foundation for Dermatology, London W1P 5HQ, UK; roderick.hay@ifd.org
*   Correspondence: ahfahal@hotmail.com or ahfahal@uofk.edu; Tel.: +249-91-234-6703

Received: 4 August 2018; Accepted: 30 August 2018; Published: 4 September 2018

Abstract: Mycetoma is a chronic infection, newly designated by the World Health Organization (WHO) as a neglected tropical disease, which is endemic in tropical and subtropical regions. It follows implantation of infectious organisms, either fungi (eumycetomas) or filamentous bacteria (actinomycetomas) into subcutaneous tissue, from where infection spreads to involve skin, bone and subcutaneous sites, leading to both health related and socioeconomic problems. In common with other NTDs, mycetoma is most often seen in rural areas amongst the poorest of people who have less access to health care. The organisms form small microcolonies that are discharged onto the skin surface via sinus tracts, or that can burrow into other adjacent tissues including bone. This paper describes the clinical features of mycetoma, as early recognition is a key to early diagnosis and the institution of appropriate treatment including surgery. Because these lesions are mostly painless and the majority of infected individuals present late and with advanced disease, simplifying early recognition is an important public health goal.

Keywords: mycetoma; clinical presentation; review

1. Introduction

Mycetoma is a unique and troubling neglected tropical disease, endemic in many tropical and subtropical areas. In addition, it is reported from different parts of the world [1,2]. It is a chronic granulomatous subcutaneous inflammatory disease that has a profound and negative impact on numerous medical, health-related and socioeconomic aspects of the lives of patients and communities in the endemic regions [3,4]. The causative organisms of mycetoma are of bacterial or fungal origin and hence these are classified as actinomycetomas and eumycetomas respectively [5,6]. Traumatic implantation of these causative organisms, which are soil and environmental inhabitants, into the subcutaneous tissue via minor trauma or injury is believed to be the route of entry in the development of mycetoma [7,8]. During the evolution of the infection, the causative organisms grow into modified localised microcolonies known as grains that are surrounded by inflammatory cells and give rise to inflammatory sinus tracts. Mycetoma is basically a localised disease; the inflammatory process usually involves the local subcutaneous tissue but it then spreads along the different tissue planes to invade the skin, deep tissues and structures and eventually the bones [9,10]. If not treated appropriately, it can lead to enormous tissue damage, disfigurement and disability that hinder the patients' normal daily activities [11,12]. Mycetoma patients are unique. They are of low socioeconomic status and health educational level, reside in remote, poor rural areas with meagre medical and health resources. Furthermore, their lesions are usually painless and hence the majority of them present late and with advanced pathology [13,14].

2. Age, Gender and Occupation in Mycetoma

No age is exempted from infection but the majority of patients are young adults in the age group of 15–30 years [15,16]. In most of the reported series, children account for 30% of the cases [17]. This has massive implications for the patients, families and communities in the endemic areas as these are the working and wage-earning members of each society and many of these drop out of education due to illness, which increases the pressure on family and community income and resources in households that are already impoverished [18,19].

Male predominance is a constant finding in mycetoma with a gender ratio of 3.7:1 [20,21]. This is commonly attributed to the greater risk of exposure to microorganisms in the soil during outdoor work-related activities. However, in mycetoma-endemic areas, females are also involved in outdoor work activities and thus other genetic or immunological factors cannot be ruled out [22,23].

Mycetoma is seen in most communities in farmers, field labourers and in herdsmen who come in contact with the land, although in endemic areas people from other occupations are affected [24,25].

The patients' photographs were all obtained following due informed consent procedure.

3. The Clinical Presentation

More than 70 microorganisms are incriminated in causing mycetoma. Nevertheless, the clinical presentation of mycetoma is almost indistinguishable regardless of the causal microorganism [26]. The triad of painless subcutaneous swelling, multiple draining sinuses and discharge that contains grains is characteristics of mycetoma. The swelling is usually firm and rounded but it may be soft, lobulated and, rarely, cystic and it is often mobile (Figure 1) [27]. Multiple secondary nodules then evolve, the nodules may suppurate and drain through multiple sinus tracts, and these sinuses may close transiently after discharge during the active phase of the disease. Prior to discharge, pustules may be visible. Fresh adjacent sinuses may open while some of the old ones may heal completely. The sinuses are connected with each other, with deep abscesses and with the skin surface (Figure 2) [28]. The discharge is usually serous, serosanguinous or purulent. During the active phase of the disease, the sinuses discharge grains, consisting of the microorganisms encapsulated in a cement-like material, melanin and other substances. The grains are believed to protect these microorganisms against host defence mechanisms, antimicrobials and antifungals [29]. The grain colour depends on the causative organism. The grains can be black, yellow, white or red and they are of variable size and consistency. In most mycetomas, they are visible to the naked eye and may be noticed by patients; the exception is actinomycetoma, due to the *Nocardia* species, in which the grains are very small and only visible under the microscope. The black grains are most commonly due to *M. mycetomatis* and related species, the red ones are due to *A. pelletierii*, the yellow to *Streptomyces somaliensis* and the white grains can be due to *A. madurae* [30]. However, black fungi may also produce grains of pale colour. Pus, exudate, the dressing gauze and biopsy material should be examined for the presence of the grains as they may give a clue to the causative organisms although the identity needs to be confirmed as visual inspection alone is not sufficiently accurate (Figure 3).

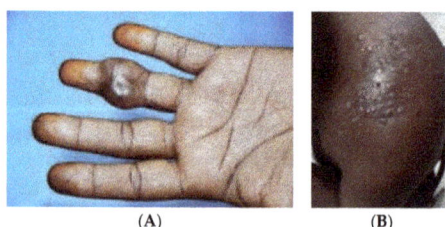

(A)   (B)

Figure 1. (**A**) A small mycetoma swelling engulfing the middle part of the left ring finger with a scar of previous surgical excision. (**B**) Multiple small nodules of *Nocardia* actinomycetoma at an earlier stage.

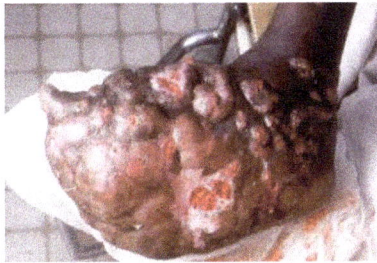

Figure 2. Massive actinomycetoma foot with multiple sinuses and discharge.

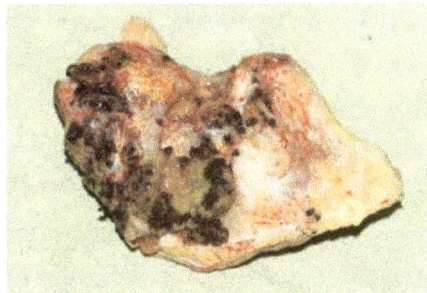

Figure 3. Surgical specimen with multiple black grains.

The onset and progress rate is more rapid with actinomycetoma than with eumycetoma. In eumycetoma, the lesion grows slowly with clearly defined margins and remains encapsulated for a long period, whereas, in actinomycetoma, the lesion is more inflammatory, more destructive and invades the bone at an earlier period; this is more evident in *A. pelletierii* actinomycetoma [31].

As the mycetoma granuloma increases in size, the skin over it becomes attached and stretched. The skin may become smooth, shiny and areas of hypo or hyperpigmentation may develop (Figure 4) [32]. In some patients, there may be areas of local hyperhidrosis confined to the mycetoma lesion itself and the skin around it. This is commonly seen with massive lesions in patients with active disease and the cause is unclear but increased local temperature due to brisk arterial circulation may a cause (Figures 5 and 6). In *Nocardia* actinomycetomas the chest wall or back is often affected and here the edges of the lesions are unclear and hard to define.

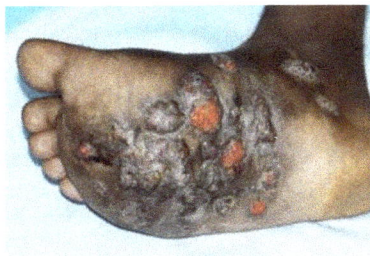

Figure 4. Foot eumycetoma with skin hyperpigmentation, multiple nodules and active sinuses.

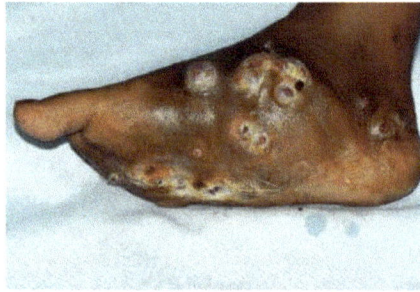

Figure 5. Foot eumycetoma with skin hyperpigmentation, multiple nodules, active sinuses discharging black grains discharge and local hyperhidrosis.

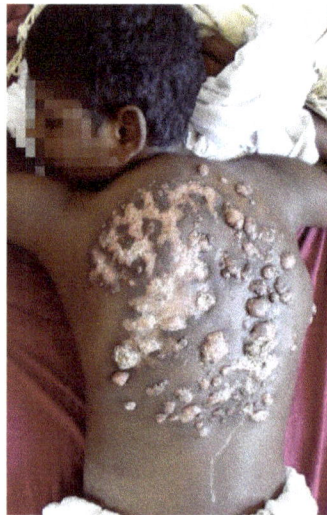

Figure 6. Massive back actinomycetoma with multiple nodules and sinuses.

In long-standing massive mycetoma lesions, dilated tortuous veins at, and proximal to, the mycetoma site are noted. They are frequently confused with varicose veins. They develop as a secondary phenomenon to accommodate the brisk venous return due to the increased arterial blood flow caused by the chronic inflammatory process at the mycetoma site (Figure 7) [33].

Unusually and for unknown reasons, the tendons and the nerves are spared until very late in the disease process; this may explain the rarity of neurological and trophic changes even in patients with long-standing mycetomas. The absence of trophic changes may be explained by the more than adequate blood supply in the mycetoma-infected area [34].

In the majority of patients, the regional lymph nodes are small and shotty. An enlarged regional lymph node is not uncommon and this may be due to secondary bacterial infection, the genuine lymphatic spread of mycetoma or it may be due to immune complex deposition as part of a local immune response to mycetoma infection [35].

In general, the infection remains localised and constitutional disturbances are rare but when they do occur they are generally due to secondary bacterial infection of the open sinus tracts and generalised immunosuppression. Cachexia and anaemia may be seen in late mycetoma. This is often due to malnutrition, sepsis and mental depression [36]. Co-morbidities in mycetoma are rare and the commonest are diabetes mellitus and hypertension, as in the general population. HIV and malignant transformation are not reported in mycetoma [30].

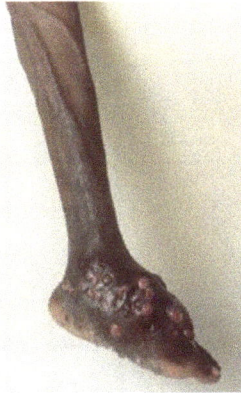

Figure 7. Massive mycetoma foot with dilated tortuous veins at and proximal to the mycetoma site.

Mycetoma is usually painless in nature; it has been suggested that the mycetoma produces substances that have an anaesthetic action. At a late stage of the disease, the pain may also become negligible due to nerve damage by the tense fibrous tissue reaction, endarteritis obliterans or poor vascularisation of the nerves [37]. Pain at the mycetoma site is reported in 20% of patients and it is commonly produced by the secondary bacterial infection or transiently when a new closed sinus is about to open onto the skin surface.

Mycetoma can produce many distortions, deformities and disabilities and that is due to structural impairment that includes bone destruction or periostitis, loss of function and disuse atrophy of the affected limb. The current treatment options are limited and suboptimal; many patients undergo repeated massive surgical excisions leading to more tissue destruction and fibrosis and disability (Figure 8) [38].

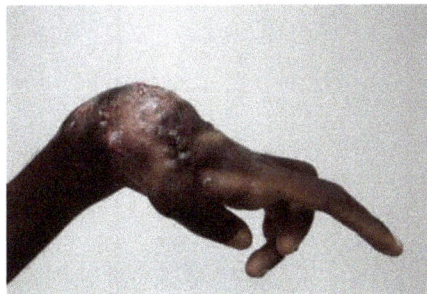

Figure 8. Hand eumycetoma with massive deformity.

4. The Site of Mycetoma

The commonest site for mycetoma is the foot (79.2%); most of the lesions are seen on the dorsal aspect of the forefoot and the left foot is affected slightly more often [39]. The hand ranks as the second commonest site (6.6%), with the right hand is more affected. This may imply a traumatic basis of the infection in this site [40]. In endemic areas, other parts of the body may be involved but less frequently, and these include the knee, arm, leg, head and neck, thigh and the perineum [41–45]. Rarer sites for eumycetomas are the chest and abdominal walls, facial bones, mandible, paranasal sinuses, eyelid, vulva, orbit and scrotum (Figures 9–11) [46–50]. *Nocardia* actinomycetomas are often found on the chest or abdominal wall. Bilateral limb mycetomas, although described, are very rare.

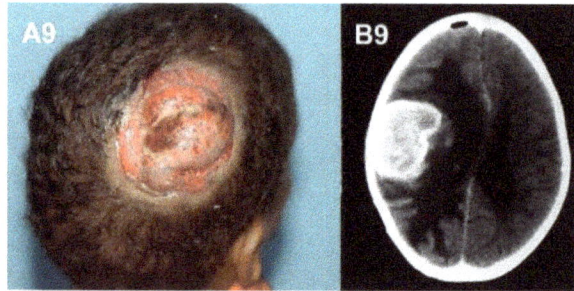

Figure 9. (A) massive head eumycetoma. (B) CT scan showing intra-cranial extension.

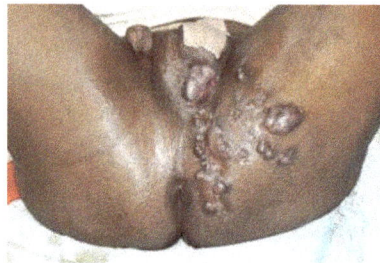

Figure 10. Massive gluteal, perineal and scrotal eumycetoma.

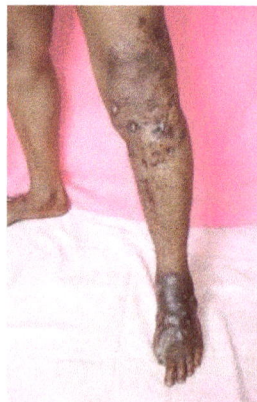

Figure 11. Massive foot actinomycetoma with leg and knee inguinal satellite lesions.

5. Mycetoma Spread

Spread along the lymphatics to the regional lymph nodes is reported and this is more frequent with actinomycetoma [12]. At the regional lymph nodes, the disease progresses; a new disease satellite lesion develops and progresses to form a massive mycetoma, and in some cases, this can cause lymphatic obstruction and lymphedema (Figure 11) [51]. Bloodstream spread in mycetoma is a rare event. It has been reported in some cases, where there was spinal cord compression and paraplegia. In these cases, the skin and subcutaneous tissue were normal and the mycetoma was an unexpected finding at surgery upon opening the spinal dura matter [52]. In these cases, the mycetoma grains were actually seen in the lumen of the intact blood vessel (Figure 12).

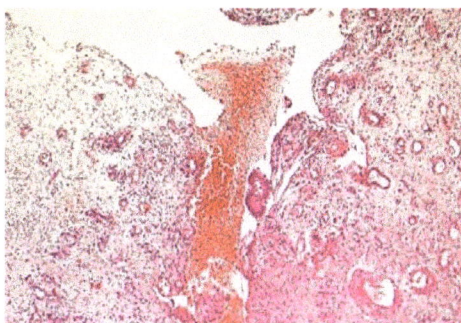

Figure 12. Photomicrograph showing *A. madurae* grains within the lumen of the intact blood vessel (H&E X 200).

6. Aggressive Mycetoma

Although mycetoma is primarily a localised disease of gradual onset and slow progress, some patients present with massive, aggressive, uncontrolled disease and most of these are fatal. In these patients, the disease progressed wildly and aggressively from the subcutaneous tissue to involve the deep organs such as the urinary bladder, pelvic organs, spinal cord, lung and other structures and resulted in fatal outcome [53–56].

Two patients with fatal eumycetoma presented with pulmonary secondaries were reported; one from the knee and the second from gluteal eumycetoma. In these patients, *Madurella mycetomatis* had progressed widely without response to the different medical and surgical treatment modalities. Vascular spread, which is a rare phenomenon in mycetoma, may explain the secondary lung lesions encountered in these patients [52,54–56].

Several cases of mycetoma of the head and neck region have reported. They proved to be serious medical and health problem, with low cure rate and were associated with grave complications and poor outcome due to intra-cranial spread [57].

Pelvic mycetoma spread has also been reported. In these cases, the urinary bladder, rectum, hip bones and other local structures were involved. The disease was complicated by multiple urinary and rectal fistulae, pathological fractures and all patients died from massive sepsis (Figure 13) [52–56].

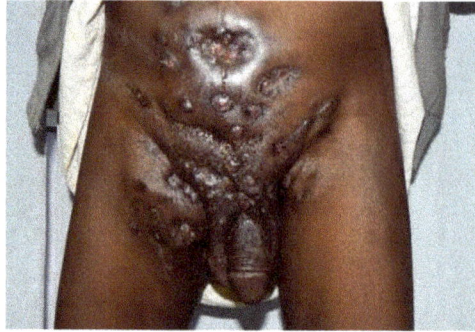

Figure 13. Massive anterior abdominal eumycetoma spreading to both inguinal regions and scrotum.

7. The Differential Diagnosis

In endemic areas, any subcutaneous mass is considered as mycetoma unless proved otherwise. The differential diagnosis of mycetoma includes thorn and foreign body granulomas, particularly in mycetoma endemic areas [57]. Also, it includes many soft tissue tumours such as Kaposi's sarcoma, fibroma, malignant melanoma or fibrolipoma and keloids [1,58]. Many dermatological conditions, such as botryomycosis, sporotrichosis and plantar or acral psoriasis, can mimic mycetoma [59]. In very early mycetomas, before the first appearance of sinuses, the lesion simply resembles a firm subcutaneous nodule, which makes recognition of the earliest signs based on a visual appearance very difficult as the differential encompasses a variety of benign and inflammatory conditions, from dermatofibromas to hypertrophic scars. The radiological features of advanced mycetoma resemble osteogenic sarcoma and bone tuberculosis (Figure 14). Primary osseous mycetoma, without overlying sinuses, is uncommon but must be differentiated from chronic osteomyelitis, osteoclastoma, bone cysts and syphilitic osteitis.

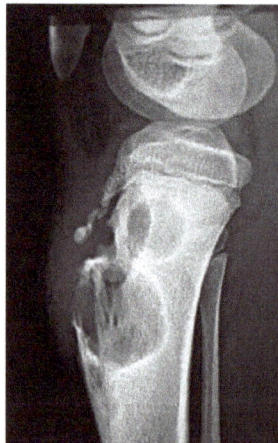

Figure 14. X-ray of thigh and knee eumycetoma showing massive soft tissue shadow, periosteal reaction and multiple bone cavities resembling osteogenic sarcoma.

This paper has concentrated on the variations in the clinical presentation of mycetomas. The currently available treatments for mycetoma are suboptimal and unsatisfactory, characterised by a low cure rate and high patient follow-up dropout and recurrence rates [49]. Furthermore, presently there are neither preventive nor control measures or programs for mycetoma. Moreover, mycetoma affects the most underprivileged population in remote areas and hence most patients present late with advanced disease. To overcome this, early case detection, which depends on detecting the visual warning signs of the disease and treatment is the only available means to prevent the numerous and serious complications of mycetoma. The first step in early case detection is meticulous clinical examination of the suspected patients, as other diagnostics tools, including direct microscopy, culture, histopathology and molecular identification, are commonly not available in mycetoma- endemic regions [60].

Author Contributions: The three authors contributed equally to this review article, and that included conceptualization, literature review, writing of original draft preparation, and review & editing.

Funding: This research received no external funding.

Conflicts of Interest: The authors declare no conflict of interest.

References

1. Fahal, A.H. Mycetoma: A thorn in the flesh. *Trans. R. Soc. Trop. Med. Hyg.* **2004**, *98*, 3–11.
2. Fahal, A.H.; Hassan, M.A. Mycetoma. *Br. J. Surg.* **1992**, *79*, 1138–1141. [CrossRef] [PubMed]
3. Bonifaz, A.; Tirado-Sánchez, A.; Calderón, L.; Saúl, A.; Araiza, J.; Hernández, M.; González, G.M.; Ponce, R.M. Mycetoma: Experience of 482 cases in a single center in Mexico. *PLoS Negl. Trop. Dis.* **2014**, *8*, e3102.
4. Ahmed, A.O.; van Leeuwen, W.; Fahal, A.; van de Sande, W.; Verbrugh, H.; van Belkum, A. Mycetoma caused by *Madurella mycetomatis*: A neglected infectious burden. *Lancet Infect. Dis.* **2004**, *4*, 566–574. [CrossRef]
5. Ahmed, A.O.A.; van de Sande, W.W.; Fahal, A.; Bakker-Woudenberg, I.; Verbrugh, H.; van Belkum, A. Management of mycetoma: Major challenge in tropical mycoses with limited international recognition. *Curr. Opin. Infect. Dis.* **2007**, *20*, 146–151. [PubMed]
6. Fahal, A.H.; van de Sandy, W.W. The epidemiology of mycetoma. *Curr. Fungal Infect. Rep.* **2012**, *6*, 320–326. [CrossRef]
7. Fahal, A.H. Mycetoma. In *Tropical Infectious Diseases. Principles, Pathogens and Practice*, 3rd ed.; Guerrant, R.L., Walker, D.H., Weller, P.F., Eds.; Elsevier: Amsterdam, The Netherlands, 2011; pp. 565–568.
8. Williams, N.S.; Bulstrode, C.; O'Connell, P.R. *Bailey and Love's Short Practice of Surgery 26E*, 26th ed.; Taylor & Francis Ltd.: London, UK, 2013; pp. 84–88.
9. Fahal, A.H. *Mycetoma: Clinico-Pathological Monograph*; University of Khartoum Press: Khurtum, Sudan, 2006; pp. 40–49.
10. Hassan, M.A.; Fahal, A.H. *Mycetoma: In Tropical Surgery*; Kamil, R., Lumbly, J., Eds.; Westminster Publication Ltd.: London, UK, 2004; pp. 30–45.
11. Fahal, A.H.; Suliman, S.H.; Gadir, A.F.A.; EL Hag, I.A.; EL Amin, F.I.; Gumaa, S.A.; Mahgoub, E.S. Abdominal wall mycetoma: An unusual presentation. *Trans. R. Soc. Trop. Med. Hyg.* **1994**, *88*, 78–80. [CrossRef]
12. Fahal, A.H.; Suliman, S.H. Clinical presentation of mycetoma. *Sudan Med. J.* **1994**, *32*, 46–66.
13. Fahal, A.H.; El Hassan, A.M.; Abdelalla, A.O.; Sheikh, H.E. Cystic mycetoma: An unusual clinical presentation of *Madurella mycetomatis*. *Trans. R. Soc. Trop. Med. Hyg.* **1998**, *92*, 66–67. [CrossRef]
14. Fahal, A.H.; EL Toum, E.A.; EL Hassan, A.M.; Gumaa, S.A.; Mahgoub, E.S. A preliminary study on the ultrastructure of *Actinomadura pelletieri* and its host tissue reaction. *J. Med. Vet. Mycol.* **1994**, *32*, 343–348. [CrossRef] [PubMed]
15. EL Hassan, A.M.; Fahal, A.H.; EL Hag, I.A.; Khalil, E.A.G. The pathology of mycetoma: Light microscopic and ultrastructural features. *Sudan Med. J.* **1994**, *32*, 23–45.
16. Fahal, A.H.; Hassan, M.A.; Sanhouri, M. Surgical treatment of mycetoma. *Sudan Med. J.* **1994**, *32*, 98–104.
17. Fahal, A.H.; EL Toum, E.A.; EL Hassan, A.M.; Gumaa, S.A.; Mahgoub, E.S. Host tissue reaction to *Madurella mycetomatis*: New classification. *J. Med. Vet. Mycol.* **1995**, *33*, 15–17. [CrossRef] [PubMed]
18. Van de Sande, W.W.; Fahal, A.H.; Goodfellow, M.; Maghoub, E.S.; Welsh, O.; Zijlstra, E.E. The merits and pitfalls of the currently used diagnostic tools in mycetoma. *PLoS Negl. Trop. Dis.* **2014**, *3*, e2918. [CrossRef] [PubMed]

19. Welsh, O.; Al-Abdely, H.M.; Salinas-Carmona, M.C.; Fahal, A.H. Mycetoma medical therapy. *PLoS Negl. Trop. Dis.* **2014**, *8*, e3218. [CrossRef] [PubMed]
20. Welsh, O.; Vera-Cabrera, L.; Welsh, E.; Salinas, M.C. Actinomycetoma and advances in its treatment. *Clin. Dermatol.* **2012**, *30*, 372–381. [CrossRef] [PubMed]
21. Mhmoud, N.A.; Ahmed, S.A.; Fahal, A.H.; de Hoog, G.S.; Gerrits van den Ende, A.H.; van de Sande, W.W. *Pleurostomophora ochracea*, a novel agent of human eumycetoma with yellow grains. *J. Clin. Microbiol.* **2012**, *50*, 2987–2994. [CrossRef] [PubMed]
22. De Hoog, G.S.; Van Diepeningen, A.D.; Mahgoub, E.S.; Van de Sande, W.W. New species of *Madurella*, causative agents of black-grain mycetoma. *Clin. Microbiol.* **2012**, *50*, 988–994. [CrossRef] [PubMed]
23. Mahgoub, E.S.; Gumaa, S.A. Ketoconazole in the treatment of eumycetoma due to *Madurella mycetomi*. *Trans. R. Soc. Trop. Med. Hyg.* **1984**, *78*, 376–379. [CrossRef]
24. Fahal, A.H.; Rahman, I.A.; El-Hassan, A.M.; EL Rahman, M.E.; Zijlstra, E.E. The efficacy of itraconazole in the treatment of patients with eumycetoma due to *Madurella mycetomatis*. *Trans. R. Soc. Trop. Med. Hyg.* **2011**, *105*, 127–132. [CrossRef] [PubMed]
25. Mahgoub, E.S.; Murray, I.G. *Mycetoma*; Medical Books Ltd.: London, UK, 1973; pp. 2–25.
26. Abbott, P.H. Mycetoma in the Sudan. *Trans. R. Soc. Trop. Med. Hyg.* **1956**, *50*, 11–24. [CrossRef]
27. Lynch, J.B. Mycetoma in the Sudan. *Ann. R. Coll. Surg. Engl.* **1964**, *35*, 319–340. [PubMed]
28. EL Moghraby, I.M. Mycetoma in Gezira. *Sudan Med. J.* **1971**, *9*, 77.
29. Mahgoub, E.S. Mycoses in the Sudan. *Trans. R. Soc. Trop. Med. Hyg.* **1977**, *71*, 184–188. [CrossRef]
30. Fahal, A.H.; Mahgoub, E.S.; EL Hassan, A.M.; Abdel-Rahman, M.E.; Alshambaty, Y.; Hashim, A.; Hago, A.; Zijlstra, E.E. A new model for management of mycetoma in the Sudan. *PLoS Negl. Trop. Dis.* **2014**, *8*, e3271. [CrossRef] [PubMed]
31. López-Martínez, R.; Méndez-Tovar, L.J.; Lavalle, P.; Welsh, O.; Saúl, A. Epidemiology of mycetoma in Mexico: Study of 2105 cases. *Gac. Med. Mex.* **1992**, *128*, 477–481. [PubMed]
32. López-Martínez, R.; Méndez-Tovar, L.J.; Bonifaz, A.; Arenas, R.; Mayorga, J.; Welsh, O.; Vera-Cabrera, L.; Padilla-Desgarennes, M.C.; Contreras Pérez, C.; Chávez, G.; et al. Update on the epidemiology of mycetoma in Mexico. A Review of 3933 cases. *Gac. Med. Mex.* **2013**, *149*, 586–592. [PubMed]
33. Ahmed, A.O.A.; Adelmann, D.; Fahal, A.H.; Verbrugh, H.A.; Van Belkum, A.; de Hoog, S.A. Environmental occurrence of *Madurella mycetomatis*, major agent of human eumycetoma in Sudan. *J. Clin. Microbiol.* **2002**, *40*, 1031–1036. [CrossRef] [PubMed]
34. Ahmed, A.O.A.; van Vianen, W.; ten Kate, M.; van de Sande, W.W.J.; Van Belkum, A. A murine model of *Madurella mycetomatis* eumycetoma. *FEMS Immunol. Med. Microbiol.* **2003**, *37*, 29–36. [CrossRef]
35. Fahal, A.H.; Azziz, K.A.A.; Suliman, S.H.; Galib, H.V.; Mahgoub, E.S. Dual infection with mycetoma and tuberculosis. *East Afr. Med. J.* **1995**, *72*, 749–750. [PubMed]
36. Fahal, A.H.; Arbab, M.A.R.; EL Hassan, A.M. Aggressive clinical presentation of mycetoma due to *Actinomadura pelletierii*. *Khartoum Med. J.* **2012**, *5*, 699–702.
37. Ibrahim, A.I.; EL Hassan, A.M.; Fahal, A.H.; van de Sande, W.W. A histopathological exploration of the *Madurella mycetomatis* grain. *PLoS ONE* **2013**, *8*, e57774. [CrossRef] [PubMed]
38. Aounallah, A.; Boussofara, L.; Ben Saïd, Z.; Ghariani, N.; Saidi, W.; Denguezli, M.; Belajouza, C.; Nouira, R. Analysis of 18 Tunisian cases of mycetoma at the Sousse hospital (1974–2010). *Bull. Soc. Pathol. Exot.* **2013**, *106*, 5–8. [CrossRef] [PubMed]
39. Dieng, M.T.; Niang, S.O.; Diop, B.; Ndiaye, B. Actinomycetomas in Senegal: Study of 90 cases. *Bull. Soc. Pathol. Exot.* **2005**, *98*, 18–20. [PubMed]
40. Marc, S.; Meziane, M.; Hamada, S.; Hassam, B.; Benzekri, L. Clinical and epidemiological features of mycetoma in Morocco. *Med. Mal. Infect.* **2011**, *41*, 163–164. [CrossRef] [PubMed]
41. Philippon, M.; Larroque, D.; Ravisse, P. Mycetoma in Mauritania: Species found, epidemiologic characteristics and country distribution. Report of 122 cases. *Bull. Soc. Pathol. Exot.* **1992**, *85*, 107–114. [PubMed]
42. Fahal, A.H.; Sharfy, A.R.A. Vulval mycetoma: A rare cause of bladder outlet obstruction. *Trans. R. Soc. Trop. Med. Hyg.* **1998**, *92*, 652–653. [CrossRef]
43. Mohamed, E.W.; Mohamed, E.N.A.; Yousif, B.M.; Fahal, A.H. Tongue actinomycetoma due to *Actinomadura madurae*: A rare clinical presentation. *J. Oral. Maxillofac. Surg.* **2012**, *70*, e622–e624. [CrossRef] [PubMed]

44. Suleiman, A.M.; Fahal, A.H. Oral eumycetoma: A rare and unusual presentation. *Oral. Surg. Oral. Med. Oral. Pathol. Oral. Radiol.* **2013**, *115*, e23–e25. [CrossRef] [PubMed]

45. Fahal, A.H.; Yagi, H.I.; EL Hassan, A.M. Mycetoma induced palatal deficiency and pharyngeal plexus dysfunction. *Trans. R. Soc. Trop. Med. Hyg.* **1996**, *90*, 676–677. [CrossRef]

46. Fahal, A.H.; Sharfi, A.R.; Sheikh, H.E.; EL Hassan, A.M. Internal fistula formation: An unusual complication of mycetoma. *Trans. R. Soc. Trop. Med. Hyg.* **1996**, *89*, 550–552. [CrossRef]

47. Mohamed, E.W.; Suleiman, H.S.; Fadella, A.I.; Fahal, A.H. Aggressive perineal and pelvic eumycetoma: An unusual and challenging problem to treat. *Khartoum Med. J.* **2012**, *5*, 771–774.

48. Hussein, A.; Ahmed, A.E.M.; Fahal, A.H.; Mahmoud, A.; Sidig, A.; Awad, K. Cervical cord compression secondary to mycetoma infection. *Sud. J. Public Health* **2007**, *2*, 112–115.

49. Zein, H.A.M.; Fahal, A.H.; Mahgoub, E.S.; EL Hassan, T.; Abdel Rahman, M.E. The predictors of cure, amputation & follow-up dropout among mycetoma patients as seen at the Mycetoma Research Centre, University of Khartoum. *Trans R. Soc. Trop. Med. Hyg.* **2012**, *106*, 639–644. [PubMed]

50. Wendy, W.J.; van de Sande, W.W.; Mahgoub, E.S.; Fahal, A.H.; Goodfellow, M.; Welsh, O. The mycetoma knowledge gap: Identification of research priorities. *PLoS Negl. Trop. Dis.* **2014**, *8*, e2667.

51. EL Hassan, A.M.; Mahgoub, E.S. Lymph node involvement in mycetoma. *Trans. R. Soc. Trop. Med. Hyg.* **1972**, *66*, 165–169. [CrossRef]

52. Arbab, M.A.; El Hag, I.A.; Abdul Gadir, A.F.; Siddik, H.E.-R. Intraspinal mycetoma: Report of two cases. *Am. J. Trop. Med. Hyg.* **1997**, *56*, 27–29. [CrossRef] [PubMed]

53. Saad, E.S.A.; Fahal, A.H. Broncho-pleuro-cutaneous fistula and pneumothorax: Rare challenging complications of chest wall eumycetoma. *PLoS Negl. Trop. Dis.* **2017**, *11*, e0005737. [CrossRef] [PubMed]

54. Mohamed, N.A.; Fahal, A.H. Mycetoma pulmonary secondaries from a gluteal eumycetoma: An unusual presentation. *PLoS Negl. Trop. Dis.* **2016**, *10*, e0004945. [CrossRef] [PubMed]

55. Mohamed, E.S.W.; Seif El Din, N.; Fahal, A.H. Multiple mycetoma lung secondaries from knee eumycetoma: An unusual complication. *PLoS Negl. Trop. Dis.* **2016**, *10*, e0004735. [CrossRef] [PubMed]

56. Scolding, P.S.; Abbas, M.A.; Omer, R.F.; Fahal, A.H. *Madurella mycetomatis*-induced massive shoulder joint destruction: A management challenge. *PLoS Negl. Trop. Dis.* **2016**, *10*, e0004849. [CrossRef] [PubMed]

57. Fahal, A.; Mahgoub, E.S.; El Hassan, A.M.; Jacoub, A.O.; Hassan, D. Head and neck mycetoma: The Mycetoma Research Centre experience. *PLoS Negl. Trop. Dis.* **2015**, *9*, e0003587. [CrossRef] [PubMed]

58. Fahal, A.; Mahgoub, E.S.; El Hassan, A.M.; Abdel-Rahman, M.E. Mycetoma in the Sudan: An update from the Mycetoma Research Centre, University of Khartoum, Sudan. *PLoS Negl. Trop. Dis.* **2015**, *9*, e0003679. [CrossRef] [PubMed]

59. Mitjà, O.; Marks, M.; Bertran, L.; Kollie, K.; Argaw, D.; Fahal, A.H. Integrated control and management of neglected tropical skin diseases. *PLoS Negl. Trop. Dis.* **2017**, *11*, e0005136. [CrossRef] [PubMed]

60. Bakhiet, S.M.; Fahal, A.H.; Musa, A.M.; Mohamed, E.S.W.; Omer, R.F.; Ahmed, E.S. A holistic approach to the mycetoma management. *PLoS Negl. Trop. Dis.* **2018**, *12*, e0006391. [CrossRef] [PubMed]

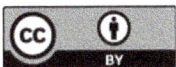

Tropical Medicine and
Infectious Disease

MDPI

Review

Control Strategies for Scabies

Daniel Engelman [1,2,3,4,*] and Andrew C. Steer [1,2,3,4]

1   Tropical Diseases, Murdoch Children's Research Institute, Parkville VIC 3052, Australia;
      Andrew.Steer@rch.org.au
2   Department of Paediatrics, University of Melbourne, Parkville VIC 3052, Australia
3   Department of General Medicine, Royal Children's Hospital, Parkville VIC 3052, Australia
4   International Alliance for the Control of Scabies, Parkville VIC 3052, Australia
*   Correspondence: Daniel.Engelman@rch.org.au; Tel.: +613-9345-5522

Received: 12 August 2018; Accepted: 3 September 2018; Published: 5 September 2018

Abstract: Scabies is a neglected tropical disease of the skin, causing severe itching and stigmatizing skin lesions. Further, scabies leads to impetigo, severe bacterial infections, and post-infectious complications. Around 200 million people are affected, particularly among disadvantaged populations living in crowded conditions in tropical areas. After almost 50 years, research into scabies control has shown great promise, particularly in highly-endemic island settings, but these findings have not been widely adopted. Newer approaches, utilizing ivermectin-based mass drug administration, appear feasible and highly effective. Inclusion of scabies in the WHO portfolio of neglected tropical diseases in 2017 may facilitate renewed opportunities and momentum toward global control. However, further operational research is needed to develop evidence-based strategies for control in a range of settings, and monitor their impact. Several enabling factors are required for successful implementation, including availability of affordable drug supply. Integration with existing health programs may provide a cost-effective approach to control.

Keywords: scabies; neglected tropical diseases; impetigo; mass drug administration; ivermectin

1. Introduction

Scabies is a skin disease caused by infestation with the mite, *Sarcoptes scabiei* var. *hominis*. The female mite, measuring less than 0.5 mm, burrows into the skin, where antigens on the exoskeleton of the mite, along with its saliva, excreta, and eggs, elicit a hypersensitivity reaction [1]. The resulting skin lesions most commonly affect the hands, wrists, ankles, and feet (Figure 1). In the vast majority of cases of common scabies (also known variably as ordinary, classical, or typical scabies) there is a low number of mites on the patient's body (5 to 15). Crusted scabies (formerly known as Norwegian scabies) is a rare form of the disease characterized by hyperinfestation with thousands to millions of mites and hyperkeratotic 'crusted' skin [2].

Transmission of scabies is predominantly via skin-to-skin contact. Transmission from bedding or clothes is rare in ordinary scabies, but can occur in crusted scabies because of its tremendous mite burden. The risk of transmission of scabies increases with higher levels of population density, reflected by the high endemicity observed in communities living in poverty with associated crowded housing conditions, and by outbreaks in in residential care facilities, prisons, schools, and refugee camps. Patients with underlying immunodeficiency from any cause, such as human immunodeficiency virus, human T-lymphotropic virus type 1 or corticosteroid treatment, or those with neurological conditions, are at an increased risk of crusted scabies [2–4].

Scabies causes considerable suffering due to the intense itch and associated scratching, leading to sleep disturbances which, in turn, impact on school and work attendance and performance, and ultimately the economic productivity of whole communities [5]. Like many infections that affect the skin, scabies is associated with social stigma and leads to social exclusion because of the appearance of the affected individual and attendant feelings of shame, as well as fears within the community of spread of infection [5,6]. Scabies can have a marked impact on quality of life measures, similar to the recognized psychological impact caused by other skin conditions such as psoriasis and vitiligo [7].

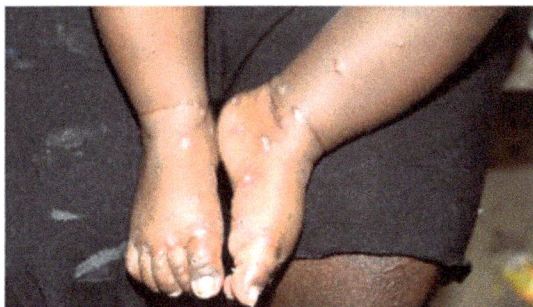

Figure 1. Infant with typical rash of scabies.

In endemic settings, scabies lesions are often super-infected with the bacteria *Streptococcus pyogenes* and *Staphylococcus aureus*. Bacterial infection occurs due to breaches in the skin barrier as a result of mite burrows and associated scratching [8], as well as direct effects of the scabies mite in downregulating host immunity and optimising conditions for bacterial growth [9,10]. These bacteria can cause local soft tissue infections such as impetigo, cellulitis, and abscesses, and can lead to life-threatening diseases including sepsis, and in the case of *S. pyogenes*, post-streptococcal glomerulonephritis [11], and possibly acute rheumatic fever (this link is epidemiologically associated but, as yet, unproven) [12,13].

This review aims to re-examine the rationale for public health control of scabies, evaluate the available evidence for scabies control interventions, and identify the barriers and future research priorities needed to develop and scale-up implementation of scabies control activities.

2. Burden of Disease

Scabies occurs worldwide, and is estimated to affect over 200 million people at any single time [14]. The highest prevalence of scabies occurs in tropical areas, especially in disadvantaged populations, and especially among children and the elderly. The Global Burden of Disease (GBD) study reported that scabies directly accounts for 0.21% of global disability-adjusted life years [15]. However, there are substantial gaps in our knowledge of the epidemiology of scabies and its complications.

First, many countries have no available data on scabies prevalence, including countries where disease burden is likely to be high, based upon known risk factors (poverty and overcrowding). For example, in a systematic review of prevalence studies of scabies published 1985 to 2015, only five sub-Saharan African countries were represented among the 48 studies included [16]. Where data do exist, they may be outdated and not representative of the current burden.

Second, routinely-collected data, and therefore GBD data, do not reflect actual disease burden. In countries where community-based prevalence survey data are available, the prevalence of scabies observed in these surveys is frequently substantially higher than the burden reported at the clinic level, and by the GBD study. For example, in the Solomon Islands, routine Ministry of Health clinic data identified 4759 cases of scabies in 2016 (total population of 584,000, corresponding to an incidence of 0.79% per year), in contrast to a detailed community-based survey in one province in the same year in which the prevalence was 19.2% [17]. This discrepancy may be because individuals within communities may not present with scabies (perhaps because it is 'normalized' or because effective treatments are often unavailable), or because there is under-diagnosis at clinics when patients do present [18].

Third, even when prevalence surveys are conducted, there is substantial heterogeneity in design and methods across studies. A key issue is the method used to diagnose scabies, which ranges from recovery of live mites by scraping of the skin, to a clinical diagnosis based on varying combinations of diagnostic features. This variability, noted even among scabies treatment trials [19], limits comparison of disease burden estimates across studies.

Fourth, there is limited evidence to determine the magnitude of the association between scabies and its complications. Available epidemiologic data suggest that, in highly endemic settings, at least 40% of impetigo lesions can be attributed to scabies, and an even higher proportion among younger children (71% in one study) [17,20–22]. The high attributable risk observed in epidemiologic studies is supported by trials of community control of scabies, as outlined below, where impetigo prevalence has been shown to fall consistently and substantially with reductions in scabies prevalence.

3. The Need for Surveillance and Control

The World Health Organization Department of Neglected Tropical Disease (NTD) Control designated scabies as an NTD for large-scale disease control action in 2017. This designation was in recognition of: (1) the large known burden and impact of scabies, justifying a global response; (2) the geographic distribution of scabies among disadvantaged populations living in tropical and subtropical regions; (3) the amenability of scabies to public health control efforts, especially noting the success of mass drug administration (MDA) for scabies (detailed below); and (4) the broad neglect of scabies across multiple research domains [23]. In 2018, the ninth meeting of the WHO NTD Strategic Technical Advisory Group Global Working Group on Monitoring and Evaluation of NTDs recognized that there is a priority need to develop resources to aid defining the global burden of scabies, and to provide guidance for countries and regions for public health approaches for scabies control, including in outbreak situations [24].

Guidance is required for assessment of disease burden at local, national and regional levels, and should include guidelines for standardised diagnosis and surveillance methodology. Consensus criteria for the diagnosis of scabies were recently developed using a four-round Delphi process among 34 international experts, under the auspices of the International Alliance for the Control of Scabies (IACS) [25]. The IACS Criteria include three levels and eight subcategories such that the criteria can be applied across a range of situations, from a dermatologist's office to a field survey in a resource-limited setting (Table 1) [26].

Table 1. Summary of 2018 IACS [1] criteria for the diagnosis of scabies [26].

Level	Criteria
A. Confirmed scabies	At least one of the following: A1: Mites, eggs or faeces on light microscopy of skin samples A2: Mites, eggs or faeces visualized on individual using high-powered imaging device A3: Mite visualized on individual using dermoscopy
B. Clinical scabies	At least one of the following: B1: Scabies burrows B2: Typical lesions affecting male genitalia B3 Typical lesions in a typical distribution and two history features
C. Suspected scabies	One of the following: C1: Typical lesions in a typical distribution and one history feature C2: Atypical lesions or atypical distribution and two history features
History features	H1: Itching H2: Close contact with an individual who has itching or typical lesions in a typical distribution
Notes:	*Diagnosis can be made at one of the three levels (A, B, or C)* *A diagnosis of clinical or suspected scabies should only be made if differential diagnoses are considered less likely than scabies.*

[1] IACS: International Alliance for the Control of Scabies.

The approach to community control for scabies is best aligned with the core strategies utilized by WHO Department of NTD Control: preventive chemotherapy using MDA, and/or innovative and intensified case management. Guidance around which approach to use will depend upon a number of factors, particularly disease burden at the community level. Therefore, feasible and accurate assessment of scabies prevalence will be crucial to inform an appropriate public health response, and also to monitor the effectiveness of this response. Below we outline the evidence to inform community control strategies for scabies, particularly MDA.

4. Community Control

The first reported public health initiatives to control scabies came from the San Blas islands (now known as the Guna Yala region) of Panama in the 1970s and 1980s. Scabies was introduced to the Guna populations and rapidly became endemic, with reported prevalences of 40–70% [27]. In a landmark series of studies, Taplin and colleagues compared approaches to scabies control in the islands. They found that treatment of all community members with 1% lindane resulted in a 98% cure rate at 10 weeks, whereas treatment of only those with clinically evident scabies had a lower effectiveness of 50% [28]. In areas where the entire community could not be treated, scabies was noted to return rapidly, leading the authors to conclude that, in those highly-endemic settings, 'treatment of individual patients without regard to community epidemiology is time consuming, and unlikely to have a significant impact in epidemic situations' [27]. Suspicion of developing mite resistance and the adverse effects profile of lindane then prompted the investigation of topical permethrin 5% for 756 residents on the island of Ticantiki. Following a MDA campaign with very high coverage, new arrivals to the island were treated and ongoing surveillance identified and treated new cases [27]. Scabies prevalence was reduced from 32% to below 2% and maintained for 3 years. Bacterial skin infection (impetigo) also declined from 32% to 1% in children without use of antibiotics. The permethrin-based MDA was well tolerated with few adverse events, but required a large project team for implementation. The team used directly observed applications, including to genital and breast areas, which may not be acceptable by some communities.

Drawing on the work in Panama, a control program commenced in five small, densely-populated islands in the Solomon Islands from 1997 to 2000 [29]. Use of topical treatments in this setting was considered 'so difficult as to be unacceptable and impractical'. Reports of the effectiveness of ivermectin for the individual and mass treatment of scabies [30], and knowledge of safety as a MDA strategy for lymphatic filariasis and onchocerciasis [31,32], led to selection of oral ivermectin as the main treatment, offered to the whole population as MDA. Permethrin 5% cream was given to children weighing less than 15 kg and pregnant women. Henceforth, we refer to this strategy of using topical treatments for ivermectin-contraindicated groups as 'ivermectin-based MDA'. Children (but not adults) were then re-examined at 6-monthly intervals and those with scabies and their household contacts were re-treated. Returned travelers and visitors were also treated, even if asymptomatic. No additional antibiotics were used. Over the three years of observation, the prevalence of scabies in children reduced from 25% to less than 1%. The proportion of children with open sores, the median number of sores, and the proportion of children with microscopic hematuria also reduced significantly. In contrast to the Panama experience, where scabies resurgence was observed after disruption of permethrin supply, when 338 residents of the same communities in the Solomon Islands were examined for scabies more than 15 years later, only a single case of scabies was found [33].

An ecological study from northern Australia aimed to reduce scabies and secondary bacterial skin infection in five remote communities from 2004 to 2007 [34]. Permethrin 5% was offered annually to all community members, but application was not directly observed. Children aged less than 15 years were screened regularly and referred for treatment if scabies or impetigo were identified. Whereas the prevalence of bacterial skin infection reduced during the project, there was little effect on scabies. A nested study found that actual use of permethrin was low, with only 44% of contacts applying the cream. Those households that did apply the cream had a much lower rate of scabies transmission [35].

The first controlled study of MDA for scabies control was conducted in Fiji in 2012. Three small island groups were randomized to one of ivermectin-based MDA (with permethrin for contraindicated groups), permethrin-based MDA, or 'standard-care' (where all community members were screened and referred for treatment if diagnosed with scabies). The trial found that at 12 months after MDA, the prevalence of scabies reduced in the ivermectin group by 94% (from 32% to 2%), in the permethrin group by 62% (42% to 16%) and in the standard-care group by 49% (37% to 19%). Once again, a considerable reduction was observed in the prevalence of impetigo without additional use of antibiotic therapy, most notably in the ivermectin group, where impetigo prevalence fell by 67% (25% to 8%).

Similar results were seen in two recent studies in the Solomon Islands. A before-and-after study evaluated a single round of ivermectin-based MDA, offered to a population of 26,000, in combination with azithromycin MDA for trachoma control. The co-administration was well tolerated with no serious adverse events [36]. A smaller study, from a different region of the Solomon Islands, reported a reduction in scabies prevalence of greater than 90%, 12 months after ivermectin-based MDA [37].

However, in a single cohort study in a remote island community of Australia, ivermectin-based MDA was less effective. Two MDA campaigns were implemented, 12 months apart, for a population of approximately 1000. Scabies prevalence fell from a baseline of 4% to less than 1%, 6 months after MDA, then increased to 9% after 12 months. A second MDA was conducted at this time, and scabies prevalence fell to 2% when measured 6 months later. Factors identified that may have contributed to the results included a lower than anticipated baseline prevalence, a highly mobile population with many new arrivals to the community after the first MDA, and a cluster of new cases associated with a case of crusted scabies.

Ivermectin-MDA programs for other NTDs also provide opportunities to study the effect on scabies [38]. In Zanzibar, Tanzania, annual MDA with ivermectin and albendazole for lymphatic filariasis from 2001–2005 resulted in a 68–98% reduction in clinic presentations for scabies [39]. However, in a recent, prospective study from the Kongwa District of Tanzania, where the baseline prevalence of scabies was 4.4%, annual ivermectin MDA for lymphatic filariasis was associated with a smaller reduction in scabies prevalence, to 2.9% after 4 years [40]. The authors concluded that a greater effect on scabies prevalence may not have been observed because of the relatively low prevalence and because only a single dose was given.

In addition to these community control strategies, there is increasing evidence of the use of MDA for management of scabies outbreaks within closed institutions such as schools, prisons, hospitals, aged care facilities and refugee and displaced person camps [30,41–43]. Scabies outbreaks in these settings are often difficult to diagnose and manage [44–46]. Ivermectin-based MDA has also been employed in the control of large-scale, open outbreaks, such as the current, drought-associated epidemic in Ethiopia, where more than one million people have been affected, although evaluation of this public health intervention is not currently available [47].

5. Outstanding Issues

The combined evidence of these control strategies reveals several common themes. First, in contrast to treating individuals and contacts, MDA strategies appear highly effective in reducing the burden of both scabies and impetigo. This strategy has been particularly successful in island communities with a very high baseline prevalence. With adequate community consultation, ivermectin-based MDA has been widely accepted by communities, well tolerated by individuals, and appeared more effective than permethrin-based MDA. Second, the benefit of MDA in communities with a lower baseline prevalence is less clear, and suggests that a different strategy may be appropriate for communities with lower prevalence (for example, less than 5%). Third, the most effective strategies have been those where active surveillance and treatment of new cases and new arrivals to the community have been incorporated, but it remains unclear to what extent these additional measures are required to ensure sustainable program success. Finally, environmental control measures (such as the washing of linen and clothing, or insecticide spraying) have not formed a component of the most successful strategies, suggesting this labor-intensive and costly strategy may not be required for community control. For control of institutional outbreaks, particularly where individuals have crusted scabies, environmental measures, if feasible, may be warranted.

Despite the promise of studies on community control for scabies, there remain several important operational questions about how their findings should be implemented, and the expected impact of such interventions. As noted, MDA appears less successful in lower-prevalence settings, and it is not clear what prevalence of scabies, or other measure, should trigger consideration of MDA. Further investigation is required to determine the optimal strategy for MDA. It is unclear whether one dose of ivermectin per MDA round is sufficient, or whether a second dose is required after 7–14 days, as is clinically recommended when using ivermectin for individual case treatment, due to its inability to kill the mite eggs [48]. The number and frequency of MDA rounds, when to stop, and duration of surveillance after stopping are all unknown. Modelling research could play an important role in this area, as for other NTDs [49–51]. The treatment of young children and pregnant women is critical for reducing transmission because these groups harbor a disproportionate burden of disease. However, because of current limitations on ivermectin use, they can only receive topical treatments, which are less practical. There is some evidence that ivermectin may be safe in these groups [52,53], but definitive research and development of pediatric-friendly formulations are needed. Further work on the feasibility and acceptability of MDA programs by communities in various settings is also required.

Standardized methods for diagnosis and mapping are required, possibly building on the 2018 IACS criteria, which need validation and testing in a variety of settings [26]. Investment into basic scientific research is required, including the development of diagnostic tests, ideally point of care tests for low-resource settings [54,55]. In lower-prevalence settings, or where MDA may be unrequired or infeasible, different strategies need to be developed and evaluated, including mass treatment of high-risk groups, or enhanced surveillance and intensified case management. Simplified, integrated clinical care pathways [56,57], and strategies such as teledermatology [58–60] may have an important role in providing high quality care to remote areas. Distinct strategies are also required for closed outbreaks in both developed and resource-limited settings. Although MDA programs do not place huge selective pressures on the microorganisms they target, ongoing monitoring for potential mite resistance to ivermectin and topical agents is important [61–64].

The impacts of scabies control programs need further evaluation, as this will inform policy makers and stakeholders of the likely health and economic benefits of the program. In particular, understanding the impact of reducing scabies and impetigo on improving quality of life and reducing downstream health complications such as skin and soft tissue infections, sepsis, and rheumatic heart disease [25]. Understanding these outcomes will facilitate cost-effectiveness evaluations in a range of settings. Research into the understanding and conception of scabies and impetigo within communities, followed by community awareness and engagement strategies, will be crucial for programmatic success.

While MDA with ivermectin appears highly effective, there are disadvantages to its use, including the apparent need for two doses, as outlined above. Moxidectin is an oral compound related to ivermectin, and was recently approved by the United States Food and Drug Administration for treatment of onchocerciasis [65]. Moxidectin has a much longer half-life than ivermectin, spanning the entire life cycle of the scabies mite [66,67]. In a preclinical treatment study using a porcine model for scabies, a single dose of moxidectin was more effective than two doses of ivermectin [68]. Clinical studies in humans are now planned, with a view to developing moxidectin as a single-dose treatment for scabies [67,69]. If clinical development is successful, moxidectin would be a very attractive option for community control of scabies because it would obviate the need for a second dose and reduce the risk of early re-infestation. Alternative topical treatments may also be required if resistance to permethrin becomes problematic [64,70].

Finally, scabies control should not occur in a vacuum. There are a number of opportunities for integration of scabies control with other NTDs, especially around the use of ivermectin [71,72]. Examples include successful co-mapping of scabies prevalence with other NTDs [17,73], and co-administration of ivermectin and azithromycin MDA with evaluation of multiple endpoints [36,37]. The roll-out of triple therapy (ivermectin, diethylcarbamazine, and albendazole) for the control of lymphatic filariasis [74,75] presents further opportunities to integrate evaluation of impact of this strategy on scabies.

6. Conclusions

In 2018, WHO recognized the need for 'a global strategy for scabies control' [24]. Such a strategy would align with the United Nations Sustainable Development Goals, including Target 3.3 to end the epidemic of NTDs (among other diseases) by 2030 [76]. Community control will be a central component of such a strategy, but broader progress will require consideration of several interrelated issues, including: engagement with key stakeholders at national, regional, and global levels to develop a coordinated, international framework; integration with existing NTD programs to leverage efficiency and cost-effectiveness of scabies control; provision of guidelines for monitoring and evaluation of programs; securement of drug supply at large scale; development of funding partnerships; and advancement of a research agenda, including operational research as outlined above, and research into improved diagnostics, new treatments (including moxidectin), and mite resistance monitoring.

Author Contributions: Conceptualization, D.E.; Writing—Original Draft Preparation, D.E. and A.C.S.; Writing—Review and Editing, D.E. and A.C.S.

Funding: This research received no external funding.

Acknowledgments: We acknowledge the contribution of Myra Hardy. The clinical photograph is provided courtesy of Daniel Mason. Informed consent was obtained and confidentiality maintained in accordance with the ethical review committee requirements.

Conflicts of Interest: The authors declare no conflict of interest.

References

1. Hay, R.J.; Steer, A.C.; Engelman, D.; Walton, S. Scabies in the developing world—Its prevalence, complications, and management. *Clin. Microbiol. Infect.* **2012**, *18*, 313–323. [CrossRef] [PubMed]
2. Chosidow, O. Clinical practices. Scabies. *New Engl. J. Med.* **2006**, *354*, 1718–1727. [CrossRef] [PubMed]
3. Davis, J.S.; McGloughlin, S.; Tong, S.Y.; Walton, S.F.; Currie, B.J. A novel clinical grading scale to guide the management of crusted scabies. *PLoS Negl. Trop. Dis.* **2013**, *7*, e2387. [CrossRef] [PubMed]
4. Walton, S.F.; Beroukas, D.; Roberts-Thomson, P.; Currie, B.J. New insights into disease pathogenesis in crusted (Norwegian) scabies: The skin immune response in crusted scabies. *Br. J. Dermatol.* **2008**, *158*, 1247–1255. [CrossRef] [PubMed]
5. Worth, C.; Heukelbach, J.; Fengler, G.; Walter, B.; Lisenfeld, O.; Feldmeier, H. Impaired quality of life in adults and children with scabies from an impoverished community in Brazil. *Int. J. Dermatol.* **2012**, *51*, 275–282. [CrossRef] [PubMed]
6. Hofstraat, K.; van Brakel, W.H. Social stigma towards neglected tropical diseases: A systematic review. *Int. Health* **2016**, *8* (Suppl. 1), i53–i70. [CrossRef]
7. Olsen, J.R.; Gallacher, J.; Finlay, A.Y.; Piguet, V.; Francis, N.A. Quality of life impact of childhood skin conditions measured using the Children's Dermatology Life Quality Index (CDLQI): A meta-analysis. *Br. J. Dermatol.* **2016**, *174*, 853–861. [CrossRef] [PubMed]
8. Steer, A.C.; Jenney, A.W.; Kado, J.; Batzloff, M.R.; La Vincente, S.; Waqatakirewa, L.; Mulholland, E.K.; Carapetis, J.R. High burden of impetigo and scabies in a tropical country. *PLoS Negl. Trop. Dis.* **2009**, *3*, e467. [CrossRef] [PubMed]

9. Swe, P.M.; Zakrzewski, M.; Kelly, A.; Krause, L.; Fischer, K. Scabies mites alter the skin microbiome and promote growth of opportunistic pathogens in a porcine model. *PLoS Negl. Trop. Dis.* **2014**, *8*, e2897. [CrossRef] [PubMed]

10. Swe, P.M.; Fischer, K. A scabies mite serpin interferes with complement-mediated neutrophil functions and promotes staphylococcal growth. *PLoS Negl. Trop. Dis.* **2014**, *8*, e2928. [CrossRef] [PubMed]

11. Hay, R.J.; Steer, A.C.; Chosidow, O.; Currie, B.J. Scabies: A suitable case for a global control initiative. *Curr. Opin. Infect. Dis.* **2013**, *26*, 107–109. [CrossRef] [PubMed]

12. Parks, T.; Smeesters, P.R.; Steer, A.C. Streptococcal skin infection and rheumatic heart disease. *Curr. Opin. Infect. Dis.* **2012**, *25*, 145–153. [CrossRef] [PubMed]

13. Thornley, S.; Marshall, R.; Jarrett, P.; Sundborn, G.; Reynolds, E.; Schofield, G. Scabies is strongly associated with acute rheumatic fever in a cohort study of Auckland children. *J. Paediatr. Child Health* **2018**, *54*, 625–632. [CrossRef] [PubMed]

14. GBD 2015 Disease and Injury Incidence and Prevalence Collaborators. Global, regional, and national incidence, prevalence, and years lived with disability for 310 diseases and injuries, 1990–2015: A systematic analysis for the Global Burden of Disease Study 2015. *Lancet* **2016**, *388*, 1545–1602. [CrossRef]

15. Karimkhani, C.; Colombara, D.V.; Drucker, A.M.; Norton, S.A.; Hay, R.; Engelman, D.; Steer, A.; Whitfeld, M.; Naghavi, M.; Dellavalle, R.P. The global burden of scabies: A cross-sectional analysis from the Global Burden of Disease Study 2015. *Lancet Infect. Dis.* **2017**, *17*, 1247–1254. [CrossRef]

16. Romani, L.; Steer, A.C.; Whitfeld, M.J.; Kaldor, J.M. Prevalence of scabies and impetigo worldwide: A systematic review. *Lancet Infect. Dis.* **2015**, *15*, 960–967. [CrossRef]

17. Mason, D.S.; Marks, M.; Sokana, O.; Solomon, A.W.; Mabey, D.C.; Romani, L.; Kaldor, J.; Steer, A.C.; Engelman, D. The prevalence of scabies and impetigo in the solomon islands: A population-based survey. *PLoS Negl. Trop. Dis.* **2016**, *10*, e0004803. [CrossRef] [PubMed]

18. Yeoh, D.K.; Anderson, A.; Cleland, G.; Bowen, A.C. Are scabies and impetigo 'normalised'? A cross-sectional comparative study of hospitalised children in northern Australia assessing clinical recognition and treatment of skin infections. *PLoS Negl. Trop. Dis.* **2017**, *11*, e0005726. [CrossRef] [PubMed]

19. Thompson, M.J.; Engelman, D.; Gholam, K.; Fuller, L.C.; Steer, A.C. Systematic review of the diagnosis of scabies in therapeutic trials. *Clin. Exp. Dermatol.* **2017**, *42*, 481–487. [CrossRef] [PubMed]

20. Romani, L.; Whitfeld, M.J.; Koroivueta, J.; Kama, M.; Wand, H.; Tikoduadua, L.; Tuicakau, M.; Koroi, A.; Ritova, R.; Andrews, R.; et al. The epidemiology of scabies and impetigo in relation to demographic and residential characteristics: Baseline findings from the Skin Health Intervention Fiji Trial. *Am. J. Trop. Med. Hyg.* **2017**, *97*, 845–850. [CrossRef] [PubMed]

21. Romani, L.; Koroivueta, J.; Steer, A.C.; Kama, M.; Kaldor, J.M.; Wand, H.; Hamid, M.; Whitfeld, M.J. Scabies and impetigo prevalence and risk factors in Fiji: A national survey. *PLoS Negl. Trop. Dis.* **2015**, *9*, e0003452. [CrossRef] [PubMed]

22. Aung, P.T.Z.; Cuningham, W.; Hwang, K.; Andrews, R.M.; Carapetis, J.R.; Kearns, T.; Clucas, D.; McVernon, J.; Simpson, J.A.; Tong, S.Y.C.; et al. Scabies and risk of skin sores in remote Australian Aboriginal communities: A self-controlled case series study. *PLoS Negl. Trop. Dis.* **2018**, *12*, e0006668. [CrossRef] [PubMed]

23. World Health Organization. Report of the Tenth Meeting of the WHO Strategic and Technical Advisory Group for Neglected Tropical Diseases. 2018. Available online: http://www.who.int/neglected_diseases/NTD_STAG_report_2017.pdf?ua=1 (accessed on 17 March 2018).

24. World Health Organization. 9th NTD-STAG Global Working Group Meeting on Monitoring and Evaluation of Neglected Tropical Diseases. 2018. Available online: http://www.who.int/neglected_diseases/events/STAG_Working_Group_on_Monitoring_Evaluation/en/ (accessed on 12 August 2018).

25. Engelman, D.; Kiang, K.; Chosidow, O.; McCarthy, J.; Fuller, C.; Lammie, P.; Hay, R.; Steer, A. Members of the International Alliance for The Control of Scabies. Toward the global control of human scabies: Introducing the International Alliance for the Control of Scabies. *PLoS Negl. Trop. Dis.* **2013**, *7*, e2167. [CrossRef] [PubMed]

26. Engelman, D.; Fuller, L.C.; Steer, A.C. Consensus criteria for the diagnosis of scabies: A Delphi study of International experts. *PLoS Negl. Trop. Dis.* **2018**, *12*, e0006549. [CrossRef] [PubMed]

27. Taplin, D.; Porcelain, S.L.; Meinking, T.L.; Athey, R.L.; Chen, J.A.; Castillero, P.M.; Sanchez, R. Community control of scabies: A model based on use of permethrin cream. *Lancet* **1991**, *337*, 1016–1018. [CrossRef]

28. Taplin, D.; Arrue, C.; Walker, J.; Roth, W.; Rivera, A. Eradication of scabies with a single treatment schedule. *J. Am. Acad. Dermatol.* **1983**, *9*, 546–550. [CrossRef]

29. Lawrence, G.; Leafasia, J.; Sheridan, J.; Hills, S.; Wate, J.; Wate, C.; Montgomery, J.; Pandeya, N.; Purdie, D. Control of scabies, skin sores and haematuria in children in the Solomon Islands: Another role for ivermectin. *Bull. World Health Organ.* **2005**, *83*, 34–42. [PubMed]

30. Leppard, B.; Naburi, A.E. The use of ivermectin in controlling an outbreak of scabies in a prison. *Br. J. Dermatol.* **2000**, *143*, 520–523. [CrossRef] [PubMed]

31. Pacque, M.; Munoz, B.; Greene, B.M.; White, A.T.; Dukuly, Z.; Taylor, H.R. Safety of and compliance with community-based ivermectin therapy. *Lancet* **1990**, *335*, 1377–1380. [CrossRef]

32. Pacque, M.C.; Dukuly, Z.; Greene, B.M.; Munoz, B.; Keyvan-Larijani, E.; Williams, P.N.; Taylor, H.R. Community-based treatment of onchocerciasis with ivermectin: Acceptability and early adverse reactions. *Bull. World Health Organ.* **1989**, *67*, 721–730. [PubMed]

33. Marks, M.; Taotao-Wini, B.; Satorara, L.; Engelman, D.; Nasi, T.; Mabey, D.C.; Steer, A.C. Long term control of scabies fifteen years after an intensive treatment programme. *PLoS Negl. Trop. Dis.* **2015**, *9*, e0004246. [CrossRef] [PubMed]

34. Andrews, R.M.; Kearns, T.; Connors, C.; Parker, C.; Carville, K.; Currie, B.J.; Carapetis, J.R. A regional initiative to reduce skin infections amongst aboriginal children living in remote communities of the Northern Territory, Australia. *PLoS Negl. Trop. Dis.* **2009**, *3*, e554. [CrossRef] [PubMed]

35. La Vincente, S.; Kearns, T.; Connors, C.; Cameron, S.; Carapetis, J.; Andrews, R. Community management of endemic scabies in remote aboriginal communities of northern Australia: Low treatment uptake and high ongoing acquisition. *PLoS Negl. Trop. Dis.* **2009**, *3*, e444. [CrossRef] [PubMed]

36. Romani, L.; Marks, M.; Sokana, O.; Nasi, T.; Kamoriki, B.; Wand, H.; Whitfeld, M.; Engelman, D.; Solomon, A.W.; Steer, A.C.; et al. Feasibility and safety of mass drug co-administration with azithromycin and ivermectin for the control of neglected tropical diseases: A single-arm intervention trial. *Lancet Glob. Health* **2018**, in press.

37. Marks, M.; Toloka, H.; Baker, C.; Kositz, C.; Asugeni, J.; Puiahi, E.; Asugeni, R.; Azzopardi, K.; Diau, J.; Kaldor, J.M.; et al. Randomised trial of community treatment with azithromycin and ivermectin mass drug administration for control of scabies and impetigo. *Clin. Infect. Dis.* **2018**, in press. [CrossRef] [PubMed]

38. Engelman, D.; Martin, D.L.; Hay, R.J.; Chosidow, O.; McCarthy, J.S.; Fuller, L.C.; Steer, A.C. Opportunities to investigate the effects of ivermectin mass drug administration on scabies. *Parasit Vectors* **2013**, *6*, 106. [CrossRef] [PubMed]

39. Mohammed, K.A.; Deb, R.M.; Stanton, M.C.; Molyneux, D.H. Soil transmitted helminths and scabies in Zanzibar, Tanzania following mass drug administration for lymphatic filariasis—A rapid assessment methodology to assess impact. *Parasit Vectors* **2012**, *5*, 299. [CrossRef] [PubMed]

40. Martin, D.; Wiegand, R.; Goodhew, B.; Lammie, P.; Mkocha, H.; Kasubi, M. Impact of ivermectin mass drug administration for lymphatic filariasis on scabies in eight villages in Kongwa District, Tanzania. *Am. J. Trop. Med. Hyg.* **2018**, in press. [CrossRef] [PubMed]

41. Cassell, J.A.; Middleton, J.; Nalabanda, A.; Lanza, S.; Head, M.G.; Bostock, J.; Hewitt, K.; Jones, C.I.; Darley, C.; Karir, S.; et al. Scabies outbreaks in ten care homes for elderly people: A prospective study of clinical features, epidemiology, and treatment outcomes. *Lancet Infect. Dis.* **2018**, *18*, 894–902. [CrossRef]

42. Agrawal, S.; Puthia, A.; Kotwal, A.; Tilak, R.; Kunte, R.; Kushwaha, A.S. Mass scabies management in an orphanage of rural community: An experience. *Med. J. Armed Forces India* **2012**, *68*, 403–406. [CrossRef] [PubMed]

43. Beeres, D.T.; Ravensbergen, S.J.; Heidema, A.; Cornish, D.; Vonk, M.; Wijnholds, L.D.; Hendriks, J.J.H.; Kleinnijenhuis, J.; Omansen, T.F.; Stienstra, Y. Efficacy of ivermectin mass-drug administration to control scabies in asylum seekers in the Netherlands: A retrospective cohort study between January 2014–March 2016. *PLoS Negl. Trop. Dis.* **2018**, *12*, e0006401. [CrossRef] [PubMed]

44. White, L.C.; Lanza, S.; Middleton, J.; Hewitt, K.; Freire-Moran, L.; Edge, C.; Nicholls, M.; Rajan-Iyer, J.; Cassell, J.A. The management of scabies outbreaks in residential care facilities for the elderly in England: A review of current health protection guidelines. *Epidemiol. Infect.* **2016**, *144*, 3121–3130. [CrossRef] [PubMed]

45. Hewitt, K.A.; Nalabanda, A.; Cassell, J.A. Scabies outbreaks in residential care homes: Factors associated with late recognition, burden and impact. A mixed methods study in England. *Epidemiol. Infect.* **2015**, *143*, 1542–1551. [CrossRef] [PubMed]

46. Mounsey, K.E.; Murray, H.C.; King, M.; Oprescu, F. Retrospective analysis of institutional scabies outbreaks from 1984 to 2013: Lessons learned and moving forward. *Epidemiol. Infect.* **2016**, *144*, 2462–2471. [CrossRef] [PubMed]

47. WHO Africa. Ethiopia-Scabies Outbreak Response in Amhara Regional State. Available online: https://www.afro.who.int/news/ethiopia-scabies-outbreak-response-amhara-regional-state (accessed on 6 July 2018).

48. Currie, B.J.; McCarthy, J.S. Permethrin and ivermectin for scabies. *New Engl. J. Med.* **2010**, *362*, 717–725. [CrossRef] [PubMed]

49. Stolk, W.A.; Walker, M.; Coffeng, L.E.; Basanez, M.G.; de Vlas, S.J. Required duration of mass ivermectin treatment for onchocerciasis elimination in Africa: A comparative modelling analysis. *Parasit Vectors* **2015**, *8*, 552. [CrossRef] [PubMed]

50. Irvine, M.A.; Stolk, W.A.; Smith, M.E.; Subramanian, S.; Singh, B.K.; Weil, G.J.; Michael, E.; Hollingsworth, T.D. Effectiveness of a triple-drug regimen for global elimination of lymphatic filariasis: A modelling study. *Lancet Infect. Dis.* **2017**, *17*, 451–458. [CrossRef]

51. Lydeamore, M.J.; Campbell, P.T.; Regan, D.G.; Tong, S.Y.C.; Andrews, R.M.; Steer, A.C.; Romani, L.; Kaldor, J.M.; McVernon, J.; McCaw, J.M. A biological model of scabies infection dynamics and treatment informs mass drug administration strategies to increase the likelihood of elimination. *Math. Biosci.* **2018**, in press. [CrossRef] [PubMed]

52. Wilkins, A.L.; Steer, A.C.; Cranswick, N.; Gwee, A. Is it safe to use ivermectin in children less than five years of age and weighing less than 15 kg? *Arch. Dis. Child* **2018**, *103*, 514–519. [CrossRef] [PubMed]

53. Gyapong, J.O.; Chinbuah, M.A.; Gyapong, M. Inadvertent exposure of pregnant women to ivermectin and albendazole during mass drug administration for lymphatic filariasis. *Trop. Med. Int. Health* **2003**, *8*, 1093–1101. [CrossRef] [PubMed]

54. Walton, S.F.; Currie, B.J. Problems in diagnosing scabies, a global disease in human and animal populations. *Am. Soc. Rev.* **2007**, *20*, 268–279. [CrossRef] [PubMed]

55. Peeling, R.W.; Boeras, D.I.; Nkengasong, J. Re-imagining the future of diagnosis of neglected tropical diseases. *Comput. Struct. Biotechnol. J.* **2017**, *15*, 271–274. [CrossRef] [PubMed]

56. Mitjà, O.; Marks, M.; Bertran, L.; Kollie, K.; Argaw, D.; Fahal, A.; Fitzpatrick, C.; Fuller, C.; Garcia-Izquierdo, B.; Hay, R.; et al. Integrated control and management of neglected tropical diseases. *PLoS Negl. Trop. Dis.* **2017**, *11*, e0005136. [CrossRef] [PubMed]

57. World Health Organization. Recognizing Neglected Tropical Diseases through Changes on the Skin: A Training Guide for Front-Line Health Workers. 2018. Available online: http://apps.who.int/iris/bitstream/handle/10665/272723/9789241513531-eng.pdf (accessed on 12 August 2018).

58. Estrada, R.; Chavez-Lopez, G.; Estrada-Chavez, G.; Paredes-Solis, S. Specialized dermatological care for marginalized populations and education at the primary care level: Is community dermatology a feasible proposal? *Int. J. Dermatol.* **2012**, *51*, 1345–1350. [CrossRef] [PubMed]

59. Hay, R.; Estrada, R.; Grossmann, H. Managing skin disease in resource-poor environments-the role of community-oriented training and control programs. *Int. J. Dermatol.* **2011**, *50*, 558–563. [CrossRef] [PubMed]

60. Faye, O.; Bagayoko, C.; Dicko, A.; Cissé, L.; Berthé, S.; Traoré, B.; Fofana, Y.; Niang, M.; Traoré, S.; Karabinta, Y.; et al. A teledermatology pilot programme for the management of skin diseases in primary health care centres: Experiences from a resource-limited country (Mali, West Africa). *Trop. Med. Infect. Dis.* **2018**, *3*, 88. [CrossRef]

61. Currie, B.J.; Harumal, P.; McKinnon, M.; Walton, S.F. First documentation of in vivo and in vitro ivermectin resistance in *Sarcoptes scabiei*. *Clin. Infect. Dis.* **2004**, *39*, e8–e12. [CrossRef] [PubMed]

62. Mounsey, K.E.; Holt, D.C.; McCarthy, J.; Currie, B.J.; Walton, S.F. Scabies: Molecular perspectives and therapeutic implications in the face of emerging drug resistance. *Future Microbiol.* **2008**, *3*, 57–66. [CrossRef] [PubMed]

63. McNair, C.M. Ectoparasites of medical and veterinary importance: Drug resistance and the need for alternative control methods. *J. Pharm Pharmacol.* **2015**, *67*, 351–363. [CrossRef] [PubMed]

64. Khalil, S.; Abbas, O.; Kibbi, A.G.; Kurban, M. Scabies in the age of increasing drug resistance. *PLoS Negl. Trop. Dis.* **2017**, *11*, e0005920. [CrossRef] [PubMed]

65. Opoku, N.O.; Bakajika, D.K.; Kanza, E.M.; Howard, H.; Mambandu, G.L.; Nyathirombo, A.; Nigo, M.M.; Kasonia, K.; Masembe, S.L.; Mumbere, M.; et al. Single dose moxidectin versus ivermectin for *Onchocerca volvulus* infection in Ghana, Liberia, and the Democratic Republic of the Congo: A randomised, controlled, double-blind phase 3 trial. *Lancet* **2018**, in press. [CrossRef]

66. Cotreau, M.M.; Warren, S.; Ryan, J.L.; Fleckenstein, L.; Vanapalli, S.R.; Brown, K.R.; Rock, D.; Chen, C.Y.; Schwertschlag, U.S. The antiparasitic moxidectin: Safety, tolerability, and pharmacokinetics in humans. *J. Clin. Pharmacol.* **2003**, *43*, 1108–1115. [CrossRef] [PubMed]

67. Mounsey, K.E.; Bernigaud, C.; Chosidow, O.; McCarthy, J.S. Prospects for moxidectin as a new oral treatment for human scabies. *PLoS Negl. Trop. Dis.* **2016**, *10*, e0004389. [CrossRef] [PubMed]

68. Bernigaud, C.; Fang, F.; Fischer, K.; Lespine, A.; Aho, L.; Dreau, D.; Kelly, A.; Sutra, J.F.; Moreau, F.; Lilin, T.; et al. Preclinical study of single-dose moxidectin, a new oral treatment for scabies: Efficacy, safety, and pharmacokinetics compared to two-dose ivermectin in a porcine model. *PLoS Negl. Trop. Dis.* **2016**, *10*, e0005030. [CrossRef] [PubMed]

69. Medicines Development for Global Health. Moxidectin Program. 2018. Available online: https://www.medicinesdevelopment.com/development-programs.htm (accessed on 3 August 2018).

70. Thomas, J.; Christenson, J.K.; Walker, E.; Baby, K.E.; Peterson, G.M. Scabies - An ancient itch that is still rampant today. *J. Clin. Pharm. Ther.* **2017**, *42*, 793–799. [CrossRef] [PubMed]

71. Engelman, D.; Fuller, L.C.; Solomon, A.W.; McCarthy, J.S.; Hay, R.J.; Lammie, P.J.; Steer, A.C. Opportunities for integrated control of neglected tropical diseases that affect the skin. *Trends Parasitol.* **2016**, *32*, 843–854. [CrossRef] [PubMed]

72. Hay, R. Skin NTDs: An opportunity for integrated care. *Trans. Royal Soc. Trop. Med. Hyg.* **2016**, *110*, 679–680. [CrossRef] [PubMed]

73. Yotsu, R.R.; Kouadio, K.; Vagamon, B.; N'Guessan, K.; Akpa, A.J.; Yao, A.; Ake, J.; Abbet, R.; Tchamba Agbor Agbor, B.; Bedimo, R.; et al. Skin disease prevalence study in schoolchildren in rural Cote d'Ivoire: Implications for integration of neglected skin diseases (skin NTDs). *PLoS Negl. Trop. Dis.* **2018**, *12*, e0006489. [CrossRef] [PubMed]

74. Thomsen, E.K.; Sanuku, N.; Baea, M.; Satofan, S.; Maki, E.; Lombore, B.; Schmidt, M.S.; Siba, P.M.; Weil, G.J.; Kazura, J.W.; et al. Efficacy, safety, and pharmacokinetics of coadministered diethylcarbamazine, albendazole, and ivermectin for treatment of bancroftian filariasis. *Clin. Infect. Dis.* **2016**, *62*, 334–341. [CrossRef] [PubMed]

75. Fischer, P.U.; King, C.L.; Jacobson, J.A.; Weil, G.J. Potential value of triple drug therapy with ivermectin, diethylcarbamazine, and albendazole (IDA) to accelerate elimination of lymphatic filariasis and onchocerciasis in Africa. *PLoS Negl. Trop. Dis.* **2017**, *11*, e0005163. [CrossRef] [PubMed]

76. Fitzpatrick, C.; Engels, D. Leaving no one behind: A neglected tropical disease indicator and tracers for the Sustainable Development Goals. *Int. Health* **2016**, *8*, i15–i18. [CrossRef] [PubMed]

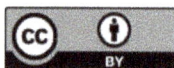

Tropical Medicine and Infectious Disease

MDPI

Review

The Skin—A Common Pathway for Integrating Diagnosis and Management of NTDs

David John Chandler *[iD] and Lucinda Claire Fuller

Dermatology Department, Brighton General Hospital, East Sussex BN2 3EW, UK; claire.fuller@nhs.net
* Correspondence: davidchandler1@nhs.net; Tel.: +44-(0)12-7366-5140

Received: 9 August 2018; Accepted: 5 September 2018; Published: 10 September 2018

Abstract: Many of the neglected tropical diseases (NTDs) have major skin manifestations. These skin-related NTDs or 'skin NTDs' cause significant morbidity and economic hardship in some of the poorest communities worldwide. We draw attention to the collective burden of skin disease and suggest that the skin be used as a platform for the integration of control activities for NTDs. The opportunities for integration are numerous, ranging from diagnosis and disease mapping to mass drug administration and morbidity management. The dermatology community has an important role to play, and will be expected to support research and control activities globally.

Keywords: integration; neglected tropical diseases; disease mapping; mass drug administration; morbidity management

---

1. Introduction

Skin and subcutaneous diseases account for substantial morbidity worldwide, with a high burden of disease in resource-poor tropical regions [1,2]. Neglected tropical diseases (NTDs) are a group of communicable diseases that are present throughout the tropical and subtropical regions of the world, where they affect the poorest and most marginalised communities. The World Health Organization (WHO) portfolio of NTDs comprises a list of 20 diseases that affect more than 2 billion people worldwide [3].

Eighteen of the twenty NTDs on the WHO list have recognised skin manifestations. In some cases, involvement of the skin is the primary manifestation of the disease; examples include Buruli ulcer, leprosy, scabies, and mycetoma. In other cases, skin involvement may be an associated clinical feature, such as the urticarial rash that can occur in schistosomiasis, soil-transmitted helminthiases, and foodborne trematodiases. The only NTDs that do not have skin manifestations are rabies and trachoma. In addition, several other diseases affecting the skin, whilst not prioritised on the WHO list, are recognised as NTDs; examples include cutaneous larva migrans, impetigo and cellulitis, podoconiosis, tropical ulcer, and tungiasis.

These skin-related NTDs or 'skin NTDs' frequently result in physical impairment and disfigurement, which can lead to life-long disability, inability to work, social stigmatisation, and discrimination. Examples of disability include permanent nerve damage and limb deformity in leprosy, advanced lymphoedema and hydrocele in lymphatic filariasis, severe itching and hanging groin in onchocerciasis, and amputation in cases of severe mycetoma. However, the true global burden of many skin NTDs is poorly understood. Data from the Global Burden of Disease Study (GBD) 2013 identified lymphatic filariasis and scabies as the 4th and 5th leading causes of morbidity out of all NTDs, resulting in 2.02 million and 1.71 million years lived with disability (YLD), respectively; however, these estimates are likely to be conservative [1,3,4].

Fungal diseases have been neglected for many years, with very little funding made available for research and control activities [5]. Consequently, high-quality data on the epidemiology and associated morbidity of superficial and deep mycoses do not exist, which makes it difficult to advocate for increased funding. The addition of this disease group to the WHO list of NTDs in 2017 should assist in raising its profile in the global health agenda; the same applies for scabies, which joined the WHO list at the same time.

The impoverishing effects of NTDs are amplified in poor and vulnerable communities; physical labour is often the main source of income, and social protection mechanisms (insurance against ill-health and disability) are not accessible [6]. In rural India, households with a family member affected by leprosy can incur catastrophic health expenditure, mostly as a result of loss of income due to chronic ill-health [7,8]. Significant health expenditure and productivity loss has also been demonstrated for other skin NTDs including podoconiosis and leishmaniasis [9–11].

Historically, disease control activities have operated within vertical programs that were set up to deal with specific priority diseases; however, these were resource intensive and inefficient. Integration offers a cost-effective and efficient approach for tackling groups of related conditions. Skin NTDs are frequently co-endemic in low-resource settings, and many of the available treatments and management strategies are beneficial for more than one condition; the skin has therefore been proposed as a common pathway to enhance the control of these neglected diseases.

From the growing literature on this subject, two key articles are worth highlighting. Engelman et al. discuss in detail many of the opportunities and challenges of integration [12]. In a paper that followed shortly after, an expert panel develop some of these ideas and offer practical advice on how to approach integration of surveillance and management activities for the skin NTDs [13].

The purpose of this review is to provide an update on the subject of skin NTDs and the opportunities for integration. We highlight examples where integration has been successful and draw attention to research questions that remain unanswered.

2. Methodology

We considered all types of publication and study design in our literature search; articles not written in English were excluded. We searched the following databases to July 2018: MEDLINE (from 1946), Embase (from 1947), and Allied & Complementary Medicine (from 1985). Core search terms included but were not limited to 'neglected tropical diseases', 'skin NTDs', 'integration', 'diagnosis', 'disease mapping', 'morbidity management', and 'mass drug administration'. We communicated with researchers active in this field to identify unpublished data and used the bibliographies of articles to expand our search.

3. Integrated Approach to Skin NTDs

An integrated approach to tackling skin NTDs offers many benefits, and the dermatology community has an important role to play in guiding this process. Integration in this context refers to combining activities for two or more diseases at the same time and in the same communities. Integration could be beneficial for several activities, from diagnosis and mapping to treatment and education, and these are discussed in more detail below.

4. Diagnosis

Skin disease is very common in resource-poor regions. Individuals frequently have more than one skin NTD, in addition to other, much more common skin conditions. Reliable diagnostic tests do not exist for many NTDs; therefore, diagnosis is based on clinical examination.

Clinical signs of skin NTDs are diverse; however, the diagnostic process can be simplified with the use of syndrome-based assessment tools. WHO have produced a training guide titled 'Recognising neglected tropical diseases through changes on the skin', which is intended to support front-line health workers without specialist knowledge of dermatology to detect skin changes suggestive of an underlying NTD [14]. Four major skin changes are identified: lumps, ulcers, swollen limbs, and patches. For each skin change there is a diagnostic flow-chart which guides the user towards a likely diagnosis and a decision on treatment or further assessment (referral).

The success of training health workers to identify skin NTDs has been demonstrated at the community level previously. Limited training of primary health care workers in Mali, focusing on leprosy and common skin diseases, resulted in significant improvements in diagnostic accuracy, appropriateness of referrals, and ability to correctly examine neurological (sensory) function, 12–18 months after the training was completed [15]. Traditional healers and those practising alternative systems of medicine are widely available in many African countries and throughout India, particularly in the rural communities, where they are easy to access and often a preferred source of treatment for health problems including leprosy [16]. Several studies have shown that it is both feasible and cost-effective to recruit traditional healers and train them to detect the signs of leprosy and refer suspected cases to specialist leprosy services [17–19]. Enhancing new case detection and avoiding delays to treatment are important goals of leprosy control. However, a recent article by Darlong et al. conducted in West Bengal, India, highlights delays to diagnosis in children with multibacillary leprosy, resulting in a significant number of cases of grade 2 disability at presentation [20]. All of the affected children in the study had leprosy-specific symptoms for more than 6 months before diagnosis, many of which involved visible skin changes such as ulceration or a skin patch. Strategies are needed to increase detection of these cases, including educational interventions that encourage earlier presentation to health services.

Integration of control activities for skin NTDs might offer further benefit by providing an operational framework through which other common (non-NTD) skin conditions can be detected and treated; however, the challenge this will provide should not be underestimated, and health workers in this setting should receive training in general dermatology. For example, it is important to appreciate that a hypopigmented skin patch has several causes, many of which are much more likely than leprosy, such as pityriasis versicolor, pityriasis alba, and achromic naevus. The importance of this particular point has been highlighted recently by several authors [21,22]. In a survey of skin NTDs, involving more than 13,000 schoolchildren aged 5 to 15 in Côte d'Ivoire, West Africa, the overall prevalence of skin disease was 25.6% [21]. Superficial mycoses were by far the most common diagnoses, and the majority of children were diagnosed with 2 or more skin conditions. Of 986 children examined by a dermatologist, the skin NTDs detected included one case of leprosy and 36 cases of scabies. Barogui and colleagues report similar findings from their experience of integrated control activities against Buruli ulcer, leprosy, and yaws in Benin, West Africa [22]. Trained health workers and community health volunteers identified 1106 patients with skin disease. Skin NTDs included only 15 cases of Buruli ulcer and 3 cases of leprosy. There were 185 suspected cases of yaws; however, these all tested negative using the point-of-care Dual Path Platform (DPP) syphilis assay.

An integrated approach to diagnosis offers the opportunity to detect multiple conditions in a single encounter. Vertical disease programs have a narrow focus and do not necessarily allow for detection and treatment of other important co-existent skin conditions. The majority of skin disease is accounted for by a few common conditions; these include bacterial skin infections (impetigo, boils), superficial mycoses, non-infective conditions such as eczema, and traumatic lesions. Algorithms for detecting and managing these skin conditions have been validated and applied in various settings and these could be applied in future integration efforts [23,24]. It would be appropriate and realistic for community-based health workers with limited dermatological training to focus on identifying and managing these common skin conditions for which relatively simple and effective treatments are available.

5. Disease Mapping and Surveillance

High-quality epidemiological data are lacking for many skin NTDs, and it is important for the success of integrated control efforts that this is addressed early. Disease mapping and identification of geographic areas of co-endemicity are important to determine disease burden and direct further research and control strategies. This step must take place before integrated management and control programmes can be planned and resources allocated. Consensus criteria for diagnosis of skin NTDs should be used, such as those available for podoconiosis [25] and, more recently, scabies [26].

Disease mapping refers to the collection of georeferenced data used to visualise the distribution and prevalence of a disease in space and time [27]. Maps are developed using a geographical information system (GIS) which allows storage, analysis, and presentation of spatial data. The African Programme for Onchocerciasis Control (APOC) was one of the earliest GIS-based mapping initiatives and has been used throughout Africa to identify priority areas for community treatment with ivermectin; APOC has also been used to map the distribution of *Loa loa* and identify areas of high prevalence where there is an increased risk of developing serious adverse events following treatment with ivermectin [28].

Integration of mapping and surveillance activities could be better suited to certain diseases, particularly those that share demographic and geographic preferences. Diseases causing lymphoedema provide a good example of where integration is suitable and where integrated mapping has been successful. Lymphoedema in the tropics has two main causes—lymphatic filariasis (LF), which is caused by infection with a parasitic nematode, predominantly *Wuchereria bancrofti*, and podoconiosis, which is caused by prolonged contact with irritant red clay soils derived from volcanic deposits.

Sime and colleagues describe their experience of the first integrated mapping of LF and podoconiosis, which captured almost 130,000 people from 1315 communities across 659 districts of Ethiopia during a 3-month period [29]. LF cases were identified by taking a blood sample and testing for circulating *Wuchereria bancrofti* antigen using an immunochromatographic card test (ICT). Podoconiosis was diagnosed clinically by excluding other causes of lymphoedema such as rheumatic heart disease, leprosy, and onchocerciasis. Smartphones were used for data collection; data were entered in real time and geographic coordinates were captured using an inbuilt geographic positioning system (GPS) function. The authors reported that using an integrated process was cost-effective and enabled rapid mapping of a larger geographical area than would otherwise have been achieved by using an individual disease survey. Recently, an integrated mapping exercise was conducted in Ethiopia, in 20 districts co-endemic for LF and podoconiosis, to identify all cases of lymphoedema [30]. More than 26,000 cases of lymphoedema and/or hydrocele were identified, and the majority of cases (>95%) had leg lymphoedema only, which could be due to LF or podoconiosis. These results will inform the planning and implementation of morbidity management and disability prevention (MMDP) services which are equally beneficial in both LF and podoconiosis.

Integrated mapping is more cost-effective than disease-specific mapping and allows for more precise mapping of co-endemic diseases and related conditions. In the Solomon Islands, Mason et al. conducted a cross-sectional study to assess the prevalence of scabies and impetigo [31], recruiting more than 1900 patients to the study; this was achieved by integrating data collection with an existing epidemiological study investigating clinical and serological markers of yaws [32].

6. Treatment

The last two decades have seen significant achievements in the control of a number of important tropical infections, including significant reductions in the prevalence of diseases such as lymphatic filariasis, guinea worm, and leprosy [33,34]. The successes of energetic vertical programmes are acknowledged; however, resource constraints have led to an increasing emphasis on integrating control activities.

Many of the opportunities for integrated treatment of skin NTDs exist for conditions that are suitable for control using mass drug administration (MDA), and, in particular, those that exhibit significant geographical overlap. Of note, seven of the most prevalent and debilitating NTDs have been the target of control efforts using integrated MDA; these include lymphatic filariasis, onchocerciasis, schistosomiasis, trachoma, and the three major soil-transmitted helminth infections (ascariasis, trichuriasis, and hookworm infection) [35]. Partnership between public and private organisations, multinational drug companies, and national ministries of health enabled the distribution of 'rapid-impact' packages of drugs throughout Africa, providing treatment for all seven of the NTDs at low cost. Ivermectin is highly effective at killing microfilariae in lymphatic filariasis and onchocerciasis, and was one of the drugs included in the rapid-impact package. Mostly due to drug company donations, it was possible to achieve a unit cost of US$0.40 per person annually, and in some cases even lower [35]. Data from the Global Burden of Disease (GBD) Study 2016 have shown considerable reductions in disease prevalence and burden (measured in DALYs) for six of the seven NTDs targeted by 'rapid-impact' integrated MDA over the last decade [36].

Ivermectin is widely recognised as a broad-spectrum antiparasitic drug, capable of killing parasites both inside and outside the body. It is particularly useful for the control of several skin NTDs. It is the treatment of choice for strongyloidiasis, and it is highly effective against scabies, pediculosis capitis, and cutaneous larva migrans [37,38]. Collateral benefits of ivermectin MDA have been observed in various settings, for example, in the lymphatic filariasis and onchocerciasis control programmes, where it was responsible for reducing the prevalence of tungiasis and scabies [38–40]. Ivermectin is also an effective treatment for gnathostomiasis and soil-transmitted helminthiasis. Improving access to low-cost generic ivermectin and broadening the licensed indications for use are some of the challenges to be addressed in order to realise the full public health potential of this drug. Studies of ivermectin MDA for scabies control have shown that the drug has a very good safety profile [41]. Although robust safety data in pregnant women and children under 5 years of age are lacking, the few published studies have failed to identify any difference in birth defects or developmental status in children born to women inadvertently treated with ivermectin during pregnancy [42–44]. Monitoring of existing ivermectin MDA programmes for safety outcomes will add to our understanding.

Moxidectin is a second-generation macrocyclic lactone related to ivermectin. It has demonstrated superior efficacy over ivermectin for the treatment of onchocerciasis [45], and recently received FDA approval (June 2018) for patients 12 years of age and older. In addition, moxidectin looks promising as a treatment for scabies. It has enhanced bioavailability (half-life of over 20 days, compared with 14 h for ivermectin) and better skin retention, meaning that a single-dose regimen may be possible [46]. Moxidectin is superior to ivermectin against the scabies mite in vitro [47]; however, clinical studies are required in order to establish suitable doses and evaluate efficacy in cases of scabies.

Integrated treatment programs can be particularly advantageous for diseases that can be treated using a single medication, as this removes the possibility of drug interactions and adverse safety events that may arise from coadministration of multiple drugs. For example, both yaws and trachoma can be targeted by mass administration of azithromycin, although the recommended doses for each are different—20 mg/kg for trachoma, and 30 mg/kg for yaws. However, a study conducted in the Solomon Islands showed that the lower dose (20 mg/kg) was effective against yaws; no active cases of yaws were identified following a single round of treatment using the lower dose in a previously endemic population [32]. This supports the argument for merging and simplifying treatment algorithms where possible and integrating mass treatment of these conditions.

On the other hand, mass treatment using more than one drug has the benefit of targeting a greater number of diseases and therefore delivering a greater impact to the health of the affected population. The effectiveness of ivermectin against highly symptomatic skin diseases such as scabies is an important factor in promoting adherence with further rounds of treatment in MDA programmes [48]; administering ivermectin together with other drugs against co-endemic skin NTDs would likely have a positive effect on overall compliance. Ivermectin and albendazole can be administered together safely, and there is evidence that they can be combined safely with other medications including azithromycin, praziquantel, and diethylcarbamazine (DEC) [49–51].

7. Morbidity Management

All of the skin NTDs have the potential to cause chronic ill-health and long term disability, even after successful treatment of the underlying cause. The patient with treated lepromatous leprosy may have disabling limb deformity and experience recurrent and prolonged episodes of immune-mediated inflammation (erythema nodosum leprosum or type 2 leprosy reaction) for many years after treatment. The patient with treated lymphatic filariasis may suffer with debilitating lymphoedema and repeated episodes of ill-health due to acute dermatolymphangioadenitis (ADLA). The dermatology community can support these patients through interventions that focus on achieving healthy skin and preventing chronic disease complications.

The burden of disease resulting from chronic complications of skin NTDs is poorly understood, and more data are needed to support political advocacy and fundraising. Efforts are being made to address this, for example, through the development of a toolkit for monitoring morbidity and disability across multiple NTDs [52]. The prototype toolkit was validated in Northeast Brazil in patients with Chagas' disease (American trypanosomiasis), leishmaniasis, leprosy, and schistosomiasis, where it was well accepted.

Community dermatology is the branch of dermatology that addresses skin health at the population level, and this is perhaps most relevant in the poorest communities where the burden of skin disease is high and skin NTDs are prevalent [53,54]. It focuses on providing low-cost interventions for the most common skin diseases, and includes strategies for managing wounds and lymphoedema that are applicable to many skin NTDs.

Simple hygiene-based interventions, typically involving daily washing of affected limbs with soap and water, are known to be effective for the management of lymphoedema in LF-endemic areas, resulting in a reduced incidence of ADLA [55]. Recent data have shown that a low-cost lymphoedema self-care package is effective in reducing the frequency and duration of ADLA in podoconiosis [56]. In this study, the package of care included instructions for foot hygiene, skin care, bandaging, exercises, and use of socks and shoes, and this was reinforced by trained members of the local community at regular monthly meetings. Patients in the treatment group experienced 4.5 fewer episodes of ADLA per person-year compared with the control group who received no intervention.

Lymphatic filariasis (LF) and podoconiosis benefit from a very similar management, and in countries where there is a high burden of both diseases, it is sensible that morbidity management activities should be integrated in order to reduce programme costs and expand coverage. Deribe and colleagues describe the successful integration of these services in Ethiopia [57], where more than 500 government-employed health workers from 24 districts were trained by lymphoedema experts on integrated morbidity management and disability prevention for LF and podoconiosis. Trained health workers follow a management algorithm and deliver a defined package of care to patients, similar to that described earlier [56], focusing on daily hygiene measures, use of emollients to restore skin function, leg elevation, exercise, use of socks and shoes, and bandaging if required. Water, sanitation, and hygiene (WASH) interventions are important for the control of other major NTDs, including trachoma, soil-transmitted helminths, and schistosomiasis [58–60], highlighting further possibilities for integrated activities particularly where diseases are co-endemic.

Self-help group interventions are beneficial in many areas of medicine, and could be a useful approach to improve health behaviours for the management of morbidity associated with skin NTDs, with the potential for empowering 'expert patients' to take a lead role. For example, women's groups practising participatory learning and action (PLA) on preventive and care-seeking behaviours are a cost-effective strategy to improve maternal and neonatal survival in low-resource settings [61]. The potential benefits for the skin NTDs are numerous, and range from improved self-care behaviours in the management of lymphoedema to earlier presentation and treatment-seeking in new cases of leprosy in children. A recent study conducted in Nepal showed that the integration of self-care for filarial lymphoedema into existing community leprosy self-help groups was feasible, and attitudes towards integration were positive [62]. Opportunities were identified for LF-affected participants to increase their knowledge of self-care and access to health services.

Stigma and social isolation are a major problem for many NTDs, not least those that have highly visible skin manifestations. The severe stigmatisation of persons affected by leprosy is well described; however, this disability extends to several other skin NTDs including lymphatic

Trop. Med. Infect. Dis. **2018**, *3*, 101

filariasis, podoconiosis, Buruli ulcer, onchocerciasis, and leishmaniasis, with similar health-related and psychosocial consequences [63]. Importantly, the reasons for stigmatisation across the different NTDs are remarkably similar; these include appearance, fear of contagion, being a burden to the family, and the inability to fulfil gender roles. It has been suggested, therefore, that integrated approaches to reduce stigmatisation may be feasible and more efficient than disease-specific interventions.

Integrated morbidity management services will also offer an opportunity to promote skin health more broadly. The GBD 2013 data on skin diseases show that dermatitis accounts for the largest global burden, with high DALY rates in many regions of the world, but particularly in central sub-Saharan Africa. The ability to recognise a failing epidermis and prescribe an emollient would be beneficial for many patients, including those with dermatitis and those affected by many of the skin NTDs.

8. Conclusions and Future Directions

The grouping together of NTDs that affect the skin draws attention to the significant burden of skin disease that occurs almost exclusively in impoverished populations in the developing world. The concept of skin NTDs is useful for a number of reasons. It facilitates the integration of control activities, from diagnostic processes to community mass drug administration. It creates a strong argument for funding for research and control activities, considering the collective burden of disease. Finally, it places the dermatology community in a strong position to help in the fight against NTDs. Dermatologists can contribute through developing appropriate clinical guidelines, training health workers, coordinating research, and guiding the design and implementation of control activities. This in turn will foster better research relationships internationally and strengthen the fields of tropical and global health dermatology. There is a growing body of literature describing experiences of integration in a variety of settings, offering explanations behind the successes and failures, and it will be important going forward to learn from these experiences. Integrated fieldwork activities, from disease mapping to mass treatment, must be well planned and supported by relevant political bodies and funding agencies. The integrated control of skin NTDs, led by the dermatology community, has the potential to strengthen health systems in resource-poor settings and improve skin health for millions of the world's most disadvantaged people.

Author Contributions: D.J.C. and L.C.F. contributed equally to all aspects of this work.

Funding: This research received no external funding.

Conflicts of Interest: The authors declare no conflict of interest.

References

1. Karimkhani, C.; Dellavalle, R.P.; Coffeng, L.E.; Flohr, C.; Hay, R.J.; Langan, S.M.; Nsoesie, E.O.; Ferrari, A.J.; Erskine, H.E.; Silverberg, J.I.; et al. Global skin disease morbidity and mortality: An update from the Global Burden of Disease Study 2013. *JAMA Dermatol.* **2017**, *153*, 406–412. [CrossRef] [PubMed]
2. Clucas, D.B.; Carville, K.S.; Connors, C.; Currie, B.J.; Carapetis, J.R.; Andrews, R.M. Disease burden and health-care clinic attendances for young children in remote Aboriginal communities of northern Australia. *Bull. World Health Organ.* **2008**, *86*, 275–281. [PubMed]
3. Herricks, J.R.; Hotez, P.J.; Wanga, V.; Coffeng, L.E.; Haagsma, J.A.; Basáñez, M.G.; Buckle, G.; Budke, C.M.; Carabin, H.; Fèvre, E.M.; et al. The Global Burden of Disease Study 2013: What does it mean for the NTDs? *PLoS Negl. Trop. Dis.* **2017**, *11*, e0005424. [CrossRef] [PubMed]
4. Hay, R.J.; Johns, N.E.; Williams, H.C.; Bolliger, I.W.; Dellavalle, R.P.; Margolis, D.J.; Marks, R.; Naldi, L.; Weinstock, M.A.; Wulf, S.K.; et al. The Global Burden of Skin Disease in 2010: An analysis of the prevalence and impact of skin conditions. *J. Investig. Dermatol.* **2014**, *134*, 1527–1534. [CrossRef] [PubMed]
5. Rodrigues, M.L.; Albuquerque, P.C. Searching for a change: The need for increased support for public health and research on fungal diseases. *PLoS Negl. Trop. Dis.* **2018**, *12*, e0006479. [CrossRef] [PubMed]

6. Houweling, T.A.J.; Karim-Kos, H.E.; Kulik, M.C.; Stolk, W.A.; Haagsma, J.A.; Lenk, E.J.; Richardus, J.H.; de Vlas, S.J.; et al. Socioeconomic inequalities in neglected tropical diseases: A systematic review. *PLoS Negl. Trop. Dis.* **2016**, *10*, e0004546. [CrossRef] [PubMed]

7. Chandler, D.J.; Hansen, K.S.; Mahato, B.; Darlong, J.; John, A.; Lockwood, D.N.J. Household costs of leprosy reactions (ENL) in rural India. *PLoS Negl. Trop. Dis.* **2015**, *9*, e0003431. [CrossRef] [PubMed]

8. Tiwari, A.; Suryawanshi, P.; Raikwar, A.; Arif, M.; Richardus, J.H. Household expenditure on leprosy outpatient services in the Indian Health System: A comparative study. *PLoS Negl. Trop. Dis.* **2018**, *12*, e0006181. [CrossRef] [PubMed]

9. Tembei, A.M.; Kengne-Ouaffo, J.A.; Ngoh, E.A.; John, B.; Nji, T.M.; Deribe, K.; Enyong, P.; Nkuo-Akenji, T.; Davey, G.; Wanji, S. A comparative analysis of economic cost of podoconiosis and leprosy on affected households in the northwest region of Cameroon. *Am. J. Trop. Med. Hyg.* **2018**, *98*, 1075–1081. [CrossRef] [PubMed]

10. Uranw, S.; Meheus, F.; Baltussen, R.; Rijal, S.; Boelaert, M. The household costs of visceral leishmaniasis care in south-eastern Nepal. *PLoS Negl. Trop. Dis.* **2013**, *7*, e2062. [CrossRef] [PubMed]

11. Lenk, E.J.; Redekop, W.K.; Luyendijk, M.; Rijnsburger, A.J.; Severens, J.L. Productivity loss related to neglected tropical diseases eligible for preventive chemotherapy: A systematic literature review. *PLoS Negl. Trop. Dis.* **2016**, *10*, 1–19. [CrossRef] [PubMed]

12. Engelman, D.; Fuller, L.C.; Solomon, A.W.; McCarthy, J.S.; Hay, R.J.; Lammie, P.J.; Steer, A.C. Opportunities for integrated control of neglected tropical diseases that affect the skin. *Trends Parasitol.* **2016**, *32*, 843–854. [CrossRef] [PubMed]

13. Mitjà, O.; Marks, M.; Bertran, L.; Kollie, K.; Argaw, D.; Fahal, A.H.; Fitzpatrick, C.; Fuller, L.C.; Izquierdo, B.G.; Hay, R.; et al. Integrated control and management of neglected tropical skin diseases. *PLoS Negl. Trop. Dis.* **2017**, *11*, e0005136. [CrossRef] [PubMed]

14. Department of Control of Neglected Tropical Diseases. *Recognizing Neglected Tropical Diseases Through Changes on the Skin: A Training Guide for Front-Line Health Workers*; WHO: Geneva, Switzerland, 2018.

15. Faye, O.; Hay, R.J.; Ryan, T.J.; Keita, S.; Traoré, A.K.; Mahé, A. A public health approach for leprosy detection based on a very short term-training of primary health care workers in basic dermatology. *Lepr. Rev.* **2007**, *78*, 11–16. [PubMed]

16. Chandler, D. Integrated care and leprosy in India: A role for indian systems of medicine and traditional health practice in the eradication of leprosy. *Curr. Sci.* **2016**, *111*, 351–355. [CrossRef]

17. Oswald, I.H. Are traditional healers the solution to the failures of primary health care in rural Nepal? *Soc. Sci. Med.* **1983**, *17*, 255–257. [CrossRef]

18. Kaur, P.; Sharma, U.C.; Pandey, S.S.; Gurmohan, S. Leprosy care through traditional healers. *Lepr. Rev.* **1984**, *55*, 57–61. [CrossRef] [PubMed]

19. Ezenduka, C.; Post, E.; John, S.; Suraj, A.; Namadi, A.; Onwujekwe, O. Cost-effectiveness analysis of three leprosy case detection methods in northern Nigeria. *PLoS Negl. Trop. Dis.* **2012**, *6*, e1818. [CrossRef] [PubMed]

20. Darlong, J.; Govindharaj, P.; Darlong, F.; Mahato, N. A study of untreated leprosy affected children reporting with grade 2 disability at a referral centre in West Bengal, India. *Lepr. Rev.* **2017**, *88*, 298–305.

21. Yotsu, R.R.; Kouadio, K.; Vagamon, B.; N'guessan, K.; Akpa, A.J.; Yao, A.; Aké, J.; Abbet, A.R.; Tchamba, A.A.; Bedimo, R.; et al. Skin disease prevalence study in schoolchildren in rural Côte d'Ivoire: Implications for integration of neglected skin diseases (Skin NTDs). *PLoS Negl. Trop. Dis.* **2018**, *12*, e0006489. [CrossRef] [PubMed]

22. Barogui, Y.T.; Diez, G.; Anagonou, E.; Johnson, R.C.; Gomido, I.C.; Amoukpo, H.; Bachirou, Z.S.; Houezo, J.G.; Saizonou, R.; Sopoh, G.E.; et al. Integrated approach in the control and management of skin neglected tropical diseases in Lalo, Benin. *PLoS Negl. Trop. Dis.* **2018**, *12*, e0006584. [CrossRef] [PubMed]

23. Mahé, A.; Faye, O.; N'Diaye, H.T.; Ly, F.; Konaré, H.; Kéita, S.; Traoré, A.K.; Hay, R. Definition of an algorithm for the management of common skin diseases at primary health care level in sub-Saharan Africa. *Trans. R. Soc. Trop. Med. Hyg.* **2005**, *99*, 39–47. [CrossRef] [PubMed]

24. Steer, A.C.; Tikoduadua, L.V.; Manalac, E.M.; Colquhoun, S.; Carapetis, J.R.; Maclennan, C. Validation of an integrated management of childhood illness algorithm for managing common skin conditions in Fiji. *Bull. World Health Organ.* **2009**, *87*, 173–179. [CrossRef] [PubMed]

25. Deribe, K.; Wanji, S.; Shafi, O.; Tukahebwa, M.E.; Umulisa, I.; Molyneux, D.H.; Davey, G. The feasibility of eliminating podoconiosis. *Bull. World Health Organ.* **2015**, *93*, 712–718. [CrossRef] [PubMed]

26. Engelman, D.; Fuller, L.C.; Steer, A.C.; International Alliance for the Control of Scabies Delphi Panel. Consensus criteria for the diagnosis of scabies: A delphi study of international experts. *PLoS Negl. Trop. Dis.* **2018**, *12*, e0006549. [CrossRef] [PubMed]

27. Brooker, S.J.; Smith, J.L. Mapping neglected tropical diseases: A global view. *Community Eye Heal.* **2013**, *26*, 32.

28. Noma, M.; Nwoke, B.E.B.; Nutall, I.; Tambala, P.A.; Enyong, P.; Namsenmo, A.; Remme, J.; Amazigo, U.V.; Kale, O.O.; Sékétéli, A. Rapid epidemiological mapping of onchocerciasis (REMO): Its application by the African Programme for Onchocerciasis Control (APOC). *Ann. Trop. Med. Parasitol.* **2002**, *96*, S29–S39. [CrossRef] [PubMed]

29. Sime, H.; Deribe, K.; Assefa, A.; Newport, M.J.; Enquselassie, F.; Gebretsadik, A.; Kebede, A.; Hailu, A.; Shafi, O.; Aseffa, A.; et al. Integrated mapping of lymphatic filariasis and podoconiosis: Lessons learnt from Ethiopia. *Parasit. Vectors* **2014**, *7*, 397. [CrossRef] [PubMed]

30. Kebede, B.; Martindale, S.; Mengistu, B.; Kebede, B.; Mengiste, A.; H/Kiros, F.; Tamiru, A.; Davey, G.; Kelly-Hope, L.A.; Mackenzie, C.D. Integrated morbidity mapping of lymphatic filariasis and podoconiosis cases in 20 co-endemic districts of Ethiopia. *PLoS Negl. Trop. Dis.* **2018**, *12*, e0006491. [CrossRef] [PubMed]

31. Mason, D.S.; Marks, M.; Sokana, O.; Solomon, A.W.; Mabey, D.C.; Romani, L.; Kaldor, J.; Steer, A.C.; Engelman, D. The prevalence of scabies and impetigo in the Solomon Islands: A population-based survey. *PLoS Negl. Trop. Dis.* **2016**, *10*, e0004803. [CrossRef] [PubMed]

32. Marks, M.; Vahi, V.; Sokana, O.; Chi, K.H.; Puiahi, E.; Kilua, G.; Pillay, A.; Dalipanda, T.; Bottomley, C.; Solomon, A.W.; et al. Impact of community mass treatment with azithromycin for trachoma elimination on the prevalence of yaws. *PLoS Negl. Trop. Dis.* **2015**, *9*, e0003988. [CrossRef] [PubMed]

33. Molyneux, D.H. 'Neglected' diseases but unrecognised successes—Challenges and opportunities for infectious disease control. *Lancet* **2004**, *364*, 380–383. [CrossRef]

34. Hotez, P.J.; Remme, J.H.F.; Buss, P.; Alleyne, G.; Morel, C.; Breman, J.G. Combating tropical infectious diseases: Report of the Disease Control Priorities in Developing Countries Project. *Clin. Infect. Dis.* **2004**, *38*, 871–988. [CrossRef] [PubMed]

35. Molyneux, D.H.; Hotez, P.J.; Fenwick, A. 'Rapid-impact interventions': How a policy of integrated control for Africa's neglected tropical diseases could benefit the poor. *PLoS Med.* **2005**, *2*, e336. [CrossRef] [PubMed]

36. Hotez, P.J.; Fenwick, A.; Ray, S.E.; Hay, S.I.; Molyneux, D.H. 'Rapid impact' 10 years after: The first 'decade' (2006-2016) of integrated neglected tropical disease control. *PLoS Negl. Trop. Dis.* **2018**, *12*, e0006137. [CrossRef] [PubMed]

37. Omura, S.; Crump, A. Ivermectin: Panacea for resource-poor communities? *Trends Parasitol.* **2014**, *30*, 445–455. [CrossRef] [PubMed]

38. Heukelbach, J.; Winter, B.; Wilcke, T.; Muehlen, M.; Albrecht, S.; de Oliveira, F.A.S.; Kerr-Pontes, L.R.; Liesenfeld, O.; Feldmeier, H. Selective mass treatment with ivermectin to control intestinal helminthiases and parasitic skin diseases in a severely affected population. *Bull. World Health Organ.* **2004**, *82*, 563–571. [PubMed]

39. Ottesen, E.A.; Hooper, P.J.; Bradley, M.; Biswas, G. The Global Programme to Eliminate Lymphatic Filariasis: Health impact after 8 years. *PLoS Negl. Trop. Dis.* **2008**, *2*, e317. [CrossRef] [PubMed]

40. Krotneva, S.P.; Coffeng, L.E.; Noma, M.; Zouré, H.G.M.; Bakoné, L.; Amazigo, U.V.; de Vlas, S.J.; Stolk, W.A. African Program for Onchocerciasis Control 1995–2010: Impact of annual ivermectin mass treatment on off-target infectious diseases. *PLoS Negl. Trop. Dis.* **2015**, *9*, e0004051. [CrossRef] [PubMed]

41. Romani, L.; Whitfeld, M.J.; Koroivueta, J.; Kama, M.; Wand, H.; Tikoduadua, L.; Tuicakau, M.; Koroi, A.; Andrews, R.; Kaldor, J.M.; et al. Mass drug administration for scabies control in a population with endemic disease. *N. Engl. J. Med.* **2015**, *373*, 2305–2313. [CrossRef] [PubMed]

42. Pacqué, M.; Muñoz, B.; Poetschke, G.; Foose, J.; Greene, B.M.; Taylor, H.R. Pregnancy outcome after inadvertent ivermectin treatment during community-based distribution. *Lancet* **1990**, *336*, 1486–1489. [CrossRef]

43. Gyapong, J.O.; Chinbuah, M.A.; Gyapong, M. Inadvertent exposure of pregnant women to ivermectin and albendazole during mass drug administration for lymphatic filariasis. *Trop. Med. Int. Health* **2003**, *8*, 1093–1101. [CrossRef] [PubMed]

44. Ndyomugyenyi, R.; Kabatereine, N.; Olsen, A.; Magnussen, P. Efficacy of ivermectin and albendazole alone and in combination for treatment of soil-transmitted helminths in pregnancy and adverse events: A randomized open label controlled intervention trial in Masindi District, Western Uganda. *Am. J. Trop. Med. Hyg.* **2008**, *79*, 856–863. [CrossRef] [PubMed]

45. Opoku, N.O.; Bakajika, D.K.; Kanza, E.M.; Howard, H.; Mambandu, G.L.; Nyathirombo, A.; Nigo, M.M.; Kasonia, K.; Masembe, S.L.; Mumbere, M.; et al. Single dose moxidectin versus ivermectin for *Onchocerca volvulus* infection in Ghana, Liberia, and the Democratic Republic of the Congo: A randomised, controlled, double-blind phase 3 trial. *Lancet* **2018**. [CrossRef]

46. Korth-Bradley, J.M.; Parks, V.; Patat, A.; Matschke, K.; Mayer, P.; Fleckenstein, L. Relative bioavailability of liquid and tablet formulations of the antiparasitic moxidectin. *Clin. Pharmacol. Drug Dev.* **2012**, *1*, 32–37. [CrossRef] [PubMed]

47. Mounsey, K.E.; Walton, S.F.; Innes, A.; Cash-Deans, S.; McCarthy, J.S. In vitro efficacy of moxidectin versus ivermectin against *Sarcoptes scabiei*. *Antimicrob. Agents Chemother.* **2017**, *61*, e00381. [CrossRef] [PubMed]

48. Ndyomugyenyi, R.; Byamungu, A.; Korugyendo, R. Perceptions on onchocerciasis and ivermectin treatment in rural communities in Uganda: Implications for long-term compliance. *Int. Health* **2009**, *1*, 163–168. [CrossRef] [PubMed]

49. Coulibaly, Y.I.; Dicko, I.; Keita, M.; Keita, M.M.; Doumbia, M.; Daou, A.; Haidara, F.C.; Sankare, M.H.; Horton, J.; Whately-Smith, C.; et al. A cluster randomized study of the safety of integrated treatment of trachoma and lymphatic filariasis in children and adults in Sikasso, Mali. *PLoS Negl. Trop. Dis.* **2013**, *7*, e2221. [CrossRef] [PubMed]

50. Mohammed, K.A.; Haji, H.J.; Gabrielli, A.F.; Mubila, L.; Biswas, G.; Chitsulo, L.; Bradley, M.H.; Engels, D.; Savioli, L.; Molyneux, D.H. Triple co-administration of ivermectin, albendazole and praziquantel in Zanzibar: A safety study. *PLoS Negl. Trop. Dis.* **2008**, *2*, e171. [CrossRef] [PubMed]

51. Thomsen, E.K.; Sanuku, N.; Baea, M.; Satofan, S.; Maki, E.; Lombore, B.; Schmidt, M.S.; Siba, P.M.; Weil, G.J.; Kazura, J.W.; et al. Efficacy, safety, and pharmacokinetics of coadministered diethylcarbamazine, albendazole, and ivermectin for treatment of bancroftian filariasis. *Clin. Infect. Dis.* **2016**, *62*, 334–341. [CrossRef] [PubMed]

52. Van 't Noordende, A.T.; Kuiper, H.; Ramos, A.N.; Mieras, L.F.; Barbosa, J.C.; Pessoa, S.M.F.; Souza, E.A.; Fernandes, T.A.; Hinders, D.C.; Praciano, M.M.; et al. Towards a toolkit for cross-neglected tropical disease morbidity and disability assessment. *Int. Health* **2016**, *8*, i71–81. [CrossRef] [PubMed]

53. Ryan, T.J. The International Society of Dermatology's Task Force for Skin Care for All: Community dermatology. *Int. J. Dermatol.* **2011**, *50*, 548–551. [CrossRef] [PubMed]

54. Kaur, P.; Singh, G. Community dermatology in India. *Int. J. Dermatol.* **1995**, *34*, 322. [CrossRef] [PubMed]

55. Stocks, M.E.; Freeman, M.C.; Addiss, D.G. The effect of hygiene-based lymphedema management in lymphatic filariasis-endemic areas: A systematic review and meta-analysis. *PLoS Negl. Trop. Dis.* **2015**, *9*, e0004171. [CrossRef] [PubMed]

56. Negussie, H.; Molla, M.; Ngari, M.; Berkley, J.A.; Kivaya, E.; Njuguna, P.; Fegan, G.; Tamiru, A.; Kelemework, A.; Lang, T.; et al. Lymphoedema management to prevent acute dermatolymphangioadenitis in podoconiosis in northern Ethiopia (GoLBeT): A pragmatic randomised controlled trial. *Lancet Glob. Heal.* **2018**, *6*, e795–803. [CrossRef]

57. Deribe, K.; Kebede, B.; Tamiru, M.; Mengistu, B.; Kebede, F.; Martindale, S.; Sime, H.; Mulugeta, A.; Kebede, B.; Sileshi, M.; et al. Integrated morbidity management for lymphatic filariasis and podoconiosis, Ethiopia. *Bull. World Health Organ.* **2017**, *95*, 652–656. [CrossRef] [PubMed]

58. Stocks, M.E.; Ogden, S.; Haddad, D.; Addiss, D.G.; McGuire, C.; Freeman, M.C. Effect of water, sanitation, and hygiene on the prevention of trachoma: A Systematic review and meta-analysis. *PLoS Med.* **2014**, *11*, e1001605. [CrossRef] [PubMed]

59. Strunz, E.C.; Addiss, D.G.; Stocks, M.E.; Ogden, S.; Utzinger, J.; Freeman, M.C. Water, sanitation, hygiene, and soil-transmitted helminth infection: A systematic review and meta-analysis. *PLoS Med.* **2014**, *11*, e1001620. [CrossRef] [PubMed]

60. Grimes, J.E.T.; Croll, D.; Harrison, W.E.; Utzinger, J.; Freeman, M.C.; Templeton, M.R. The relationship between water, sanitation and schistosomiasis: A systematic review and meta-analysis. *PLoS Negl. Trop. Dis.* **2014**, *8*, e3296. [CrossRef] [PubMed]

61. Seward, N.; Neuman, M.; Colbourn, T.; Osrin, D.; Lewycka, S.; Azad, K.; Costello, A.; Das, S.; Fottrell, E.; Kuddus, A.; et al. Effects of women's groups practising participatory learning and action on preventive and care-seeking behaviours to reduce neonatal mortality: A meta-analysis of cluster-randomised trials. *PLoS Med.* **2017**, *14*, e1002467. [CrossRef] [PubMed]
62. Pryce, J.; Mableson, H.E.; Choudhary, R.; Pandey, B.D.; Aley, D.; Betts, H.; Mackenzie, C.D.; Kelly-Hope, L.A.; Cross, H. Assessing the feasibility of integration of self-care for filarial lymphoedema into existing community leprosy self-help groups in Nepal. *BMC Public Health* **2018**, *18*, 201. [CrossRef] [PubMed]
63. Hofstraat, K.; van Brakel, W.H. Social Stigma Towards Neglected Tropical Diseases: A systematic review. *Int. Health* **2016**, *8*, i53–i70. [CrossRef] [PubMed]

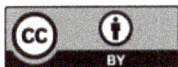

Tropical Medicine and Infectious Disease

MDPI

Communication

The Development of a Mobile Application to Support Peripheral Health Workers to Diagnose and Treat People with Skin Diseases in Resource-Poor Settings

Liesbeth F. Mieras [1,*] , **Anna T. Taal** [1], **Erik B. Post** [2], **Alcino G. Z. Ndeve** [3] **and Colette L. M. van Hees** [4]

1   Technical Department, Netherlands Leprosy Relief, 1090 HA Amsterdam, The Netherlands;
    A.Taal@Leprastichting.nl
2   Challenge TB, KNCV Tuberculosis Foundation, Jakarta 12870, Indonesia; Erik.Post@KNCVtbc.org
3   Technical Department, Netherlands Leprosy Relief, Maputo, Mozambique; AlcinoNdeve@nlrmoz.org
4   Department of Dermatology, Erasmus Medical Centre, 3000 CA Rotterdam, The Netherlands;
    C.vanHees@ErasmusMC.nl
*   Correspondence: L.Mieras@Leprastichting.nl; Tel.: +31-20-59-50-528

Received: 27 July 2018; Accepted: 10 September 2018; Published: 15 September 2018

Abstract: The high prevalence of skin diseases in resource-poor settings, where health workers with sufficient knowledge of skin diseases are scarce, calls for innovative measures. Timely diagnosis and treatment of skin diseases, especially neglected tropical diseases (NTDs) that manifest with skin lesions, such as leprosy, is crucial to prevent disabilities as well as psychological and socioeconomic problems. Innovative technological methods like telemedicine and mobile health (mHealth) can help to bridge the gap between the burden of skin diseases and the lack of capable staff in resource-poor settings by bringing essential health services from central level closer to peripheral levels. Netherlands Leprosy Relief (NLR) has developed a mobile phone application called the 'SkinApp', which aims to support peripheral health workers to recognize the early signs and symptoms of skin diseases, including skin NTDs, and to start treatment promptly or refer for more advanced diagnostic testing or disease management when needed. Further research is needed to determine how greatly mHealth in general and the SkinApp in particular can contribute to improved health outcomes, efficiency, and cost-effectiveness.

Keywords: skin diseases; mobile phone application; NTDs; dermatology; mHealth; leprosy

1. Introduction

1.1. Short Communication

This article is written as a short communication, describing the ongoing development process of a mobile phone application that supports peripheral health workers in diagnosing and treating skin diseases in resource-poor settings.

1.2. Epidemiology of Skin Diseases in Low- and Middle-Income Countries

It is known that skin diseases are highly prevalent, particularly in resource-poor areas, where children are disproportionally affected—though there is a lack of systematically-collected data supporting this [1,2]. The epidemiology of skin diseases varies per country and within countries, but available data show that in rural areas, usually more than 50% and sometimes as much as 80% of the population has a skin condition; especially in areas endemic for conditions like scabies, onchocerciasis or tinea capitis [1]. The Global Burden of Disease (GBD) Study 2013 indicated that skin conditions were the fourth leading cause of disability worldwide [3].

Neglected topical diseases (NTDs) that manifest in skin lesions like leprosy and lymphatic filariasis (see Table 1) are among the skin diseases that often cause disabilities such as permanent wounds, contractures, and advanced lymphedema. Timely diagnosis and treatment can prevent permanent disabilities, but skin NTDs are usually not the most prevalent skin diseases, and are therefore more likely to be missed by health workers with limited or no dermatology training.

Skin conditions are usually not fatal, but it is important to recognize those that may be, such as blistering diseases. They can also be a sign of an underlying medical condition that might be life-threatening, such as HIV/AIDS. In view of the HIV/AIDS epidemic, the importance of dermatology cannot be underestimated, as 90% of HIV/AIDS patients develop a skin problem (see Table 1) during the course of their illness, and often initially present with a skin condition [4].

Table 1. Skin Diseases in The SkinApp. NTD: neglected tropical disease.

Common Skin Diseases	NTDs Manifesting in Skin Lesions	HIV-Related Skin Diseases	Others
Acne [1]	Buruli ulcer [1]	Angular cheilitis [1]	Albinism
Atopic eczema [1]	Cutaneous leishmaniasis [1]	Herpes simplex [1]	Blistering diseases
Contact eczema [1]	Leprosy [1]	Herpes zoster [1]	Creeping eruption
Impetigo [1]	Lymphatic filiariasis [1]	Kaposi sarcoma [1]	Vitiligo
Pityriasis versicolor [1]	Mycetoma	Molluscum contagiosum [1]	
Psoriasis	Onchocerciasis [1]	Oral candidiasis [1]	
Seborrhoeic eczema [1] (*)	Podoconiosis	Pruritic papular eruption [1]	
Tinea capitis [1]	Scabies [1]		
Tinea corporis [1] (*)	Yaws		

[1] Diseases included since the first version of the SkinApp. (*) also HIV-related.

1.3. Psycological and Socioeconomic Burden

Physical problems caused by skin conditions can lead to deterioration of the quality of life. Additionally, skin diseases often cause psychological problems such as anxiety, depression, and exclusion. A study in Colombia to determine the impact of skin diseases on the quality of life found that even the most localized or asymptomatic skin lesion leads to a disruption at some level of patient wellness [5]. The high visibility of skin diseases contributes to the likelihood of stigmatization, and may even result in unemployment [6]. Skin diseases can negatively impact productivity at school and work, while a considerable amount of household money has to be spent on treatment that is often ineffective due to insufficient availability of health workers with basic dermatology training at the peripheral level [7]. The economic impact of accessing care and rehabilitation services can be substantial, especially when the condition is chronic or leads to disabilities [8].

1.4. Capacity Gap

Studies have shown that a minimum of 10% of the consultations at peripheral healthcare level relates to common skin diseases [9,10]. Unfortunately, healthcare workers often lack the knowledge and skill to diagnose and treat skin diseases due to lack of training [7,9]. There is a need to bridge the gap between the prevalence of skin conditions at community level and the availability of capable staff in peripheral health facilities. An increased capacity to diagnose and treat skin diseases will contribute to the timely diagnosis and treatment of skin diseases in general, and skin NTDs in particular, and thus to the prevention of chronic conditions and disabilities.It will also contribute to timely and appropriate referral. Seth et al. call for increased efforts to address this problem, especially in low-resource settings, using recent innovations to help provide dermatological care to underserved regions in a cost-effective manner [11].

2. Mobile Health (mHealth)

2.1. Technologies to Support Dermatology Services

There are various innovative ways to enhance the quality of peripheral dermatology care. These include, but are not limited to, technological methods such as telemedicine, artificial intelligence, and mobile health (mHealth). In teledermatology, telecommunication technologies are used to exchange information regarding skin conditions over distances that a patient would otherwise have to travel [12]. The two main methods are: 'real-time' (synchronous) videoconferencing teledermatology, when the patient and dermatologist meet simultaneously in different locations; and 'store-and-forward' (asynchronous) teledermatology, in which images are transmitted electronically to a consulting dermatologist [13]. A significant limitation regarding teledermatology is the need for a dermatologist that can be consulted when required. Additional limitations for real-time teledermatology are the need for a stable internet connection and the costs for the necessary infrastructure.

Artificial intelligence can be used to make a computer-based algorithm that is able to make diagnostic decisions regarding skin conditions to a good degree of accuracy [12]. However, these techniques are still in development and only available for a limited number of skin diseases [14].

2.2. mHealth to Improve Peripheral Services forSkin Diseases

mHealth refers to the use of mobile communication devices to support health system needs. It can be made available by and for resource managers and health workers, as well as community members, patients, and their caregivers. It can also be used for management purposes, data collection and reporting, decision support, training, emergency referrals, alerts, and supervision [15,16]. In Labrique's paper on mHealth innovations as health system strengthening tools, the focus is on mHealth applications as point of care decision support for health workers to enhance their capability in diagnosing, treating, and referring people with skin diseases [16]. A systematic review on the feasibility and effective use of mHealth strategies by frontline health workers in developing countries concluded that these tools are potentially an effective means to promote the shifting of essential health services to lower cadres of health workers, but that a balance between the technical requirements and the cost of a system is a vital factor in the scalability of such solutions [17].

There are many mobile phone applications concerning skin diseases. As of August 2017, more than 520 dermatology-related mobile phone applications are available in the Google Play Store and the Apple App Store [18]. The majority of these applications are developed for clinical use such as teledermatology consultation, as self-surveillance and self-diagnosis aids, or as general dermatology references [18,19]. General dermatology reference applications range from an information source for patients to a comprehensive guide for health professionals [19]. Teledermatology is an effective method, as it provides consultations for health professionals in remote and resource-poor areas [20,21]. Some teledermatology applications cover a broad range of diseases, such as 'Dermassistance', which combines a mobile phone application with the use of teledermatology (https://www.dermassistance.es/). There is also a variety of disease-specific applications available. In the field of leprosy, for example, there is an initiative aimed at the early recognition of leprosy using image recognition through neural network technology by the Vellore Institute of Technology (http://preleprosy.com/), but this is still in development.

2.3. Development of NLR SkinApp

To increase the capability of peripheral health workers in resource-poor settings to diagnose and treat skin diseases and thus strengthen the health system, the Netherlands Leprosy Relief (NLR) developed an application suitable for Android and Apple devices. To our knowledge, no other similar mobile phone application is available. The aim was not only to support health workers to better serve a large proportion of their patients with common skin diseases, but also to enhance the detection and treatment of less common skin diseases, such as leprosy. Knowing that correct diagnosis and timely treatment help to prevent disabilities, the use of the SkinApp can contribute to reduced suffering caused by dermatological conditions.

The SkinApp uses an algorithm to support the process of diagnosis. It was inspired by the algorithm developed by Mahé for the management of common skin diseases at the primary healthcare level [22,23]. It contains descriptions of skin diseases, supporting photos, as well as treatment and referral advice. The selected skin diseases are a combination of commonly occurring skin diseases, skin diseases that may lead to mortality, HIV/AIDS related skin diseases [24,25], and NTDs manifesting in skin lesions prevalent in sub-Saharan African countries [8,26].

The development of the NLR SkinApp went through three stages: (1) a pilot project using a paper-based algorithm in Nigeria [23]; (2) a pilot of the first version of the mobile phone application in 2015 in Zambezia Province, Mozambique; and (3) an implementation project in Nampula Province, Mozambique, 2017–2018. During all three stages, several dermatology experts with experience in resource-poor areas generously contributed to the content, narrative, and imagery, and provided feedback.

The study in Nigeria was a prospective pilot study to assess the performance of first-line healthcare providers using a paper-based algorithm to support their diagnosis and treatment of seven skin diseases. In this study, 19 patent medicine vendors and 12 traditional healers assessed a total of 4147 patients with skin lesions, and their diagnoses and treatment choices were validated by two independent dermatologists. Overall, the first-line healthcare providers using the algorithm correctly diagnosed and treated or referred 82% of patients presenting with skin lesions. Adding pictorial images of signs and symptoms was believed to further improve the algorithm [23]. On the basis of these findings, it was decided to start the development of a mobile phone application.

In the first version of the SkinApp, which was tested in Zambezia Province, in Mozambique, 21 diseases were included in the algorithm: eight common skin diseases, six NTDs that manifest in skin lesions, and seven HIV/AIDS-related skin diseases (see Table 1). The pilot project was set up to determine the user-friendliness of the application and to identify points for improvement This was done by observing and interviewing SkinApp users through semi-structured interview guides and focus group discussions. The health workers—consisting of one physician, four medical technicians and five nurses—said that they used the application in cases where the diagnosis was clear but the treatment was unknown; whenever they were in doubt; to read through signs and symptoms from diseases in their differential diagnosis; and, when necessary, to go through the algorithm step by step to see if they could come to a diagnosis. They also used the app as a training tool, going through it in their free time. The main findings were that (1) smartphone ownership is very common among health workers in Zambezia; (2) the SkinApp was easy to use after a short introduction about its functionalities; (3) not all skin diseases in the application were relevant in the context of Zambezia Province (e.g., Buruli ulcer); (4) the treatment advice was clear, but not all treatment options were available at the peripheral level in Zambezia Province; (5) a teledermatology function would enhance the usefulness of the application.

Based on the results of the pilot and advancing insight, a second version of the SkinApp was developed. While the first version presented possible diagnoses with a description of signs, symptoms, and treatment advice, the second version aligned much better with the clinical validation of a patient with a skin disease. This was achieved by integrating an improved algorithm that starts with signs and symptoms and their location on a body map, and leads to the most likely diagnosis and treatment advice. In the second version, a number of diseases and supporting photos were added. A feedback button was inserted, which could be developed into a teledermatology function if required. The second version of the SkinApp was implemented in Nampula Province in 2017–2018. A WhatsApp group was formed for SkinApp users to meet the need for a teledermatology option. This enabled them to consult with an experienced Mozambican dermatologist, if needed, though an internet connection is required. Findings from the implementation project confirmed that the SkinApp is more easily accessible than literature and books, and that it is easy to operate. The narrative and illustrative content were considered clear. However, a glossary explaining dermatological terminology would help to improve intelligibility. Adding a reporting option was also mentioned as a possible improvement. These findings helped to further improve the user-friendliness of the SkinApp, but these pilots did not address the performance of the SkinApp as a diagnostic tool.

On the basis of the experiences with the SkinApp in Mozambique and the feedback received from involved dermatologists, a third version has since been developed. Its performance is currently being validated. The third version contains a total number of 29 skin diseases (see Table 1), an improved algorithm, a glossary with frequently-used terminology, and a section on treatment options for frequently-seen skin conditions (broken skin and dry skin).

The second version of the NLR SkinApp is currently available in English and Portuguese for mobile devices with Android as well as iOS operating systems through the Google Play Store (SkinApp) and the Apple App Store (as Skin_App) respectively, free of charge. Once downloaded, the SkinApp can be used offline.

The third version will be released once the current validation study is completed. The validation study is done in clinical settings under appropriate ethical and statistical guidelines. It encompasses concordance testing of the photos used in the application. The accuracy of the SkinApp will be assessed by comparing the diagnosis made by peripheral health workers using the SkinApp, to the diagnosis made by experienced dermatologists. Further evaluation of the use of the third version is planned for in several African countries. The capacity of the health workers to diagnose and treat skin diseases at baseline will be compared to their capacity two years after the introduction of the use of the SkinApp. Furthermore, a comparison will be made between the detection and treatment of skin diseases—specifically neglected tropical diseases—before and after the introduction of the SkinApp.

Once validated, the NLR SkinApp will be made available for use in other countries, where it can be modified to the context by changing the language, adapting the included skin diseases to those prevalent in the area, and using country-specific photos and treatment advices.

3. Discussion and Conclusions

Agarwal et al. conducted a systematic review entitled 'Evidence on feasibility and effective use of mHealth strategies by frontline health workers in developing countries' [17]. They found that mHealth strategies for peripheral health workers in low-resource countries are potentially an effective means to promote the shifting of essential health services to peripheral levels. What is not known about mHealth strategies is whether they contribute to improved health outcomes, efficiency, or cost-effectiveness. Additional research is needed to determine the added value of mHealth in general, and the SkinApp in particular.

One of the success factors for the adoption of mobile tools identified by Agarwal et al. was the involvement of the health workers throughout the development and implementation process [17]. The SkinApp has been developed in three stages, during which the input of peripheral health workers regarding the use of the SkinApp was obtained. Some of their requests have not yet been integrated into the newest version of the SkinApp, such as the desire for data collection and a teledermatology option. Once the third version of the SkinApp is validated, these functionalities could be added to the application. However, in order to maximize user-friendliness, the aim is to limit the size of the application in megabytes. Furthermore, options to send and receive information not only require an internet connection, but will also need a network of professionals to process the information received and prepare information to be sent. This will increase the cost of the necessary technical support as well as human resources, while a balance between technical requirements and the cost of the system is a vital factor in the scalability of such solutions [17]. The success of an mHealth intervention also depends on the existence of an mHealth platform to facilitate not only the adoption of the tool, but also to guarantee a sustained effective use.

There is a clear need to address the mismatch between the burden of skin diseases at the community level in resource-poor areas and the capability of peripheral health workers to diagnose, treat, and refer people with skin diseases, including skin NTDs. mHealth in general and the NLR SkinApp in particular can help to bridge this gap. The technical requirements and costs to ensure the sustainability of these innovative approaches are likely to increase, especially upon usage in different countries, which requires context-specific adaptation such as the use of the local language and alignment with the epidemiological situation. Therefore, more research is needed to gather evidence on the health outcomes and (cost-) effectiveness of mHealth for skin diseases, including skin NTDs, to ensure a wider use in support of peripheral health workers.

Author Contributions: Conceptualization: E.B.P., C.L.M.v.H, A.T.T., L.F.M.; investigation: A.G.Z.N.; project administration: E.B.P., A.G.Z.N., A.T.T, L.F.M.; writing—original draft: L.F.M.; writing—review and editing: E.B.P., C.L.M.v.H., A.T.T., L.F.M.

Funding: This research received no external funding.

Acknowledgments: We are grateful for the valuable comments and suggestions from experienced dermatologists in various stages of development of the SkinApp: Ben Naafs, Koos Sanders, Claire Fuller, Tahir Dahiru and others, and we would like to thank the teams in Nigeria and Mozambique and Marloes Frijters for the fieldwork related to the development of the SkinApp.

Conflicts of Interest: The authors declare no conflicts of interest.

References

1. Hay, R.; Fuller, L. The assessment of dermatological needs in resource-poor regions. *Int. J. Dermatol.* **2011**, *50*, 552–557. [CrossRef] [PubMed]
2. Vos, T.; Allen, C.; Arora, M.; Barber, R.; Bhutta, Z.; Brown, A.; Carter, A.; Casey, D.; Charlson, F.; Murray, C.; et al. Global, regional, and national incidence, prevalence, and years lived with disability for 310 diseases and injuries, 1990–2015: A systematic analysis for the Global Burden of Disease Study 2015. *Lancet* **2016**, *388*, 1545–1602. [CrossRef]
3. Hay, R.; Johns, N.; Williams, H.; Bolliger, I.; Dellavalle, R.; Margolis, D.; Marks, R.; Naldi, L.; Weinstock, M.; Wulf, S.; et al. The global burden of skin disease in 2010: An analysis of the prevalence and impact of skin conditions. *J. Investig. Dermatol.* **2014**, *134*, 1527–1534. [CrossRef] [PubMed]
4. Hu, J.; McKoy, K.; Papier, A.; Klaus, S.; Ryan, T.; Grossman, H.; Masenga, E.J.; Sethi, A.; Craft, N. Dermatology and HIV/AIDS in Africa. *J. Glob. Infect. Dis.* **2011**, *3*, 275–280. [PubMed]
5. Sanclemente, G.; Burgos, C.; Nova, J.; Hernández, F.; González, C.; Reyes, M.; Córdoba, N.; Arévalo, Á.; Meléndez, E.; Colmenares, J.; et al. The impact of skin diseases on quality of life: A multicenter study. *Actas Dermosifiliogr.* **2017**, *108*, 244–252. [CrossRef] [PubMed]
6. Barankin, B.; DeKoven, J. Psychosocial effect of common skin diseases. *Can. Fam. Physician* **2002**, *48*, 712–716. [PubMed]
7. Figueroa, J.; Fuller, L.; Abraha, A.; Hay, R. Dermatology in southwestern Ethiopia: Rationale for a community approach. *Int. J. Dermatol.* **1998**, *37*, 752–758. [CrossRef] [PubMed]
8. Mitjà, O.; Marks, M.; Bertran, L.; Kollie, K.; Argaw, D.; Fahal, A.; Fitzpatrick, C.; Fuller, L.; Garcia Izquierdo, B.; Hay, R.; et al. Integrated control and management of neglected tropical skin diseases. *PLoS Negl. Trop. Dis.* **2017**, *11*, e0005136. [CrossRef] [PubMed]
9. Mahe, A.; N'Diaye, H.; Bobin, P. The proportion of medical consultations motivated by skin diseases in the health centers of Bamako (Republic of Mali). *Int. J. Dermatol.* **1997**, *36*, 185–186. [CrossRef] [PubMed]
10. Odueko, O.M.; Onayemi, O.; Oyedeji, G.A. A prevalence survey of skin diseases in Nigerian children. *Niger. J. Med.* **2001**, *10*, 64–67. [PubMed]
11. Seth, D.; Cheldize, K.; Brown, D.; Freeman, E. Global burden of skin disease: Inequities and innovations. *Curr. Dermatol. Rep.* **2017**, *6*, 204–210. [CrossRef] [PubMed]

12. Surovi, N.A.; Kiber, A.; Kashem, A.; Babi, K.N. Study and Development of Algorithm of Different Skin Diseases Analysis Using Image Processing Method. Available online: http://www.alliedacademies.org/articles/study-and-development-of-algorithm-of-different-skin-diseases-analysis-using-image-processing-method.html (accessed on 26 June 2018).

13. Desai, B.; McKoy, K.; Kovarik, C. Overview of international teledermatology. *Pan Afr. Med. J.* **2010**, *6*, 3. [CrossRef] [PubMed]

14. Yadav, N.; Narang, V.; Shrivastava, U. Skin diseases detection models using image processing: A survey Utpal Shrivastava. *Int. J. Comput. Appl.* **2016**, *137*, 34–39.

15. WHO. Classification of Digital Health Interventions v1.0. World Health Organization. Available online: http://www.who.int/reproductivehealth/publications/mhealth/classification-digital-health-interventions/en/ (accessed on 26 June 2018).

16. Labrique, A.; Vasudevan, L.; Kochi, E.; Fabricant, R.; Mehl, G. mHealth innovations as health system strengthening tools: 12 common applications and a visual framework. *Glob. Health Sci. Pract.* **2013**, *1*, 160–171. [CrossRef] [PubMed]

17. Agarwal, S.; Perry, H.; Long, L.; Labrique, A. Evidence on feasibility and effective use of mHealth strategies by frontline health workers in developing countries: Systematic review. *Trop. Med. Int. Health* **2015**, *20*, 1003–1014. [CrossRef] [PubMed]

18. Flaten, H.K.; Claire, C.S.; Schlager, E.; Dunnick, C.A.; Dellavalle, R.P. Growth of mobile applications in dermatology 2017 update. *Dermatol. Online J.* **2018**, *24*, 13.

19. Brewer, A.C.; Endly, D.C.; Henley, J.; Amir, M.; Sampson, B.P.; Moreau, J.F.; Dellavalle, R.P. Mobile applications in dermatology. *JAMA Dermatol.* **2013**, *149*, 1300–1304. [CrossRef] [PubMed]

20. Lipoff, J.B.; Cobos, G.; Kaddu, S.; Kovarik, C.L. The Africa Teledermatology Project: A retrospective case review of 1229 consultations from sub-Saharan Africa. *J. Am. Acad. Dermatol.* **2015**, *72*, 1084–1085. [CrossRef] [PubMed]

21. Nguyen, A.; Tran, D.; Uemura, M.; Bardin, R.L.; Shitabata, P.K. Practical and sustainable teledermatology and teledermatopathology: Specialty care in Cameroon Africa. *J. Clin. Aesthet. Dermatol.* **2017**, *10*, 47–56. [PubMed]

22. Mahe, A.; Faye, O.; N'Diaye, H.T.; Ly, F.; Konare, H.; Keita, S.; Traore, A.K.; Hay, R. Definition of an algorithm for the management of common skin diseases at primary health care level in sub-Saharan Africa. *Trans. Soc. Trop. Med. Hyg.* **2005**, *99*, 39–47. [CrossRef] [PubMed]

23. Taal, A.; Hussaini, T.; Gayus, B.; Dahiru, T.; Post, E. First-line health care provider performance in the management of common skin diseases using an algorithmic approach as a diagnostic tool in Kano State, Nigeria. *Res. Rep. Trop. Med.* **2015**, *6*, 85–94. [CrossRef]

24. Van Hees, C.; Naafs, B. *Common Skin Diseases in Africa, an Illustrated Guide*, 3rd ed.; Stichting Troderma: Voorburg, The Netherlands, 2014.

25. Kousa, M.; Sanders, C. HIV Related Skin Diseases and Sexually Transmitted Infections. Available online: https://www.ntvg.nl/artikelen/hiv-related-skin-diseases-and-sexually-transmitted-infections-africa/volledig (accessed on 29 June 2018).

26. WHO. Neglected Tropical Diseases. Available online: http://www.who.int/neglected_diseases/en/ (accessed on 16 July 2018).

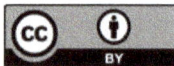

Tropical Medicine and Infectious Disease

MDPI

Review

Polymerase Chain Reaction (PCR) as a Potential Point of Care Laboratory Test for Leprosy Diagnosis—A Systematic Review

Sushma Tatipally [1], Aparna Srikantam [1,*] and Sanjay Kasetty [2]

[1] LEPRA Society, Blue Peter Public Health and Research Centre, Cherlapally, Hyderabad 501301, Telangana, India; sushma@leprahealthinaction.in

[2] Formerly at LEPRA Society, Blue Peter Public Health and Research Centre, Cherlapally, Hyderabad 501301, Telangana, India; sanjay.kasetty@gmail.com

* Correspondence: aparna@leprahealthinaction.in; Tel.: +91-40-27264547

Received: 20 July 2018; Accepted: 23 September 2018; Published: 1 October 2018

Abstract: Leprosy is an infectious disease caused by *Mycobacterium leprae* and mainly affects skin, peripheral nerves, and eyes. Suitable tools for providing bacteriological evidence of leprosy are needed for early case detection and appropriate therapeutic management. Ideally these tools are applicable at all health care levels for the effective control of leprosy. This paper presents a systematic review analysis in order to investigate the performance of polymerase chain reaction (PCR) vis-à-vis slit skin smears (SSS) in various clinical settings and its potential usefulness as a routine lab test for leprosy diagnosis. Records of published journal articles were identified through PubMed database search. Twenty-seven articles were included for the analysis. The evidence from this review analysis suggests that PCR on skin biopsy is the ideal diagnostic test. Nevertheless, PCR on SSS samples also seems to be useful with its practical value for application, even at primary care levels. The review findings also indicated the necessity for improving the sensitivity of PCR and further research on specificity in ruling out other clinical conditions that may mimic leprosy. The *M. leprae*-specific repetitive element (RLEP) was the most frequently-used marker although its variable performance across the clinical sites and samples are a matter of concern. Undertaking further research studies with large sample numbers and uniform protocols studied simultaneously across multiple clinical sites is recommended to address these issues.

Keywords: leprosy; leprosy diagnosis; PCR; slit skin smears; point of care test; skin biopsy; early diagnosis

---

1. Introduction

Leprosy is an infectious disease caused by *Mycobacterium leprae* and mainly affects skin, peripheral nerves, and eyes [1–3]. Leprosy has long-term consequences on the structure and function of the peripheral nerves leading to disabilities in limbs, which impact on the socioeconomic well-being of the affected individuals [4]. Despite three decades of effective treatment with multidrug therapy (MDT), leprosy persists as a public health problem in many regions of the world [5]. Each year 300,000 people are newly diagnosed with leprosy worldwide; half are reported from India [6]. Despite the World Health Organization (WHO) declaring the elimination of leprosy as a public health problem in the year 2000, new leprosy cases still continue to occur in India with an annual incidence of around 135,000 cases [7]. There is evidence that many more patients still go undetected due to various reasons including social stigma attached to the disease, which hinders health-care-seeking behavior among affected persons [8]. Hence it is imperative to widen the scope and accuracy of leprosy detection for early identification before the consequences of nerve damage have set in [9]. The current standard diagnosis of leprosy is mostly based on clinical evaluation of patients, except in a few settings where the microscopy of slit skin smears (SSS) for acid-fast bacilli and/or histopathological examination (HPE) of skin biopsies are being used as additional tests [10]. Clinical manifestations of leprosy are determined by patient immune responses to *Mycobacterium leprae*. Leprosy patients are classified by the Ridley–Jopling classification on the basis of the morphology, type, and number of skin lesions, as well as nerve involvement supplemented by the bacterial index (BI) and histopathological examination. The Ridley–Jopling types are tuberculoid (TT), borderline tuberculoid (BT), borderline (BB), borderline lepromatous (BL), lepromatous leprosy (LL), pure neural (PN) and indeterminate (I) [11].

The current operational classification of leprosy used by WHO is based on number of skin lesions; patients with less than five lesions are classified as paucibacillary (PB) and more than five as multibacillary (MB) leprosy. However, this classification, merely based on the number of lesions, may not always hold good for specific treatment strategies, as it has been frequently demonstrated that acid-fast bacilli (AFB) are present in cases clinically classified as PB. Such PB patients with active lesions may potentially be transmitting *M. leprae* to their contacts unless they are treated appropriately [12]. Hence there has been an emphasis on bringing back the laboratory diagnostic component into routine practice [13]. The two traditional tests *viz.* SSS and HPE of biopsies, though still holding well in terms of convenience of usage, have their own inherent limitations. SSS is relatively low in sensitivity and includes the risk of subjective errors of microscopic examination, whereas the HPE has the limitations of long turnaround time and technically demanding laboratory procedures [14]. Hence it is very important to develop diagnostic strategies involving highly sensitive laboratory tests for early detection of leprosy. Suitable tools for providing bacteriological evidence of leprosy are needed for early case detection and appropriate therapeutic management of leprosy. Ideally these tools are applicable at all health care levels for effective control of leprosy.

Molecular diagnosis by nucleic acid amplification test (NAAT) is an emerging science in the clinical management of infectious diseases. Polymerase chain reaction (PCR) is one of the most popular NAAT currently being used for the diagnosis of infectious diseases [15]. Routine clinical use of NAAT has been well established in tuberculosis and other mycobacterial diseases. NAAT has almost replaced the conventional lab diagnostic tests in TB and has become the most widely used test at all levels of health care [16]. Such molecular diagnosis has not yet been practiced in the case of leprosy. PCR nevertheless has been popularly used for drug resistance testing and molecular typing of leprosy but never so far for the routine clinical diagnosis [17,18]. Given the potential use of this very important test, there is a need for a scientific analysis of the effectiveness of PCR for lab diagnosis of leprosy in correlation with the current standards. This evidence is envisaged to help the formulation of better policies for diagnosis and treatment of leprosy. With this background, the present systematic review analysis has been conducted in order to investigate the performance of PCR vis-à-vis SSS in various clinical settings and its potential usefulness as a routine lab test for leprosy diagnosis.

2. Materials and Methods

2.1. Study Design

The study is a systematic review analysis to assess the usefulness of PCR for the laboratory diagnosis of leprosy. The review has been carried out with the purpose of accruing evidence on the performance of PCR in correlation with clinical classification of leprosy and standard laboratory diagnostic tests. The highlights from the review are envisaged to be useful in addressing the gaps in the existing systems and recommending better strategies for the future application of PCR during routine clinical diagnosis of leprosy. The protocol has been prepared based on Preferred Reporting Items for Systematic reviews and Meta-Analyses (PRISMA) guidelines for systematic review analysis [19].

2.2. Data Search

Records of published journal articles were identified through searching the PubMed database [20]. Journal articles published until April 2018 were included. The data search was conducted between 15 March 2018 to 4 May 2018. All field searches for PCR and leprosy yielded 924 articles, which were filtered to 812 with Medical Subject Heading (MeSH) terms *Mycobacterium leprae*, leprosy, Hansen's disease, laboratory diagnosis, biomarkers, PCR, SSS examination, and biopsies (protocol furnished as Figure 1). Out of 924, 715 full text articles were shortlisted. Twenty-seven of the 715 articles were included for the analysis based on these inclusion criteria: the study should have involved PCR as one of the tests for leprosy diagnosis or confirmation along with one other standard test such as SSS or biopsy and PCR tests conducted on (any) biological (clinical) samples. Exclusion criteria included articles published in a language other than English, articles which did not have free full text available, PCR used for purposes other than leprosy diagnosis, such as PCR used as a test for drug resistance, molecular typing, or where the PCR test was not used on clinical samples.

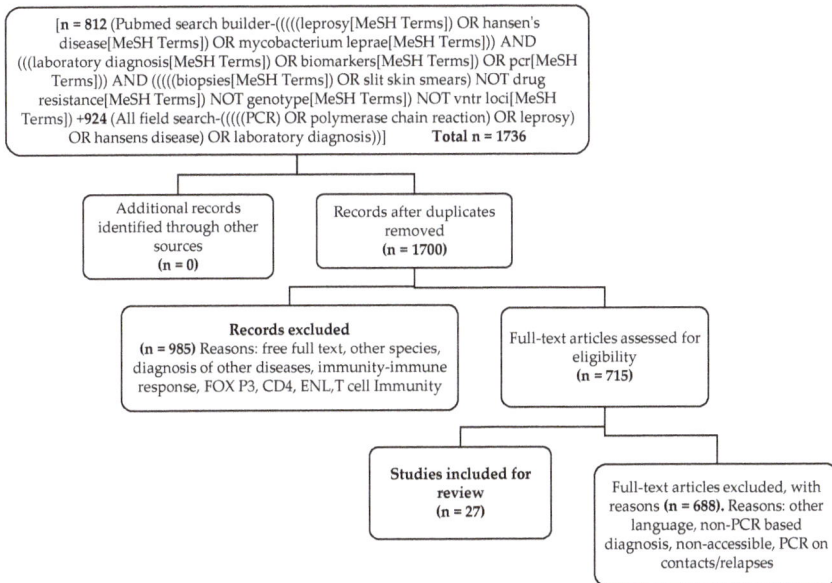

Figure 1. Flow chart detailing review steps (PRISMA guidelines).

2.3. Data Extraction

Each study was reviewed for the number of patients screened for leprosy diagnosis, mode of diagnosis including clinical examination and lab tests. Laboratory tests were further stratified into bacteriological examination by microscopy (AFB) and molecular tests (PCR) or histopathological examination (biopsy/HPE), clinical characteristics of the patients screened including PB/MB and nature of the clinical samples collected for lab diagnosis. Data on PCRs conducted on contacts/treated relapsed patients were excluded from the analysis. Percentage of positive results (sensitivity) for AFB microscopy and PCR were tabulated with reference to the clinical class of leprosy, AFB, and type of clinical sample used. Mean PCR positivity vis-à-vis genetic markers and the method of PCR used were also calculated.

2.4. Definitions of Some of the Data Terms Used in the Review

Report: Each individual paper included in the analysis is considered as one report;

Assay: PCR on each sample type and/or each gene marker from each report was considered as an independent assay;

Gene Marker: each genetic marker used for specific amplification of *M. leprae* DNA from clinical specimens;

PCR Method: laboratory technique of PCR used for amplifying the DNA targeting the *M. leprae* genetic markers.

2.5. Data Analysis

Data extraction has been carried out in such a way that PCR on each sample type and/or each gene marker was considered as an independent assay. Some of the papers reported PCR in one or more samples and/or one or more gene targets. Hence there were 38 assay resulting from the total of 27 papers that were reviewed. The matrix of published articles with types of lab tests conducted, types of samples used for testing, % PCR positivity, % AFB positivity on various samples, gene markers and/or PCR methods are tabulated for comparative analysis (Table 1). Mean and range are extracted for number of samples tested, percentage positivity of AFB, PCR for each clinical class, clinical specimen, PCR marker used, and PCR method used.

3. Results

3.1. Basic Clinical and Geographical Information

The review included published papers on PCR in new leprosy cases, along with clinical and conventional lab diagnostic tests. Out of 1700 papers screened, 27 papers qualified for the criteria of inclusion (flow chart, Figure 1). Out of the 27, nine were on leprosy patients from India, seven from Brazil, five from Bangkok, two from Philippines and one each from China, Ethiopia, Nepal, and Vietnam. Most of the reports included testing on clinically-diagnosed leprosy cases for confirming the laboratory test findings, limiting the scope of analysis for estimating only the sensitivity of the diagnostic tests. Most of those analyzed were reported based on either AFB microscopy on SSS or biopsies as the conventional lab standard test for comparing the PCR results.

3.2. Analysis

The average number of study subjects across the reports was 96 (range 20–439). Eighteen out of the 27 reports classified patients as PB and MB leprosy. Twenty-four (63%) out of 38 assays studied were less than 100 patients and 14 (37%) included more than 100 patients (Table 1). Seventeen out of 27 reports (62.9%) were based on a single PCR marker and nine (33%) used more than one marker; one (3.7%) used four markers. Three (8%) studies reported PCR results of a single marker on multiple samples (data not shown).

3.3. Clinical Classification vs. Sensitivity of AFB and PCR

Twenty-eight of the 38 of the total assays reported PCR on PB cases (six included data on AFB microscopy) (data not shown). Mean positivity for PCR was 48% (range 07–81) and AFB microscopy was 23% (range 1.7–35). Out of 38 assays, 26 reported PCR on MB leprosy cases and data on AFB was available for 17/26. Mean positivity for PCR was 77% (range 17–100) and AFB microscopy 59% (range 15–100) in reports on MB leprosy cases. Mean positivity for PCR was 44% (range 13–93) and AFB microscopy was 30% (range 10–86), if the total number of cases was not segregated as PB and MB (Table 2), indicating that PCR has only an incremental value over microscopy for bacteriological diagnosis of leprosy. Our observation on positivity of microscopy and PCR in PB leprosy cases reiterates the necessity to revise the current leprosy classification and treatment criteria. This also indicates that on an average 19% of cases were wrongly classified as PB (if only skin lesions were considered) and would have been missed treatment, had they not been tested with AFB and 10% more if PCR had not been used.

As expected, PCR turned out to be the most sensitive test for bacteriological confirmation on MB cases. Given the fact that MB leprosy lesions most frequently contain *M. leprae*, the mean PCR positivity in MB cases should have been more; however, the data suggests a lower average. This could have been due to technical bias due to errors in clinical sample collection and/or laboratory testing. These issues need to be addressed through development of robust clinical and lab protocols based on evidence from large multicentric studies through uniform study methodology.

A few reports included PCR results stratified for Ridley-Jopling classes of leprosy. Azevedo et al., 2017 [13] reported PCR across the spectrum, with percentage of PCR positivity as TT-21/38 (55.2%); BT-20/21 (95.2%); BB-18/18 (100%); BL-12/12 (100%); LL-13/13 (100%). In another recent report Chaitanya et al., 2017, reported the results for a multiplex PCR as indeterminate 31/41 (75.6%) TT-03/03 (100%); BT- 40/42 (95.2%); BB-03/03 (100%); BL-58/59 (98%); LL-70/72 (97%). PCR showed a good additional value in diagnosing TT and indeterminate cases, which are traditionally known to be negative for AFB on microscopy. This indicates that PCR could be a better test in classifying bacillary-positive cases than smear and microscopy [21].

3.4. Clinical Specimens and PCR

De Wit et al. (1993) reported on the utility of PCR for detection of *M. leprae* in nasal swab specimens amplifying the 531-bp *pra* gene, demonstrating 79.6% positivity of PCR [22]. Kyeong-Han Yoon reported PCR on slit skin samples, which was subsequently reported by many others [23–28]. PCR on biopsies has been reported by Wichitwechkarn et al. (1995), with a mean PCR positivity of 66% and subsequently by many others. We found that biopsy was the most common specimen to have been tested for PCR of *M. leprae* [13,21,29–37] (Table 1).

Out of 38 protocols studied, the majority (20) were based on skin biopsy (53%) followed by SSS (13, 34%); the rest of the samples included nerve biopsy, blood, and urine. AFB positivity in SSS has been 36% (range 18–69) and skin biopsy 44% (range 10–85). Likewise, PCR positivity on slit skin and biopsy was 61% (range 18–93) and 70% (range 46–93), respectively (Table 2). Since the skin biopsy and SSS happen to be the most frequent clinical samples collected for leprosy diagnosis, we tried to analyze the usefulness of PCR in the two samples. PCR seems to be more sensitive than microscopy in both the type of samples (SSS and biopsies), although skin biopsies have demonstrated significantly higher sensitivity to both microscopy and PCR as compared to SSS (Table 2). The reason could be the presence of a lesser number of bacilli in SSS than those in biopsy. The data suggests that PCR on skin biopsy seems to be the most sensitive test for demonstrating *M. leprae* bacilli. Nevertheless, with 62% sensitivity, PCR on SSS seems to be a better test when compared to microscopy (36%). Given the inherent limitations of skin biopsy such as the invasive nature of collection and technical expertise needed for test reporting, PCR on SSS samples with an average sensitivity of 62% seems to be more practical for application at primary care levels.

Apart from these two conventional specimens, researchers also studied *M. leprae* PCR on other unconventional samples. Caleffi et al. (2012) used PCR, amplifying a 151-bp PCR fragment of the *M. leprae pra* gene in urine samples. Thirty four of the 73 (46.58%) leprosy patients studied were positive for PCR [38]. Tiwari et al. (2017) evaluated PCR in nerve biopsy specimens of 35 pure neuritic leprosy cases. AFB was positive in 13 (37.14%) cases and PCR positivity was observed in 22 (62.86%) cases [39]. A study involved 43 newly-diagnosed leprosy patients, where quantitative PCR was carried out on whole blood samples (PCR positivity—13.95%) in comparison with SSS of the ear lobe (microscopy—30.23%; PCR positivity—41.86%) [40]. It is interesting to note that even urine and blood samples could be used for PCR testing. These reports suggest that blood and urine, although less sensitive on PCR than SSS, may still be considered as potential specimens, owing to the convenience of sample collection at all levels of health care. Future research for generating more evidence on usefulness of PCR on urine and blood, both in terms of sensitivity and feasibility for a point of care test would be promising.

Table 1. Data showing different studies involving conventional and molecular diagnosis of leprosy using different samples.

Sl. No.	Type of Sample	PCR Type	Marker/Gene	No. of Patients Studied	Smear Microscopy			PCR				First Author	Study Location/Country	Reference No.
					No. Tested	No. Positive	%	No. Tested	No. Positive	%	p Value			
1	Skin biopsy	Conventional PCR	RLEP	102	102	63	61.76	102	59	57.84	NA	Michelle de Campos Soriani Azevedo	Brazil	[13]
2	Skin biopsy	Multiplex PCR	RLEP	220	220	122	55.45	220	164	74.55	p < 0.05	V Sundeep Chaitanya	India	[21]
3	Skin biopsy	Multiplex PCR	M-PCR	220	220	122	55.45	220	205	93.18	NA	V Sundeep Chaitanya	India	[21]
4	Nasal swabs	Conventional PCR	531 bp fragment	103	0	0	0	103	82	79.61	NA	Madeleine Y. L. de Wit	Philippines	[22]
5	SSS	Conventional PCR	372 bp fragment	102	102	62	60.78	102	95	93.14	NA	Kyeong-Han Yoon	Philippines	[23]
6	Skin biopsy	Conventional PCR	372 bp	102	102	87	85.29	102	95	93.14	NA	Kyeong-Han Yoon	Philippines	[23]
7	SSS	in situ PCR	530 bp fragment	25	25	5	20	25	18	72	p = 0.01	R Kamal	India	[24]
8	SSS	Conventional PCR	RLEP	73	73	17	23.29	73	56	76.71	p < 0.001	R Kamal	India	[25]
9	SSS	Multiplex PCR	372&201 bp	439	439	223	50.8	439	371	84.51	NA	Surajita Banerjee	India	[26]
10	SSS	Conventional PCR	RLEP	50	50	9	18	50	36	72	NA	Shraddha Siwakoti	Nepal	[27]
11	SSS	Conventional PCR	PCR-LP	91	91	21	23.08	91	22	24.18	NA	Flaviane Granero Maltempe	Brazil	[28]
12	SSS	Conventional PCR	PCR-P	91	91	21	23.08	91	17	18.68	p > 0.05	Flaviane Granero Maltempe	Brazil	[28]
13	SSS	Conventional PCR	pra gene	53	0	0	0	53	17	32.08	NA	Jesdawan Wichitwechkaran	Bangkok	[29]
14	Skin biopsy	Conventional PCR	pra gene	53	0	0	0	53	35	66.04	NA	Jesdawan Wichitwechkaran	Bangkok	[29]
15	Skin biopsy	RT-PCR	16S rRNA	50	50	33	66	50	41	82	NA	Mekonnen Kurabachew	Ethiopia	[30]

Table 1. *Cont.*

Sl. No.	Type of Sample	PCR Type	Marker/Gene	No. of Patients Studied	Smear Microscopy			PCR			p Value	First Author	Study Location/Country	Reference No.
					No. Tested	No. Positive	%	No. Tested	No. Positive	%				
16	Nasal mucosal biopsies	RT-PCR	16S rRNA	60	60	24	40	60	47	78.33	NA	Benjawan Phetsuksiri	Bangkok	[31]
17	Skin biopsy	Conventional PCR	RLEP	110	110	43	39.09	110	81	73.64	NA	Isabela Maria Bernardes Goulart	Brazil	[32]
18	Skin biopsy	Conventional PCR	372 bp	110	110	43	39.09	110	58	52.73	NA	Isabela Maria Bernardes Goulart	Brazil	[32]
19	Skin biopsy	qPCR	16S rRNA	69	69	0	0	69	53	76.81	NA	Pham Dang Bang	Vietnam	[33]
20	Skin biopsy	qPCR	RLEP	47	0	0	0	47	38	80.85	NA	Alejandra Nóbrega Martinez	Brazil	[34]
21	Skin biopsy	qPCR	16S rRNA	47	0	0	0	47	24	51.06	NA	Alejandra Nóbrega Martinez	Brazil	[34]
22	Skin biopsy	qPCR	*sodA*	47	0	0	0	47	22	46.81	NA	Alejandra Nóbrega Martinez	Brazil	[34]
23	Skin biopsy	qPCR	85B	47	0	0	0	47	26	55.32	NA	Alejandra Nóbrega Martinez	Brazil	[34]
24	Skin biopsy	Multiplex PCR	372bp &201 bp	165	165	84	50.91	165	111	67.27	NA	Abu Hena Hasanoor Reja	India	[35]
25	Skin biopsy	qPCR	RLEP & 372 bp fragment	51	51	18	35.29	51	38	74.51	p > 0.05	Wen Yan	China	[36]
26	Skin biopsy	Nested PCR	RLEP &372 bp fragment	51	51	18	35.29	51	37	72.55	NA	Wen Yan	China	[36]
27	Skin biopsy	Conventional PCR	530 bp fragment	55	55	9	16.36	55	40	72.73	NA	Mohammad Shah Alam	Bangladesh	[37]
28	Urine	Conventional PCR	*pra* gene	73	73	0	0	73	34	46.58	p > 0.05	K.R. Caleffi	Brazil	[38]

Table 1. *Cont.*

Sl. No.	Type of Sample	PCR Type	Marker/Gene	No. of Patients Studied	Smear Microscopy			PCR			p Value	First Author	Study Location/Country	Reference No.
					No. Tested	No. Positive	%	No. Tested	No. Positive	%				
29	Nerve biopsy	Conventional PCR	375 bp fragment	35	35	13	37.14	35	22	62.86	NA	Vandana Tiwari	India	[39]
30	SSS	qPCR	16S rRNA	43	43	13	30.23	43	18	41.86	NA	Rafael Silva Gama	Brazil	[40]
31	blood	qPCR	16S rRNA	43	0	0	0	43	6	13.95	NA	Rafael Silva Gama	Brazil	[40]
32	SSS	Multiplex PCR	372 bp fragment	164	164	65	39.63	164	135	82.32	$p < 0.0001$	Surajita Banerjee	India	[41]
33	SSS	qPCR	16S rRNA	66	66	36	54.55	66	52	78.79	NA	Janisara Rudeeaneksin	Bangkok	[42]
34	Skin biopsy	in situ PCR	530 bp fragment	20	20	2	10	20	12	60	NA	R. Dayal	India	[43]
35	SSS	Conventional PCR	*pra* gene	122	122	49	40.16	122	86	70.49	$p < 0.001$	Kowit Kampirapap	Bangkok	[44]
36	Skin biopsy	Conventional PCR	RLEP	180	180	122	67.78	180	114	63.33	$p < 0.0001$	V Sundeep Chaitanya	India	[45]
37	Skin biopsy	Conventional PCR	ML1545	180	180	122	67.78	180	164	91.11	NA	V Sundeep Chaitanya	India	[45]
38	SSS	Conventional PCR	372 bp fragment	52	52	36	69.23	52	36	69.23	NA	Lucas Gomes Patrocinio	Brazil	[46]

Table 2. Details of assay—clinical classification, clinical sample vs. smear microcopy and polymerase chain reaction (PCR) positivity.

Classification	No. of Assay (Reports) Studied	Average Number of Patients/Samples Tested (Range)	No. of Assay Reported the AFB Microscopy	%AFB Positivity Mean (Range)	No. of Assay Reported PCR Tests	%PCR Positivity
Bacillary Load						
Paucibacillary	28	37.07 (7–234)	6	25.18 (1.75–35.29)	28	48.63 (7.69–81)
Multibacillary	27	61.40 (12–205)	17	62.25 (15.38–100)	27	79.65 (17.39–100)
Clinical samples						
Slit skin samples	14	101 (25–439)	12	37.73 (18–69.23)	14	60.71 (18.68–93.14)
Skin biopsy	20	96.3 (20–220)	14	48.96 (10–85.29)	20	70.27 (46.81–93.18)

3.5. Gene Markers—PCR Sensitivity

Various published reports on PCR in leprosy diagnosis studied a spectrum of gene markers as PCR targets on various clinical samples by multiple laboratory methods. There were twelve different markers used for PCR testing (Table 1). RLEP and 16S rRNA are the most frequent markers used, with PCR sensitivity ranging between 57% and 80% for RLEP and from 13% to 82% for 16S rRNA. RLEP seems to be the most sensitive marker for detecting *M. leprae* DNA, although its variable performance across the assays needs to be further addressed (Table 3). The sensitivity of RLEP PCR varied between samples, between clinical settings, and also between studies of the same authors. Martinez et al. (2011) reported highest RLEP sensitivity (81%) as compared to other three PCR markers [34]. Maltempe et al. (2016) reported RLEP PCR on SSS to be equally sensitive as AFB smear microscopy (24%) [28], which is the lowest (data not shown). Yan et al. (2014) reported at least 72% of RLEP PCR positivity as compared to 35% on smear microscopy of paraffin-embedded biopsies among PB leprosy cases [36]. The observations paved the way for exploring more evidence on RLEP PCR, the most frequently used and promising marker, for reasons of its variable performance and opportunities for improving its effectiveness. It was also observed that multiplexing RLEP with other markers yielded better results (data not shown), indicating the necessity for undertaking more studies in this direction, with large sample numbers and uniform protocols simultaneously studied across multiple clinical sites. The data also suggested that the highest mean positivity with any of the markers so far reported seems to be only 71%, which needs to be improved if PCR is to be used as a robust test for diagnosing leprosy. Since DNA extraction is one of the critical steps in any PCR-based diagnosis, it is logical to look into impact of role of DNA extraction procedures on PCR outcomes. We observed that most of the assays reviewed were based on the standard DNA extraction protocols such as phenol:chloroform method. We did not find any specific protocol associated with a higher PCR sensitivity (data not shown). None of the assays had reported the use of DNA extraction controls, which could have validated the sample processing procedure.

Table 3. PCR markers and methods vs. sensitivity.

	Number of Assays Studied (n = 38)	Highest Positivity (%PCR)	Lowest Positivity (%PCR)
Gene markers			
RLEP	9	80.85	57.84
16S rRNA	10	82	13.95
Method of PCR			
Conventional	19	93.14	18.68
Multiplex	6	93.18	67.27
Q-PCR	6	80.85	13.95
RT-PCR	5	74.5	82

There should be more research exploring better markers and suitable lab protocols for increasing the sensitivity of PCR for detecting *M. leprae*. Advancing scientific knowledge and an omics approach should throw some light on identifying such novel markers and developing them into robust PCR test modules for point-of-care diagnostic testing in leprosy.

3.6. Method of PCR vs. PCR Sensitivity

Out of 27 reports reviewed, 19 were based on conventional PCR, 6 were on quantitative real time PCR (qPCR), 4 on multiplex PCR and 2 were on reverse transcriptase PCR (RT-PCR) assays. Researchers have employed various PCR techniques for molecular diagnosis of *M. leprae* from SSS, skin biopsy, blood and urine samples. Conventional PCR targeting a single gene has been found to be the most frequently reported method. Several authors have used conventional PCR on slit skin, biopsy, urine, blood [27,37–40]. On the other hand, few studies have utilized multiplex PCR on slit skin and biopsies, amplifying more than one target sequence, at the same level of laboratory settings as conventional PCR [21,26,35,41]. There are also reports on methods such as quantitative PCR, RT-PCR and in situ PCR, which are based on advanced laboratory facility and studies have reported RT-PCR on skin biopsies, SSS and nasal biopsies [30,31,33,36,42]. Real-time quantitative (q-PCR) PCR technique was used by Martinez et al. (2011) and Gama et al. (2018) [34,40]. Yan et al. (2014) studied the nested PCR technique using two sets of primers to apply two different *M. leprae*-specific gene fragments from paraffin-embedded skin biopsy specimens [36]. Dayal et al. (2005) and Kamal et al. (2010) reported in situ PCR [24,43].

From the above analyzed assay, the highest percentage of PCR sensitivity was observed using multiplex PCR technique (82%) followed by RT-PCR (78%) and conventional PCR (63%). These two techniques seem to be very useful PCR techniques in the rapid diagnosis of *M. leprae*. This observation indicates that even a simple PCR but with more than one marker and appropriate technical protocol could do better in picking up *M. leprae* DNA from clinical samples. This in turn indicates the usefulness of simple PCR-based tests for bacteriological diagnosis of leprosy even with a modestly-equipped laboratory facility, although RT-PCR carries a technical advantage over simple PCR by providing quantitative estimate.

The review analysis found that no individual *M. leprae* gene marker has been associated with higher sensitivity. However, using more than one marker in a multiplex format of conventional PCR seem to have yielded significantly higher mean positivity and hence could be a better choice (Table 3). Almost all studies reported in this review have studied techniques based on traditional laboratory-based PCRs, since the evidence gathered through this review suggests that it is more important to have appropriate protocols and robust markers for PCR sensitivity than sophisticated technology. Recent advancements in molecular methods has enhanced the capability of detection and characterization of infectious diseases. PCR is one of the techniques of molecular diagnosis that has great benefits and enhances advancements in rapid diagnosis. There are many simple point of care (POC) PCRs such as the LAMP test and Xpert TB available for diseases like TB, HIV, and malaria etc. [47–52]. Developing one or more of the existing markers into such POC platforms should be the goal of future research in molecular diagnosis of leprosy. Developing such point-of-care, easy-to-use PCR modules could have potential application at all healthcare levels. This addresses the issue of access to healthcare for persons affected by leprosy or those at risk of developing leprosy. Increasing access to healthcare leads to early detection of leprosy and prevention of consequences—the most important aspects of leprosy control. Hence it is envisaged that further research on PCR in leprosy include investigating various markers for the usefulness of point-of-care testing.

4. Conclusions

The evidence from this review analysis suggests that PCR on a skin biopsy is the ideal diagnostic test. Nevertheless, PCR on SSS samples also seems to be useful with its practical value for application at primary healthcare levels. Future research for better evidence on the usefulness of PCR on other samples such as urine and blood are recommended to avoid collecting slit skin/biopsy samples, which are relatively more invasive. Our observation on positivity of AFB microscopy and PCR in PB leprosy cases reiterates the necessity to revise the current leprosy classification and treatment criteria based merely on the number of skin lesions. PCR could be a better test in classifying bacillary positive cases than smear microscopy. Having said that, our review findings indicate the necessity for improving the sensitivity of PCR and further research on specificity is required in ruling out other clinical conditions that may mimic leprosy. Development of robust clinical and lab protocols based on evidence from large multicenter studies through uniform study methodology might be of great help in addressing the sensitivity and specificity issues. We found that no individual *M. leprae* gene marker has been associated with higher PCR sensitivity, indicating the need for more evidence for robust markers. However, using more than one marker in a multiplex format of conventional PCR seems to have

Trop. Med. Infect. Dis. **2018**, *3*, 107

yielded significantly higher PCR positivity and hence could be a better choice. RLEP, although the most frequent marker used, showed variable performance across the clinical sites, and samples are a matter of concern. Combining it with other markers in a multiplex PCR format might work. Multiplexing more than one target *M. leprae* gene might also help to address this issue. Undertaking more studies of this nature, with large sample numbers and uniform protocols simultaneously studied across multiple clinical sites would be useful. In addition, there should be more research exploring better markers for increasing sensitivity of PCR for detecting *M. leprae*. Advancing scientific knowledge and omics approach should throw some light on the identification of such novel markers and developing them into robust PCR test modules for point-of-care diagnostic testing in leprosy.

Limitations of This Systematic Review Analysis

The present review has been mainly based on the reports available on the PubMed database and did not include any other databases due to the time and resource constraints. This might have led to a selection bias of papers published only on PubMed. We did not gather any other types of information sources such as unpublished data, data from ongoing studies from various researchers, which could perhaps have made our observations stronger. The data from records mainly comprising clinically-diagnosed leprosy cases, except one record, meant that we were unable to estimate test specificity. Analysis included data only on new patients. However, the authors would like to address the other two important applications of PCR, namely for contact screening and treatment monitoring through separate independent reviews. We limited the analysis to systematic review only and did not attempt meta-analysis due to heterogeneity of the data. This review could not elicit any significant evidence on usefulness of any specific marker for PCR, due to either limited number of studies or limited number of samples. Further studies with large sample sizes with existing or new markers are warranted to enhance evidence on this particular aspect.

Author Contributions: A.S.: Conceived the idea, formed the review group, prepared the review protocols, data analysis, manuscript writing, review, approval of the manuscript; S.T.: Data collection, manuscript writing, reading of individual review papers; S.K.: reading of individual review papers, manuscript writing.

Funding: This research received no external funding.

Acknowledgments: LEPRA-Blue Peter Public Health and Research Center is core funded by Lepra, UK. S.T. is supported under ICMR grant No. AMR/IN/113/2017-ECD-II. Authors are thankful for the assistance provided by Pramilesh Suryavanshi for his initial contributions during the protocol preparation and Chakrapani Chatla for his assistance during data analysis and critical review.

Conflicts of Interest: Authors have no competing interests of any sort while bringing out this review analysis.

References

1. Noordeen, S.K. The epidemiology of leprosy. In *Leprosy*; Hastings, R.C., Ed.; Churchill Livingstone, Produced by Longman Group Ltd.: Hong Kong, China, 1985; pp. 15–30.
2. Dockrell, H.M. *Leprosy*, 3rd ed.; Bryceson, A.D.M., Pfaltzgraff, R.E., Eds.; Churchill Livingstone: Edinburgh, UK, 1990; p. 240, ISBN 0-443-03373-0.
3. Lockwood, D.N.J. Leprosy. *Medicine* **2005**, *33*, 26–29. [CrossRef]
4. Van Brakel, W.H.; Sihombing, B.; Djarir, H.; Beise, K.; Kusumawardhani, L.; Yulihane, R.; Kurniasari, I.; Kasim, M.; Kesumaningsih, K.I.; Wilder-Smith, A. Disability in people affected by leprosy: The role of impairment, activity, social participation, stigma and discrimination. *Glob. Health Action.* **2012**, *5*. [CrossRef] [PubMed]
5. World Health Organization. *Global Target Attained, Remaining Endemic Countries Pose Greatest Challenge*; Press Release, WHA/2; WHO: Geneva, Switzerland, 2002.
6. World Health Organization. *The Global Leprosy Strategy 2016–2020: Accelerating towards a Leprosy-Free World*; WHO: Geneva, Switzerland, 2016.
7. World Health Organization. Global leprosy update, 2016: Accelerating reduction of disease burden. *Wkly. Epidemiol. Rec.* **2017**, *92*, 501–520.

8.   Sermrittirong, S.; van Brakel, W.H. Stigma in leprosy: Concepts, causes and determinants. *Lepr. Rev.* **2014**, *85*, 36–47. [PubMed]

9.   Duthie, M.S.; Truman, R.W.; Goto, W.; O'Donnell, J.; Hay, M.N.; Spencer, J.S.; Carter, D.; Reed, S.G. Insight toward early diagnosis of leprosy through analysis of the developing antibody responses of *Mycobacterium leprae*-infected armadillos. *Clin. Vaccine Immunol.* **2011**, *18*, 254–259. [CrossRef] [PubMed]

10.   Veena, S.; Kumar, P.; Shashikala, P.; Gurubasavaraj, H.; Chandrasekhar, H.R. Significance of histopathology in leprosy patients with 1–5 skin lesions with relevance to therapy. *J. Lab. Physicians* **2011**, *3*, 21–24. [CrossRef] [PubMed]

11.   Lockwood, D.N.; Nicholls, P.; Smith, W.C.; Das, L.; Barkataki, P.; van Brakel, W.; Suneetha, S. Comparing the clinical and histological diagnosis of leprosy and leprosy reactions in the INFIR cohort of Indian patients with multibacillary leprosy. *PLoS Negl. Trop. Dis.* **2012**, *6*, e1702. [CrossRef] [PubMed]

12.   Fischer, M. Leprosy—An overview of clinical features, diagnosis, and treatment. *J. Dtsch. Dermatol. Ges.* **2017**, *15*, 801–827. [CrossRef] [PubMed]

13.   Lastória, J.C.; Abreu, M.A. Leprosy: A review of laboratory and therapeutic aspects—Part 2. *An. Bras. Dermatol.* **2014**, *89*, 389–401. [CrossRef] [PubMed]

14.   Azevedo, M.C.; Ramuno, N.M.; Fachin, L.R.; Tassa, M.; Rosa, P.S.; Belone, A.F.; Diorio, S.M.; Soares, C.T.; Garlet, G.P.; Trombone, A.P. qPCR detection of *Mycobacterium leprae* in biopsies and slit skin smear of different leprosy clinical forms. *Braz. J. Infect. Dis.* **2017**, *21*, 71–78. [CrossRef] [PubMed]

15.   Speers, D.J. Clinical applications of molecular biology for infectious diseases. *Clin. Biochem. Rev.* **2006**, *27*, 39–51. [PubMed]

16.   Niemz, A.; Boyle, D.S. Nucleic acid testing for tuberculosis at the point-of-care in high-burden countries. *Expert Rev. Mol. Diagn.* **2012**, *12*, 687–701. [CrossRef] [PubMed]

17.   Martinez, A.N.; Talhari, C.; Moraes, M.O.; Talhari, S. PCR-based techniques for leprosy diagnosis: From the laboratory to the clinic. *PLoS Negl. Trop. Dis.* **2014**, *8*, e2655. [CrossRef] [PubMed]

18.   Male, M.M.; Rao, B.G.; Chokkakula, S.; Kasetty, S.; Rao, P.V.R.; Jonnalagada, S.; Reddy, A.M.; Srikantam, A. Molecular screening for primary drug resistance in *M. leprae* from newly diagnosed leprosy cases from India. *Lepr. Rev.* **2016**, *87*, 322–331.

19.   Moher, D.; Liberati, A.; Tetzlaff, J.; Altman, D.G.; Group, P. Preferred reporting items for systematic reviews and meta-analyses: The PRISMA statement. *Ann. Intern. Med.* **2009**, *151*, 264–269. [CrossRef] [PubMed]

20.   Canese, K.; Weis, S. PubMed: The Bibliographic Database. In *The NCBI Handbook [Internet]*, 2nd ed.; National Center for Biotechnology Information (US): Bethesda, MD, USA, 2013.

21.   Chaitanya, V.S.; Cuello, L.; Das, M.; Sudharsan, A.; Ganesan, P.; Kanmani, K.; Rajan, L.; Ebenezer, M. Analysis of a novel multiplex polymerase chain reaction assay as a sensitive tool for the diagnosis of indeterminate and tuberculoid forms of leprosy. *Int. J. Mycobacteriol.* **2017**, *6*, 1–8. [CrossRef] [PubMed]

22.   De Wit, M.Y.; Douglas, J.T.; McFadden, J.; Klatser, P.R. Polymerase chain reaction for detection of *Mycobacterium leprae* in nasal swab specimens. *J. Clin. Microbiol.* **1993**, *31*, 502–506. [PubMed]

23.   Yoon, K.H.; Cho, S.N.; Lee, M.K.; Abalos, R.M.; Cellona, R.V.; Fajardo, T.T., Jr.; Guido, L.S.; Dela Cruz, E.C.; Walsh, G.P.; Kim, J.D. Evaluation of polymerase chain reaction amplification of mycobacterium leprae-specific repetitive sequence in biopsy specimens from leprosy patients. *J. Clin. Microbiol.* **1993**, *31*, 895–899. [PubMed]

24.   Kamal, R.; Natrajan, M.; Katoch, K.; Katoch, V.M. Evaluation of diagnostic role of in situ PCR on slit-skin smears in pediatric leprosy. *Indian J. Lepr.* **2010**, *82*, 195–200. [PubMed]

25.   Kamal, R.; Dayal, R.; Gaidhankar, K.; Biswas, S.; Gupta, S.B.; Kumar, N.; Kumar, R.; Pengoria, R.; Chauhan, DS.; Katoch, K.; et al. RLEP PCR as a definitive diagnostic test for leprosy from skin smear samples in childhood and adolescent leprosy. *Indian J. Lepr.* **2016**, *88*, 193–197.

26.   Banerjee, S.; Sarkar, K.; Gupta, S.; Mahapatra, P.S.; Gupta, S.; Guha, S.; Bandhopadhayay, D.; Ghosal, C.; Paine, S.K.; Dutta, R.N.; et al. Multiplex PCR technique could be an alternative approach for early detection of leprosy among close contacts—A pilot study from India. *BMC Infect. Dis.* **2010**, *10*, 252. [CrossRef] [PubMed]

27.   Siwakoti, S.; Rai, K.; Bhattarai, N.R.; Agarwal, S.; Khanal, B. Evaluation of polymerase chain reaction (PCR) with slit skin smear examination (SSS) to confirm clinical diagnosis of leprosy in eastern Nepal. *PLoS Negl. Trop. Dis.* **2016**, *10*, e0005220. [CrossRef] [PubMed]

28. Maltempe, F.G.; Baldin, V.P.; Lopes, M.A.; Siqueira, V.L.D.; de Lima Scodro, R.B.; Cardoso, R.F.; Caleffi-Ferracioli, K.R. Critical analysis: Use of polymerase chain reaction to diagnose leprosy. *Braz. J. Pharm. Sci.* **2016**, *52*. [CrossRef]

29. Wichitwechkarn, J.; Karnjan, S.; Shuntawuttisettee, S.; Sornprasit, C.; Kampirapap, K.; Peerapakorn, S. Detection of *Mycobacterium leprae* infection by PCR. *J. Clin. Microbiol.* **1995**, *33*, 45–49. [PubMed]

30. Kurabachew, M.; Wondimu, A.; Ryon, J.J. Reverse transcription-PCR detection of *Mycobacterium leprae* in clinical specimens. *J. Clin. Microbiol.* **1998**, *36*, 1352–1356. [PubMed]

31. Phetsuksiri, B.; Rudeeaneksin, J.; Supapkul, P.; Wachapong, S.; Mahotarn, K.; Brennan, P.J. A simplified reverse transcriptase PCR for rapid detection of *Mycobacterium leprae* in skin specimens. *FEMS Immunol. Med. Microbiol.* **2006**, *48*, 319–328. [CrossRef] [PubMed]

32. Goulart, I.M.; Cardoso, A.M.; Santos, M.S.; Goncalves, M.A.; Pereira, J.E.; Goulart, L.R. Detection of *Mycobacterium leprae* DNA in skin lesions of leprosy patients by PCR may be affected by amplicon size. *Arch. Dermatol. Res.* **2007**, *299*, 267–271. [CrossRef] [PubMed]

33. Bang, P.D.; Suzuki, K.; Phuong le, T.; Chu, T.M.; Ishii, N.; Khang, T.H. Evaluation of polymerase chain reaction-based detection of *Mycobacterium leprae* for the diagnosis of leprosy. *J. Dermatol.* **2009**, *36*, 269–276. [CrossRef] [PubMed]

34. Martinez, A.N.; Ribeiro-Alves, M.; Sarno, E.N.; Moraes, M.O. Evaluation of qPCR-based assays for leprosy diagnosis directly in clinical specimens. *PLoS Negl. Trop. Dis.* **2011**, *5*, e1354. [CrossRef] [PubMed]

35. Reja, A.H.; Biswas, N.; Biswas, S.; Dasgupta, S.; Chowdhury, I.H.; Banerjee, S.; Chakraborty, T.; Dutta, P.K.; Bhattacharya, B. Fite-Faraco staining in combination with multiplex polymerase chain reaction: A new approach to leprosy diagnosis. *Indian J. Dermatol. Venereol. Leprol.* **2013**, *79*, 693–700. [CrossRef] [PubMed]

36. Yan, W.; Xing, Y.; Yuan, L.C.; De Yang, R.; Tan, F.Y.; Zhang, Y.; Li, H.Y. Application of RLEP real-time PCR for detection of *M. leprae* DNA in paraffin-embedded skin biopsy specimens for diagnosis of paucibacillary leprosy. *Am. J. Trop. Med. Hyg.* **2014**, *90*, 524–529. [CrossRef] [PubMed]

37. Alam, M.S.; Shamsuzzaman, S.M.; Mamun, K.Z. Demography, clinical presentation and laboratory diagnosis of leprosy by microscopy, histopathology and PCR from Dhaka city in Bangladesh. *Lepr. Rev.* **2017**, *88*, 122–130.

38. Caleffi, K.R.; Hirata, R.D.; Hirata, M.H.; Caleffi, E.R.; Siqueira, V.L.; Cardoso, R.F. Use of the polymerase chain reaction to detect *Mycobacterium leprae* in urine. *Braz. J. Med. Biol. Res.* **2012**, *45*, 153–157. [CrossRef] [PubMed]

39. Tiwari, V.; Malhotra, K.; Khan, K.; Maurya, P.K.; Singh, A.K.; Thacker, A.K.; Husain, N.; Kulshreshtha, D. Evaluation of polymerase chain reaction in nerve biopsy specimens of patients with Hansen's disease. *J. Neurol. Sci.* **2017**, *380*, 187–190. [CrossRef] [PubMed]

40. Gama, R.S.; Gomides, T.A.R.; Gama, C.F.M.; Moreira, S.J.M.; de Neves Manta, F.S.; de Oliveira, L.B.P.; Marcal, P.H.F.; Sarno, E.N.; Moraes, M.O.; Garcia, R.M.G.; et al. High frequency of *M. leprae* DNA detection in asymptomatic household contacts. *BMC Infect. Dis.* **2018**, *18*, 153. [CrossRef] [PubMed]

41. Banerjee, S.; Biswas, N.; Kanti Das, N.; Sil, A.; Ghosh, P.; Hasanoor Raja, A.H.; Dasgupta, S.; Kanti Datta, P.; Bhattacharya, B. Diagnosing leprosy: Revisiting the role of the slit-skin smear with critical analysis of the applicability of polymerase chain reaction in diagnosis. *Int. J. Dermatol.* **2011**, *50*, 1522–1527. [CrossRef] [PubMed]

42. Rudeeaneksin, J.; Srisungngam, S.; Sawanpanyalert, P.; Sittiwakin, T.; Likanonsakul, S.; Pasadorn, S.; Palittapongarnpim, P.; Brennan, P.J.; Phetsuksiri, B. LightCycler real-time PCR for rapid detection and quantitation of *Mycobacterium leprae* in skin specimens. *FEMS Immunol. Med. Microbiol.* **2008**, *54*, 263–270. [CrossRef] [PubMed]

43. Dayal, R.; Singh, S.P.; Mathur, P.P.; Katoch, V.M.; Katoch, K.; Natrajan, M. Diagnostic value of in situ polymerase chain reaction in leprosy. *Indian J. Pediatr.* **2005**, *72*, 1043–1046. [CrossRef] [PubMed]

44. Kampirapap, K.; Singtham, N.; Klatser, P.R.; Wiriyawipart, S. DNA amplification for detection of leprosy and assessment of efficacy of leprosy chemotherapy. *Int. J. Lepr. Other Mycobact. Dis.* **1998**, *66*, 16–21. [PubMed]

45. Sundeep Chaitanya, V.; Das, M.; Eisenbach, T.L.; Amoako, A.; Rajan, L.; Horo, I.; Ebenezer, M. *Mycobacterium leprae* specific genomic target in the promoter region of probable 4-alpha-glucanotransferase (ML1545) gene with potential sensitivity for polymerase chain reaction based diagnosis of leprosy. *Int. J. Mycobacteriol.* **2016**, *5*, 135–141. [CrossRef] [PubMed]

Trop. Med. Infect. Dis. **2018**, *3*, 107

46. Patrocínio, L.G.; Goulart, I.M.; Goulart, L.R.; Patrocinio, J.A.; Ferreira, F.R.; Fleury, R.N. Detection of *Mycobacterium leprae* in nasal mucosa biopsies by the polymerase chain reaction. *FEMS Immunol. Med. Microbiol.* **2005**, *44*, 311–316. [CrossRef] [PubMed]

47. Boehme, C.C.; Nabeta, P.; Henostroza, G.; Raqib, R.; Rahim, Z.; Gerhardt, M.; Sanga, E.; Hoelscher, M.; Notomi, T.; Hase, T.; et al. Operational feasibility of using loop-mediated isothermal amplification for diagnosis of pulmonary tuberculosis in microscopy centers of developing countries. *J. Clin. Microbiol.* **2007**, *45*, 1936–1940. [CrossRef] [PubMed]

48. Boehme, C.C.; Nabeta, P.; Hillemann, D.; Nicol, M.P.; Shenai, S.; Krapp, F.; Allen, J.; Tahirli, R.; Blakemore, R.; Rustomjee, R.; et al. Rapid molecular detection of tuberculosis and rifampin resistance. *N. Engl. J. Med.* **2010**, *363*, 1005–1015. [CrossRef] [PubMed]

49. Mori, Y.; Notomi, T. Loop-mediated isothermal amplification (LAMP): A rapid, accurate, and cost-effective diagnostic method for infectious diseases. *J. Infect. Chemother.* **2009**, *15*, 62–69. [CrossRef] [PubMed]

50. Lawn, S.D.; Nicol, M.P. Xpert® MTB/RIF assay: Development, evaluation and implementation of a new rapid molecular diagnostic for tuberculosis and rifampicin resistance. *Future Microbiol.* **2011**, *6*, 1067–1082. [CrossRef] [PubMed]

51. Arora, D.R.; Maheshwari, M.; Arora, B. Rapid point-of-care testing for detection of HIV and clinical monitoring. *ISRN AIDS* **2013**, *2013*, 287269. [CrossRef] [PubMed]

52. Kim, S.; Nhem, S.; Dourng, D.; Ménard, D. Malaria rapid diagnostic test as point-of-care test: Study protocol for evaluating the VIKIA® Malaria Ag Pf/Pan. *Malar. J.* **2015**, *14*, 114. [CrossRef] [PubMed]

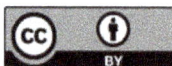

*Tropical Medicine and
Infectious Disease*

MDPI

Article

Investigation of a Scabies Outbreak in Drought-Affected Areas in Ethiopia

Wendemagegn Enbiale [1,*] and Ashenafi Ayalew [2]

[1] Dermatology and Venerology, Bahir Dar University, P.O. Box 1996, Bahir Dar, Ethiopia
[2] Amhara Regional Health Bureau, P.O. Box 744, Amhara, Ethiopia; ashunets@gmail.com
* Correspondence: wendaab@gmail.com; Tel.: +251-911034612

Received: 10 September 2018; Accepted: 25 October 2018; Published: 29 October 2018

Abstract: The impact of the severe drought in Ethiopia, attributed to El Niño weather conditions, has led to high levels of malnutrition that have, in turn, increased the potential for disease outbreaks. In 2015, Ethiopia faced a scabies outbreak in drought-affected areas where there was a shortage of safe water for drinking and personal hygiene. Following a house-to-house census to assess the prevalence of scabies, a detailed study was conducted looking at the disease burden. Following the outbreak report, training was provided on scabies identification and management for zonal and district health officials from administrative districts affected by the drought (nutritional hot-spot *woredas*). The training was cascaded down to the health extension workers in the affected areas. Screening and management guidelines and protocols were also distributed. House-to-house data collection was undertaken by 450 health extension workers (HEWs) to assess the prevalence of scabies. The HEWs used a simplified reporting tool. Subsequently, data were collected and validated in two zones and six *woredas* from 474 participants who had been diagnosed with scabies using a standardized questionnaire. This was designed to look at the specificity of the diagnosis of scabies, age distribution, severity, duration of illness, secondary infection and other sociodemographic variables as preparation for mass drug administration (MDA). The HEWs screened 1,125,770 people in the 68 districts in Amhara Region and a total of 379,000 confirmed cases of scabies was identified. The prevalence in the different districts ranged from 2% to 67% and the median was 33.5% [interquartile range (IQR) 19–48%]. 49% of cases were school-aged children. The detailed study of 474 individuals who were recorded as scabies cases revealed that the specificity of the diagnosis of scabies by the HEWs was 98.3%. The mean duration of illness was 5 months (SD of ± 2.8). One third of patients were recorded as having severe illness, 75.1% of cases had affected family members, and 30% of affected children were noted to have secondary bacterial infection. Eleven percent of the students had discontinued school due to scabies or/and drought and 85% of these had secondary bacterial infection. These community-based data serve as reliable proxy indicators for community-based burden assessment of the scabies epidemic. This study will also provide a good basis for advocating the use of a community-level clinical diagnostic scheme for scabies using an algorithm with a simple combination of signs and symptoms in resource-poor settings.

Keywords: scabies; outbreak; drought; emergency state

---

1. Background

Scabies is a common public health problem, globally affecting about 200 million people. It is a particular problem where there is social disruption, overcrowding, and where personal hygiene is poor. Immunosuppression, poor nutritional status, and dementia are also risk factors for scabies [1–3]. Natural disasters, war, and poverty lead to overcrowding and have been associated with increased rates of transmission [4].

Scabies is caused by an ecto-parasitic infestation of the skin by the human itch mite, *Sarcoptes scabiei* var. *hominis* [1]. It usually spreads by direct, prolonged, skin-to-skin contact with an infested individual. The main effect of scabies is debilitating itching, leading to scratching, which in turn is followed by breakdown of the barrier function of the skin and complications due to bacterial infection, ranging from impetigo, abscesses, and cellulitis, to more serious conditions such as septicemia and glomerulonephritis, leading to renal failure and rheumatic heart disease [1,4].

1.1. Drought

The data from The International Disaster Database indicate that in Africa more than 40 million people were affected by drought in 2015–2016. Following the 2015–2016 El-Niño event, which affected many countries globally, Ethiopia experienced drought and extreme water shortage across large parts of the country. This has further limited access to water for personal hygiene and basic sanitation for many individuals, especially those in rural communities, leading to a great increase in the risk of communicable diseases like scabies and diarrheal diseases [5].

Most definitions of drought describe it as a prolonged period of abnormally low rainfall, leading to a shortage of water. The effects of drought are critically dependent on both context and vulnerability of the underlying population. The development and severity of the drought depends on the background level of water use, which may also influence the timing of the onset, duration, and end of the drought, as well as the social, economic, and administrative infrastructures which address the consequences of water deficit. The impact on health is particularly dependent on the socio-economic environment that, in turn, has a direct impact on the resilience of the population. Poor health, poverty, and conflict are additional contributing factors that exacerbate the impact of drought [6,7].

1.2. Government Priorities/Political Setting

Following official acknowledgment by the Ethiopian government of a food crisis in July 2015, the Federal Ministry of Health established a command post spearheaded by the Public Health Emergency Management (PHEM) directorate. In September 2015, the Amhara Regional State PHEM announced the first report of a scabies epidemic [8]. To validate the diagnosis, a team of field epidemiologists and a dermatologist visited three of the areas where the claim had emerged. The experts collected data from three health centers and six health posts in addition to visiting households that had been previously diagnosed with scabies at local health facilities. The experts concluded that scabies was the major active public health problem affecting the community, with the status of an outbreak [9].

Prior to September 2015, the regular review of drought-related public health emergencies, in both federal and regional PHEM disease surveillance systems, focused solely on malnutrition, diarrheal diseases, measles, malaria, and meningitis; however, there was no consideration of skin-related conditions. A recent literature review by Anderson and Davies has shown that El Niño has been associated with increases in the occurrence of sun-related skin diseases and certain vector-borne and waterborne diseases [10]. Despite outbreak reports in some parts of the country [8], scabies was not included in either the list of reportable diseases or the weekly reports.

After the first visit to some of the affected zones and a review of information regarding the burden of the problem, the inspection team advocated the inclusion of scabies as a separate item on the weekly surveillance list for the Federal Ministry of Health and Regional Health Bureau. Since October 2015, scabies has been included as one of the reportable diseases in the drought affected areas. The weekly PHEM surveillance reports revealed that scabies was becoming significantly more extensive than its more usual occurrence as sporadic clinical cases, and was now a public health concern affecting wider geographic areas and population groups, especially in the *woredas* most severely affected by drought and malnutrition. Hence, it required public mobilization and public health emergency interventions. The report revealed that the Amhara, Tigray, and Oromia regions had the highest burdens of scabies in Ethiopia.

The extent of the drought and the increased number of water-scarce *woredas* with limited access to water sanitation and hygiene (WASH) interventions, further worsened the spread of the disease and its severity among the vulnerable. From the November 2015 harvest season assessment, the number of nutritional hot-spot *woredas* increased to 429, involving a total population of nearly 49 million. That same month, the public health emergency management task force received a report that the number of severely affected *woredas* in Amhara, Tigray, and Oromia had reached 32, and despite the limited surveillance program for scabies, the estimated total number of cases reached more than 250,000 with prevalence of at least 15% in some districts [6].

In October 2015, following the national government elections, prominent officials at all levels of the administration attended an official meeting. The researchers used this as an opportunity to present the preliminary data of the burden of scabies and the recommended action to be taken by the relevant officials (zonal and *woreda* administrators, zonal and *woreda* health office officers, heads of the Regional Health Bureau, and other officials) and to advocate for region wide evidence generation in preparation for the intervention.

A systematic review of scabies prevalence studies published between 1985 and 2015, included only five African countries, highlighting the paucity of prevalence data in Africa [11]. This house-to-house census and validation study of scabies provides a unique opportunity to ascertain community prevalence. Such data is more reliable than health facility-based data which generally underestimates prevalence, as individuals within communities may not present with scabies (perhaps because it is 'normalized') or because there is under-diagnosis or lack of effective treatments at clinics [12].

2. Methods

The outbreak assessment developed in two stages.

2.1. Phase 1

Following one-day face-to-face training on data recording, diagnosis, and management of scabies along with other relevant conditions for district health officials and the subsequent cascading of training to the front line care workers or health extension workers, a house-to-house census was undertaken in all the 68 hotspot *woredas* (districts) in the Amhara region (Figure 1).

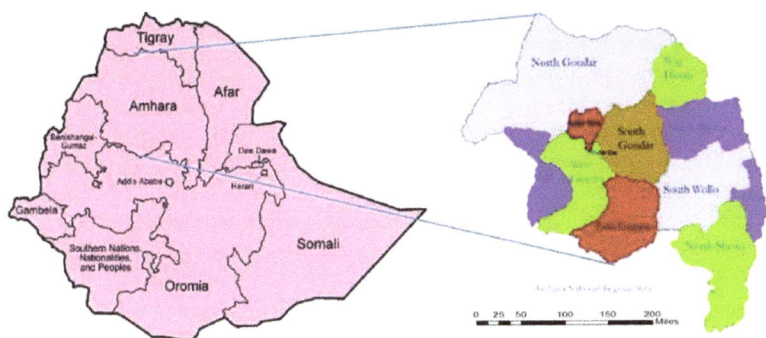

Figure 1. Amhara regional State, Ethiopia (2015/2016).

A cross-sectional house-to-house census was performed, identifying scabies cases and contacts based on regional scabies identification and management guidelines in the Amhara region as preparation for the developing a scabies outbreak control program [7]. The census was performed in all households of the previously identified 68 hot-spot districts. The sites were selected by the Regional Health Bureau and PHEM team from the routine weekly report (districts in the region that have reported scabies). In each household, all family members were screened. The study period was from October to November 2015.

The census was conducted as part of the Regional Health Bureau screening in preparation for a community-based scabies control program. The local HEW, supervised by health officers/BSc nurses from nearby health centers, registered each resident by name, age, and sex and each resident was screened for scabies. Age groups were defined as follows: <2 years, 2 to 18 years, >18 years.

Each participant was examined by a HEW trained in scabies diagnosis and treatment. The diagnosis of scabies was based on the clinical case definition (Table 1). In addition to scabies screening, the census was used for the integrated assessment of pre-determined drought-related health problems (malnutrition, measles, diarrheal diseases, meningitis, malaria, and scabies). The screening of drought related pre-determined diseases by the health extension workers in relation to scabies had, up to this point, used only a limited set of information variables to identify cases of scabies and their contacts in each district.

Table 1. Clinical case definition of scabies and contact [7].

Scabies	Presence of itching with typical lesions on hands, inter-digital, and/or genitalia and/or itching and close contact with an individual who has itching or typical lesions in a typical distribution.
Contact	A contact is a person who does not fulfill the clinical criteria for infestation with scabies (above) or a person without signs and symptoms consistent with scabies, who has had direct contact (particularly prolonged, direct, skin-to-skin contact) with a suspected or confirmed case in the two months preceding the onset of scabies signs and symptoms in the index case

The data were analyzed and results are presented using descriptive statistics. Scabies prevalence in the different age group and districts was calculated. In addition, statistical analysis was performed with SPSS 10.0 for Windows (SPSS Inc., Chicago, IL, USA). The median, interquartile range (IQR) and odds ratio (OR) were calculated and the p-value derived.

2.2. Phase 2

This study, performed between 16 October and 2 December 2015, was undertaken primarily to validate the data collected by the HEW and secondly to obtain an understanding of associated factors of the scabies epidemic. The study population was residents identified as cases in the house-to-house census. From the two zones, six districts with an estimated population of 600,000 were selected using clustered sampling techniques. The sample size was determined using a single proportion formula with consideration of the scabies median prevalence from the house-to-house census (33.5%) with a confidence level of 97% in the two zones. The reporting forms of the HEWs were used to select 474 cases. The inclusion criteria included those patients who have been identified as a case of scabies by the HEWs and the selection was performed with simple random sampling using the registration form. The team invited each patient to the village health post for a dermatology review including history, full body physical examination, and a standardized questionnaire which was completed by the dermatologist. The questionnaire included socio-demographic details of cases and additional variables such as presence of itching, severity of infestation, duration of illness and presence of secondary bacterial infection. The diagnosis of scabies was made clinically using the standardized case definition for the study (Table 1).

For clinical purposes, the severity of scabies was defined by the number of skin lesions and the presence or absence of crust. Mild: when the number of scabies associated skin lesions (papules, excoriation, and pustule) was less than or equal to ten. Moderate: The number of scabies associated skin lesions were between 10 and 50 lesions. Severe: when the number of scabies associated skin lesions were equal to or greater than 50 or the presence of scabies-associated crust. Secondary infection was defined by the presence of pustules and/or yellowish crusts.

Trop. Med. Infect. Dis. **2018**, 3, 114

The study received ethical approval on 14 September 2015 from the Regional Health Bureau as part of its operational research (reference number R.T.T/1/63107). A written support letter was received from the Regional Health Bureau to enlist the cooperation of the Zonal Health offices. Permission was subsequently also secured from the zonal and district health offices. The data collectors obtained verbal consent from each participant or his/her guardians. Written consent was obtained from patients who had images recorded.

The data was analyzed and results presented using descriptive statistics.

3. Results

3.1. Phase 1

The field based house-to-house survey using HEWs in the Amhara Region screened 1,125,770 individuals from October to November 2015 in 68 districts (Figure 2). A total of 379,000 confirmed cases were found. Overall, 195,665 (51.6%) of the patients were female and (60%) of confirmed cases were below 18 years of age. Children and young adults under 18 years old were 2.5 times more at risk in developing scabies (Table 2).

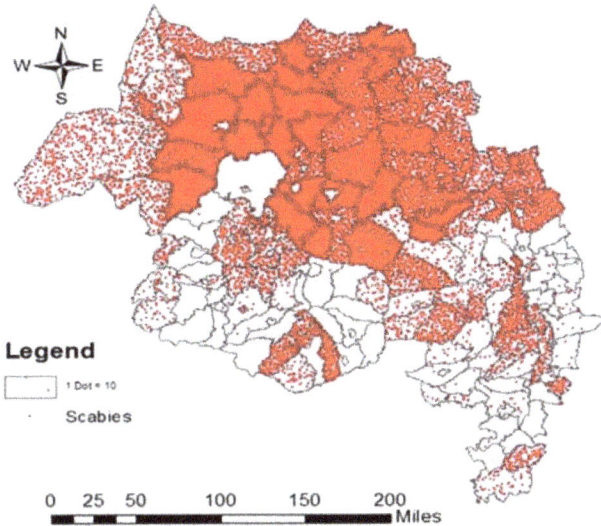

Figure 2. Scabies distribution in in Amhara Region, Ethiopia (2015–2016).

Table 2. Prevalence of scabies and bivariate analysis of demographic factors based on a house-to-house census in Amhara Region, Ethiopia (October 2015).

Variable	Total (N)	Affected (n)	Prevalence	OR *	p Value
Sex					
Female	585,400	195,665	33.4	Ref	Ref
Male	540,370	183,335	33.9	1.05	0.8
Total	1,125,770	379,000	33.7		
Age group (years) **					
<2	60,792	27,909	45.9	2.5	0.01
2 to 18	518,980	249,535	48.1	2.4	0.01
>18	545,998	101,556	18.6		

* Odds Ratio. ** Age groups were defined as follows: <2 years, 2 to 18 years, >18 years.

The scabies prevalence in the 68 districts ranged from 2% to 67% with a median prevalence of 33.5 (IQR 19–48%).

3.2. Phase 2

Of the 474 subjects enrolled in the 'detailed' study, 466 (98.3%) were confirmed to have scabies by a dermatologist (expert control group), which meant that the clinical diagnosis of the HEWs achieved a level of agreement with this control group of 98.3% (Figure 3). The index cases of the epidemic have been traced in both areas to the students in traditional church schools suggesting that these groups are important as sources of the infestation and in continued community transmission.

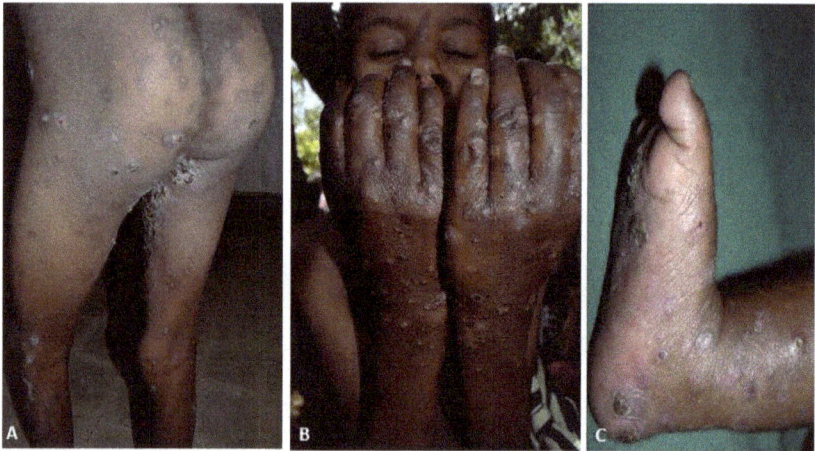

Figure 3. (**A**) Extensive crusting papules, excoriation with post-inflammatory hyperpigmentation in a 34-year-old female. (**B**) Pustules, crusts, and erosion in 12-year-old boy. (**C**) Pustules, crusts, and erosions in a 2-year-old female.

The majority (66.9%) of the scabies cases in this part of the study were in males, although the gender ratio varied with age. The proportion of males was by far the highest (113 or 87%) in those aged 18 years and above.

The median age of those affected was 10 years. The highest proportion of cases was found in those between 2 and 18 years old. 182 (39%) of the total number of cases were of school age and, of these, 63% were currently attending school, 15% never attended school, 11% had discontinued schooling prior to the drought and scabies outbreak and another 11% had discontinued their education as a result of scabies and the drought.

In the same validation study, all cases (466) had scabies skin lesions and all cases reported itching (itching and classic skin lesion are two case definitions used for scabies). The median number of lesions was found to be 10 to 49 (moderate). Approximately a quarter (116) of the cases had a history of a skin sore, of whom 94 (81%) had encrusted sores (Figure 3A). There were 14 (3%) cases with crusted scabies (Table 3).

The median duration of illness was 5 months, ranging from 0.5 to 12 months. Approximately one quarter (116) developed a secondary bacterial infection; the secondary bacterial infection rate was highest among those aged between 2 and 18 years (Table 4). On the other hand there was no significant difference in gender-specific bacterial infection rates (25% and 26% for females and males respectively). The bacterial infection rate among the school age group was 40% (Figure 3B). The rate was significantly higher 85% (95% CI of 79–91 and $p < 0.001$) among those who had dropped-out of school.

Table 3. Clinical signs and symptoms of scabies cases in the Amhara region, Ethiopia (2015).

Variables	N (%)
Sign and symptom	
Itching	466 (100%)
Classic scabies lesion	466 (100%)
Bacterial infection	116 (25%)
Crusted scabies	14 (3%)
Severity of the skin lesion	
Mild	13 (28%)
Moderate	191 (41%)
Severe	144 (31%)

Table 4. Scabies secondary bacterial infection rate by age, Amhara region, Ethiopia (2015).

Variable	Scabies Cases (N)	Infection (N)	Infection % (95% CI)	Odds Ratio	p Value
<2 years	46	7	15.2 (11.8–18.2)	1.8	0.012
2–18 years	288	101	35.1 (29.3–40.9)	4.2	<0.001
>18 years	132	11	8.3 (6.9–9.7)	Ref.	
Total	466	119	25.5 (21.3–29.7)		

4. Discussion

This regional census documenting cases of scabies and the cross-sectional validation study for the intervention campaign, documents the burden of community-based scabies in Ethiopia. This survey was noteworthy in screening the highest number of cases ever reported in the literature and, at the same time, in documenting the largest number of scabies cases. Other cross-sectional community-based studies in relatively large populations have been reported: (1) in Malawi in a village with a population of 61,735 where the prevalence was 0.7%; and (2) in Cambodia in 13 villages with a population of 14,843 where the prevalence was 4.3% [13–17]. As a community-based study the median prevalence in our survey was much larger and the range much wider (2% to 67%). This is supported by previous reports that the prevalence of scabies in community-based surveys is frequently higher than the burden reported in the Global Burden of Disease study (GBD) or reports from routine clinic data [12,18].

Even though there is no evidence on a cause and effect association, the scabies outbreak occurred following the 2015–2016 El Nino drought. In contrast, the study by Andersen et al. reported scabies to be one of the dermatological problems with a significant decrease in incidence related to El Nino [10].

Hay et al., in their review of scabies in the developing world, noted that 'the attack rate is probably equal between the sexes, and the differences in prevalence reported in some studies are probably attributable to confounding factors', which was also confirmed in this large population census [19]. Seventy-three percent of infestations were registered in those under the age 18, which correlates with the impression that in developing countries, scabies is much more common among preschool children than adolescents and rates significantly decreased in mid-adulthood [20,21].

The burden of this scabies epidemic was compounded by the high rate of secondary bacterial infection, with 30% of school-age children presenting with mild to severe secondary bacterial infection, in agreement with another population based study in the Solomon Islands [22]. This survey will strengthen the data that show that scabies infestations are an important risk factor for bacterial infection of the skin [23,24].

The key conclusions are, firstly that this community based data will serve reliable proxy indicators for the burden of the scabies epidemic in communities. Secondly this study also reaffirmed the idea that community level clinical diagnosis of scabies by community health workers using a simplified diagnostic algorithm has the potential to address the scabies burden in resource poor settings [25,26].

Finally this study will also serve as a sizeable input for the WHO's 'global strategy for scabies control' [27].

There are potential limitations in this study which are listed as follows:

1. The study used an aggregated report of the census with a limited data set (scabies case, contact, age, and sex) which could be a limitation of the study, especially for risk factor analysis.
2. In the house-to-house census of scabies cases, the examining HEWs had no other relevant experience apart from the one-day training described, which may have led to missed cases. The validation study focused only on specificity of the diagnosis.
3. Both in the census and in the validation study, the diagnosis of scabies and impetigo was made on the basis of clinical history and skin examination alone. Skin scrapings for direct microscopy or other confirmatory tests were not used.

Despite these limitations, the population survey and validation study have provided important new data about the extent of scabies in communities in northern Ethiopia and has registered the highest number of scabies cases ever reported in a single outbreak.

Author Contributions: W.E. contributed substantially to the conception and design of the house-to-house survey and validation study, the acquisition of data, the analysis and interpretation. He also drafted the article, provided final approval of the version to publish and agreed to be accountable for all aspects of the work in ensuring that questions related to the accuracy or integrity of any part of the work are appropriately investigated and resolved. A.A. contributed substantially to the design of house-to-house survey, the acquisition of data and the analysis. He also gave critical revision of the article, provided final approval of the version to publish and agreed to be accountable for all aspects of the work in ensuring that questions related to the accuracy or integrity of any part of the work are appropriately investigated and resolved.

Funding: The house-to-house census is funded by Amhara Regional Health Bureau and the validation study is funded by St Paul Hospital Millennium Medical College.

Acknowledgments: We would like to thank Amhara Regional Health bureau for taking the leadership position and giving us all the necessary support for the implementation of the survey. Many thanks also for L. Claire Fuller and Roderick Hay from International Foundation for Dermatology for their support from encouragement for the writing and language editing of the manuscript.

Conflicts of Interest: The authors declare no conflicts of interest.

References

1. Hicks, M.I.; Elston, D.M. Scabies. *Dermatol. Ther.* **2009**, *22*, 279–292. [CrossRef] [PubMed]
2. Heukelbach, J.; Feldmeier, H. Scabies. *Lancet* **2006**, *367*, 1767–1774. [CrossRef]
3. Ugbomoiko, U.; Oyedeji, S.; Babamale, O.; Heukelbach, J. Scabies in resource-poor communities in Nasarawa State, Nigeria: Epidemiology, clinical features and factors associated with infestation. *Trop. Med. Infect. Dis.* **2018**, *3*, 59. [CrossRef] [PubMed]
4. World Health Organization. *Epidemiology and Management of Common Skin Diseases in Children in Developing Countries*; WHO: Geneva, Switzerland, 2005; Available online: whqlibdoc.who.int/hq/2005/WHO_FCH_CAH_05.12_eng.pdf (accessed on 23 July 2018).
5. WHO. *El Nino and Health*; WHO Report 2016; WHO: Geneva, Switzerland, 2016; Available online: who_el_nino_and_health_global_report_21jan2016.pdf (accessed on 4 June 2017).
6. *EM-DAT: The OFDA/CRED International Disaster Database*; Universite Catholique de Louvain: Brussels, Belgium. Available online: http://www.emda.be/result-disaster-profiles?disgroup=natural&period=1900%242012&dis_type=Drought&Submit=Display+Disaster+Profile (accessed on 4 June 2017).
7. UNISDR. *Global Assessment Report on Disaster Risk Reduction: Revealing Risk, Redefining Development*; United Nations International Strategy for Disaster Reduction: Geneva, Switzerland, 2011.
8. *Scabies Outbreak Preparedness and Response Plan*; FMOH: Addis Ababa, Ethiopia, 2015; Available online: www.humanitarianresponse.info (accessed on 23 July 2018).
9. *Interim-Guideline for Multi Sectorial Scabies Outbreak Emergency Response*; FMOH: Addis Ababa, Ethiopia, 2015.

10. Andersen, L.K.; Davis, M.D. The effects of the El Nino Southern Oscillation on skin and skin-related diseases: A message from the International Society of Dermatology Climate Change Task Force. *Int. J. Dermatol.* **2015**, *54*, 1343–1351. [CrossRef] [PubMed]

11. Romani, L.; Steer, A.C.; Whitfeld, M.J.; Kaldor, J.M. Prevalence of scabies and impetigo worldwide: A systematic review. *Lancet Infect. Dis.* **2015**, *15*, 960–967. [CrossRef]

12. Engelman, D.; Andrew, I.D.; Steer, C. Control strategies for scabies. *Trop. Med. Infect. Dis.* **2018**, *3*, 98. [CrossRef] [PubMed]

13. Accorsi, S.; Barnabas, G.A.; Farese, P.; Padovese, V.; Terranova, M.; Racalbuto, V.; Morrone, A. Skin disorders and disease profile of poverty: Analysis of medical records in Tigray, northern Ethiopia, 2005-2007. *Trans. R. Soc. Trop. Med. Hyg.* **2009**, *103*, 469–475. [CrossRef] [PubMed]

14. Landwehr, D.; Keita, S.M.; Pönnighaus, J.M.; Tounkara, C. Epidemiologic aspects of scabies in Mali, Malawi, and Cambodia. *Int. J. Dermatol.* **1998**, *37*, 588–590. [CrossRef] [PubMed]

15. Carapetis, J.R.; Connors, C.; Yarmirr, D.; Krause, V.; Currie, B.J. Success of a scabies control program in an Australian aboriginal community. *Pediatr. Infect. Dis. J.* **1997**, *16*, 494–499. [CrossRef] [PubMed]

16. Nair, B.K.; Joseph, A.; Kandamuthan, M. Epidemic scabies. *Indian J. Med. Res.* **1977**, *65*, 513–518. [PubMed]

17. Dos Santos, M.M.; Amaral, S.; Harmen, S.P.; Joseph, H.M.; Fernandes, J.L.; Counahan, M.L. The prevalence of common skin infections in four districts in Timor-Leste: A cross-sectional survey. *BMC Infect. Dis.* **2010**, *10*, 61–66. [CrossRef] [PubMed]

18. Karimkhani, C.; Colombara, D.V.; Drucker, A.M.; Norton, S.A.; Hay, R.; Engelman, D.; Steer, A.; Whitfeld, M.; Naghavi, M.; Dellavalle, R.P. The global burden of scabies: A cross-sectional analysis from the Global Burden of Disease Study 2015. *Lancet Infect. Dis.* **2017**, *17*, 1247–1254. [CrossRef]

19. Hay, R.J.; Steer, A.C.; Engelman, D.; Walton, S. Scabies in the developing world—Its prevalence, complications, and management. *Clin. Microbiol. Infect.* **2012**, *18*, 313–323. [CrossRef] [PubMed]

20. Burkhart, C.G.; Burkhart, C.N.; Burkhart, K.M. An epidemiologic and therapeutic reassessment of scabies. *Cutis* **2000**, *65*, 233–240. [PubMed]

21. Kouotou, E.A.; Nansseu, J.R.N.; Sieleunou, I.; Defo, D.; Bissek, A.C.Z.K.; Ndam, E.C.N. Features of human scabies in resource-limited settings: The Cameroon case. *BMC Dermatol.* **2015**, *15*, 12. [CrossRef] [PubMed]

22. Mason, D.S.; Marks, M.; Sokana, O.; Solomon, A.W.; Mabey, D.C.; Romani, L.; Engelman, D. The prevalence of scabies and impetigo in the Solomon Islands: A population-based survey. *PLoS Negl. Trop. Dis.* **2016**, *10*, e0004803. [CrossRef] [PubMed]

23. Swe, P.M.; Zakrzewski, M.; Kelly, A.; Krause, L.; Fischer, K. Scabies mites alter the skin microbiome and promote growth of opportunistic pathogens in a porcine model. *PLoS Negl. Trop. Dis.* **2014**, *8*, e2897. [CrossRef] [PubMed]

24. Romani, L. The AIM study: A field trial of co-administration of azithromycin and ivermectin mass drug administration (MDA), CRF skin examination clinical record form, version 1, 2015. Available online: https://kirby.unsw.edu.au/project/aim-study (accessed on 23 July 2018).

25. Mahé, A.; Faye, O.; N'Diaye, H.T.; Ly, F.; Konare, H.; Keita, S.; Hay, R. Definition of an algorithm for the management of common skin diseases at primary health care level in sub-Saharan Africa. *Trans. R. Soc. Trop. Med. Hyg.* **2005**, *99*, 39–47. [CrossRef] [PubMed]

26. Steer, A.C.; Tikoduadua, L.V.; Manalac, E.M.; Colquhoun, S.; Carapetis, J.R.; Maclennan, C. Validation of an integrated management of childhood illness algorithm for managing common skin conditions in Fiji. *Bull WHO* **2009**, *87*, 173–179. [CrossRef] [PubMed]

27. World Health Organization. 9th NTD-STAG Global Working Group Meeting on Monitoring and Evaluation of Neglected Tropical Diseases. 2018. Available online: http://www.who.int/neglected_diseases/events/STAG_Working_Group_on_Monitoring_Evaluation/en/ (accessed on 12 August 2018).

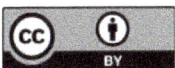

Tropical Medicine and Infectious Disease

MDPI

Article

In Situ Diagnosis of Scabies Using a Handheld Digital Microscope in Resource-Poor Settings—A Proof-of-Principle Study in the Amazon Lowland of Colombia

Hollman Miller [1], Julian Trujillo-Trujillo [2] and Hermann Feldmeier [3,*]

[1] Public Health Service, Vaupes Department, Mitú 97001, Colombia; hollmanmiller@gmail.com
[2] Department of Neglected Tropical Diseases, Ministry of Health and Social Protection, Bogotá 110311, Colombia; trujillotrujillojulian@gmail.com
[3] Institute of Microbiology and Infection Immunology, Campus Benjamin Franklin, Charité—University Medicine Berlin, corporate member of Freie Universität Berlin, Humboldt-Universität zu Berlin and Berlin Institute of Health, 12203 Berlin, Germany
* Correspondence: hermann.feldmeier@charite.de

Received: 31 July 2018; Accepted: 24 October 2018; Published: 2 November 2018

Abstract: Scabies is a neglected tropical disease associated with important morbidity. The disease occurs worldwide and is particularly common in resource-poor communities in the Global South. A validated technique for the diagnosis of scabies in resource-poor settings does not exist. The objective of the study was to determine the practicability and accuracy of handheld digital microscopy in three indigenous communities in the Amazon lowland of Colombia, where scabies is the most common parasitic skin disease. One-hundred-and-eleven children and adults from three indigenous communities with a presumptive diagnosis of scabies were examined clinically by using a handheld digital microscope placed directly on the skin. The microscopical identification of a mite was verified by an "experienced mother", a woman who had acquired the skills to diagnose scabies as part of traditional Amerindian medicine. The "experienced mother" removed the parasite with a fine needle and placed it on a flat surface in order to enable its direct examination with the digital microscope. Using digital microscopy, scabies was diagnosed in 24 out of 111 participants and confirmed by the extraction of a *Sarcoptes* mites from the acarine eminence. A characteristic tunnel (burrow) with or without mite could be clearly identified irrespective of the degree of pigmentation of the skin. Besides, digital microscopy revealed pathological characteristics of scabies hitherto unknown and impossible to be seen in dermoscopy, such as partially or totally obliterated tunnels, tunnels with multiple entry or exit points, circumscribed hyperpigmentation around obliterated tunnels and mites secluded in a nodule. This proof-of-principle study demonstrated the accurate diagnosis of scabies by handheld digital microscopy in patients with pigmented skin and the feasibility of this technique in resource-poor settings.

Keywords: scabies; diagnosis; digital handheld microscope; resource-poor setting; Amerindian communities; Amazon lowland

---

1. Introduction

Scabies, a parasitic skin disease caused by the mite *Sarcoptes scabiei* var. *hominis*, causes considerable morbidity through both direct effects and secondary bacterial infection [1–4]. Scabies provokes intense itch, severely affecting sleep and quality of life [5,6]. The disease occurs worldwide and is particularly common in resource-poor communities in the countries of the Global South [7,8]. In developing countries, children bear the highest disease burden, with an average prevalence of

5–10% [3,5]. In countries with a tropical climate, prevalences are up to 25% in the general population with >40% in some communities in the South Pacific and northern Australia [8–11].

As scabies can mimic a spectrum of skin diseases of infectious and non-infectious etiology, its clinical diagnosis requires experience. Clinical manifestations may differ between babies, children and adults [12,13], but also may vary between settings [14,15] and in the tropics, bacterial superinfection can further complicate the diagnosis [4,8,16]. How to diagnose scabies best in resource-poor settings in endemic areas is still a matter of debate [17]. Usually, the diagnosis is based on a case definition with unknown specificity and sensitivity [3,18]. To enable effective case management in the countries of the Global South, a diagnostic method is needed which is accurate and appropriate in people with moderately to intensely pigmented skin.

Sarcoptes mites can only be identified with certainty using a substantial magnification. We, therefore, decided to use a handheld digital video microscope allowing a magnification of up to 200-fold which, e.g., enables to reliably detect movements of the intestine and contractions of the heart of another skin parasite, *Tunga penetrans* [19]. This parasite is embedded in the lower strata of the epidermis and is difficult to identify even in unpigmented skin. The same technique was also used to diagnose myiasis caused by *Dermatobia hominis*, and trombiculid chigger mites (Hollman Miller, unpublished observation 2017). Here we show that (i) *Sarcoptes* mites can be reliably detected inside the tunnel they have created; (ii) tunnels vary considerably in shape, length and structure; and (iii) if a mite is present, it is almost always located in the acarine eminence at the end of the tunnel (burrow).

2. Material and Methods

2.1. Study Area and Population

The study was performed in Vaupes Department in the Amazon lowland of Colombia. The department has a surface of about 54,000 km^2. The population mainly consists of indigenous people of various ethnicities. They live in small communities along the Vaupes, Apaporis and Isana River and its affluents. Vaupes is covered with dense rain forest and most communities are only accessible by boat. Mitú, the capital of Vaupes Department, is situated at Latitude: 1°15′28″ North and Longitude: 70°14′04″ West with an altitude of 158 m above sea level. The climate is tropical the whole year round.

Scabies is the most common skin disease in the Amazon lowland of Colombia. Prevalence is in the order of 2% in the general population and 80% of the cases are children (Hollman Miller, unpublished observation 2017). Other important parasitic skin diseases are tungiasis, myiasis and cutaneous leishmaniasis. Prior to the present study, no control measures for scabies were undertaken in the area.

2.2. Study Design and Data Collection

The study was performed in the indigenous communities Cariya (N 0°22′22″, W 70°07′46.6″) and Santa Catalina (N 0°21′51.55″, W 70° 5′52.80″), situated along the Tiquié river, as well as in Barrio 12 de octubre, at the periphery of Mitú (N 01°14′00.4″, W 70°14′01.9″) between January and May 2017. Communities were selected on the basis of information from local health personnel that scabies seemed to be frequent and that they were accessible from Mitú by boat or car. In each community, individuals with a presumptive diagnosis of scabies were eligible, independent of their age.

In indigenous communities in the Amazon lowland of Colombia, scabies is traditionally diagnosed and treated by an experienced mother ("mujer experimentada"). These are women without medical training who have learned to diagnose scabies with the naked eye as a part of traditional Amerindian medicine, usually from their mothers. The experienced mother carefully inspects the patient's skin and looks for the presence of a pearly vesicle (*vesicula perlada*) which reflects the entry point of a mite into the skin [20] (Figure 1). Pearly vesicles are whitish and translucent, have a diameter of 0.5 to 3 mm and have a soft resistance against pressure (Figure 2A,B). They are frequently decapitated by scratching and then look like an excoriation. Once the experienced mother has identified a pearly vesicle or its remains, she looks for the acarine eminence (*eminencia acarina*), an oval elevation of the skin with a pearlescent appearance at the limit of visibility (0.3 × 0.4 mm) [20]. By experience, the experienced mother knows that the mite is located in the acarine eminence, usually at short distance to a pearly vesicle (Figure 3). When an experienced mother has identified an acarine eminence, she removes the mite from the corneal layer with the help of a sharp thorn or a sharpened piece of hard wood—a method performed in the Americas for hundreds of years [21] {We had very severe itching in the knuckles and on the back of our hands. The missionary told us, these were *Aradores* (farmers) that dig into the skin. (...) They sent for a mulatto woman who prided herself to be able to [diagnose and heal] all the little beasts that dig into man's skin, the Nigua, the Nuche, the Coya and the Arador; (*Sarcoptes* mite) She heated the tip of a small splinter of very hard wood by the lamp and pierced it in the furrows visible on the skin. After a long search she announced (...) that there was already an *Arador*. I saw a small round sack at the top of the splinter, (...). Because I had the skin full of *Aradores* on both hands, I ran out of patience with the operation, which had lasted well into the night. (...). (Von Humboldt, Südamerikanische Reise, Ullstein Publisher, Berlin, reprint of original, 1979, p. 348)} Hence, in traditional Amerindian medicine, the identification of the acarine eminence is the prerequisite for treatment of scabies.

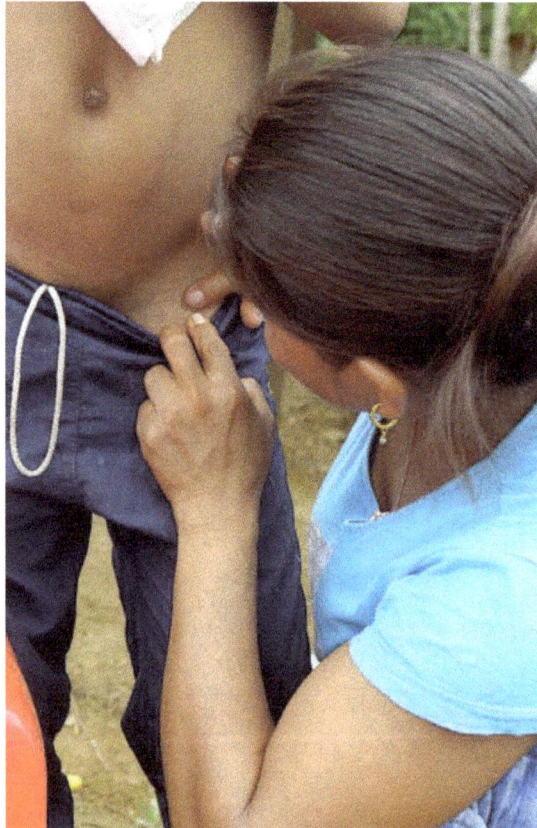

Figure 1. Experienced mother examining the skin of a child for the presence of a pearly vesicle.

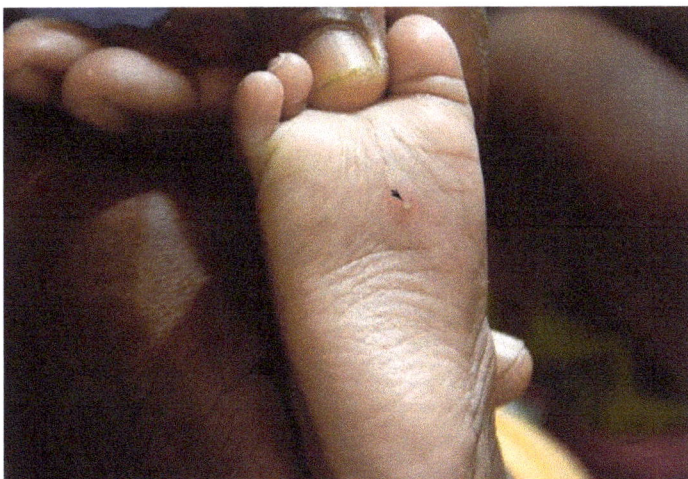

(A)

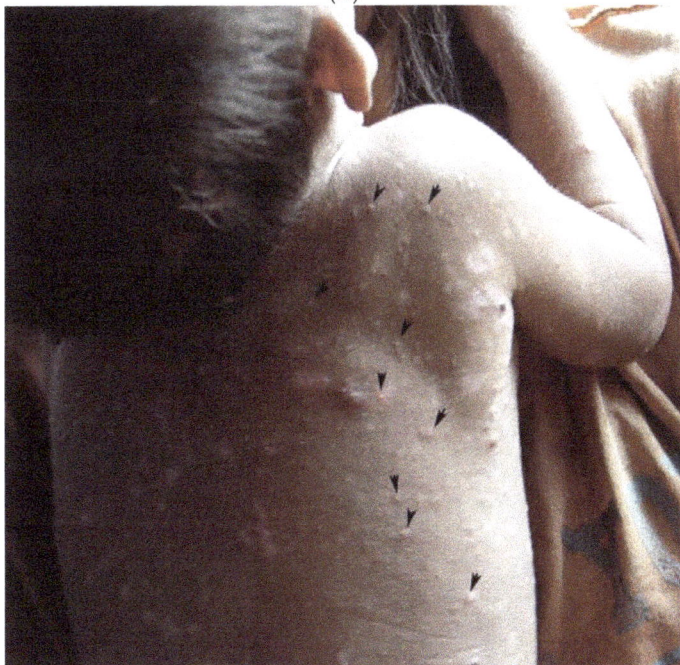

(B)

Figure 2. (**A**) A pearly vesicle at the sole of the foot (arrow). (**B**). Multiple pearly vesicles on the back of a child with severe scabies (arrows).

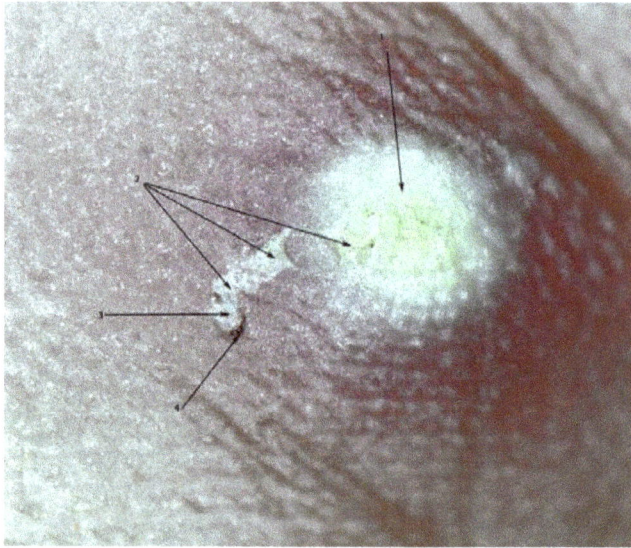

Figure 3. Pearly vesicle (1) and acarine eminence linked by a tunnel (2). The mite is situated at the end of the tunnel with its dorsal part turned towards the surface of the skin (3). The delta-wing sign is clearly visible (4). Photo by digital microscopy; magnification 30-fold.

Community health workers were informed about the arrival of the health team a couple of days in advance. Individuals with itchy lesions of the skin were asked to present themselves at a designated place in the morning and in the afternoon. No active search for cases was performed. After the medical history had been taken, the skin was examined macroscopically. Thereafter, the digital handheld microscope (dnt DigiMicro Mobile 5 Megapixel handheld microscope; Drahtlose Nachrichtentechnik GmbH, Dietzenbach, Germany) was placed directly on the skin and suspicious lesions were examined one by one, first using a 10-fold magnification followed by 30-fold magnification to identify the morphological characteristics of *Sarcoptes* mites (Figure 4A,B). Each lesion was scrutinized for the presence of a tunnel (intact, in the process of obliteration or totally obliterated), the presence of a mite inside a tunnel as well as the presence of faecal pellets or eggs. Other characteristics systematically looked for were the acarine eminence and the pearly vesicle [22,23], the presence of coagulated blood inside or around a tunnel (as an indicator of micro-haemorrhage induced by scratching); exfoliation or desquamation of the corneal layer (as an indicator of repeated scratching); and circumscript hyper-pigmented areas, visible only microscopically.

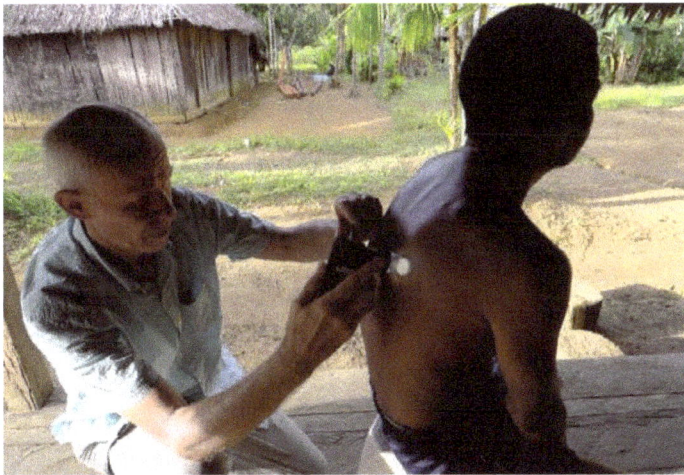

(A)

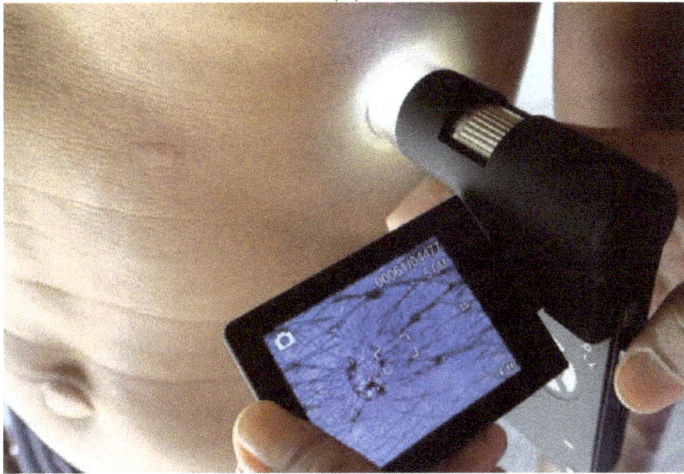

(B)

Figure 4. (A) Examination of the skin with the digital handheld microscope. **(B)** Examination of the skin with the digital handheld microscope, close-up.

Pathological findings were photographed, stored on an SD-card inside the microscope and transferred to a computer at the end of the day.

When a mite was detected in an acarine eminence by digital microscopy, the "experienced mother" was asked to remove it with a sterile entomological spin of #3 size and to place it on flat surface, such as a finger nail (Figure 5A,B) to confirm microscopy results. Using the video function of the microscope it was attempted to identify mites moving inside a tunnel or on the surface of the skin.

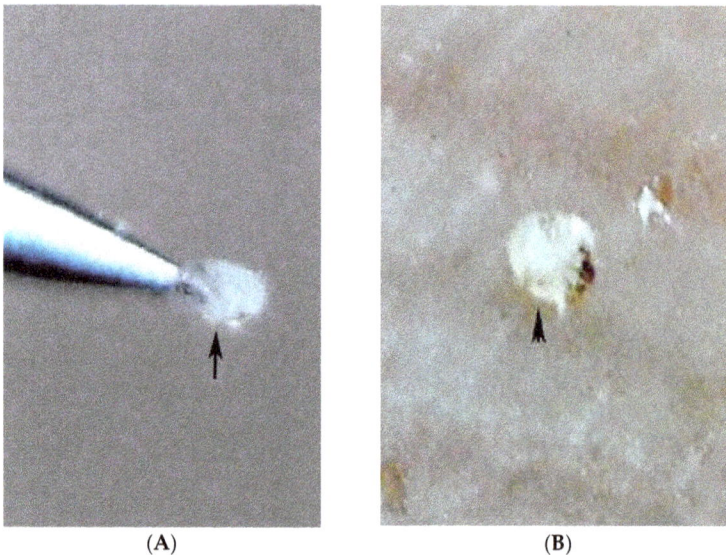

Figure 5. (**A**) *Sarcoptes* mite being extracted with a sterile needle by an experienced mother; magnification 70-fold. (**B**) Dorsal view of a mite extracted by the experienced mother from an acarine eminence; the hyperpigmented area of the anterior part of the mite corresponds to the delta-wing sign as seen in the dermatoscope; magnification 90-fold.

2.3. Diagnosis

Scabies was suspected if a patient showed a suspicious skin alteration accompanied by itching for at least 2 weeks. The following skin alterations were considered suspicious: presence of characteristic primary lesions (papules, crusted papules, vesicles, nodules) with or without the presence of secondary lesions (excoriation of the skin, secondary bacterial infection) that were obviously not associated with other dermatological conditions. Bacterial superinfection was diagnosed when pustules, suppuration or an abscess were present.

Diagnosis of scabies was defined as detection of the morphological characteristics of a mite in an acarine eminence by digital microscopy and subsequent confirmation by the extraction of the parasite; or if faecal pellets were identified inside a tunnel by digital microscopy.

2.4. Treatment

After diagnosis, the patient was treated with 200 µg/kg ivermectin orally, followed by a second dose after 1 week. Children <5 years and pregnant and lactating women were treated topically with sulfur in petrolatum 8%, once a day for 3 days [23]. Ivermectin and sulfur in petrolatum are standard treatments of scabies recommended by the Colombian Ministry of Health.

3. Results

The demographic characteristics of the study participants are summarized in Table 1. All participants had pigmented skin. Scabies was diagnosed in 24 out of 111 participants (21.6%). The frequency of cases was highest in Cariya (54.5%), and considerably lower in Santa Catalina and Barrio 12 de Octubre (15.6 and 20.4% of study participants, respectively). Sixteen of the 24 patients (66%) were children younger than 10 years of age. The clinical characteristics of the patients are depicted in Table 2.

Table 1. Demographic characteristics of participants.

Community	Number of Participants	Age in Years Median (Range)	Males/Females	Scabies Diagnosed [a] (%)
Cariyá	11	29 (3–88)	4/7	6 (54.5)
Santa Catalina	51	19 (2–71)	28/23	8 (15.7)
Barrio 12 de Octubre	49	12 (3 months–77)	21/28	10 (20.4)
Total	111	15 (3 months–88)	53/58	24 (21.6)

[a] see Material and Methods.

Table 2. Clinical characteristics of 24 patients with scabies.

Characteristics	Frequency (n/%)
Number of topographic areas affected	
1–5	10/(41.6%)
6–10	13/(54.1%)
>10	1/(4.31%)
Appearance of lesions (weeks ago)	
<4 weeks	6/(25.0%)
4–12 weeks	14/(58.3%)
>12 weeks	4/(16.6%)
Type of lesion [a]	
Papule	23/(95.8%)
Vesicle	16/(66.6%)
Nodule	2/(8.3%)
Crusted lesion [b]	15/(62.5%)
Excoriation/desquamation	19/(79.1%)
Bacterial superinfection [c]	15/(62.5%)

[a] Multiple classifications possible. [b] Crust developed on top of vesicle or papule. [c] Pustule, suppuration.

In 23 cases, a mite was identified in an acarine eminence. In one case, a mite was detected in the middle of a tunnel without an acarine eminence (Table 3). Pearly vesicles were observed in 17 cases, usually in a short distance of a few mm to an acarine eminence (Figure 6A,B). Frequently, only the residues of a pearly vesicle were visible (Figure 6C).

Table 3. Findings by digital microscopy in 24 scabies patients [a].

Characteristics [b]	Frequency (n/%)
Tunnel without mite	8/(33.7%)
Tunnel with mite	24/(100%)
Tunnel with mite present in the acarine eminence	23/(95.8%)
Tunnel with mite in the middle of the tunnel	1
Tunnel with faecal pellets	8/(33.3%)
Partially or totally obliterated tunnel	16/(66.7%)
Extraction of mite by experienced mother	24/(100%) [c]
Pearly vesicle surrounded by erythema	17/(70.8%)
Circumscribed hyperpigmentation	22/(91.6%)
Micro-haemorrhagia	4/(16.6%)
Excoriation/desquamation of the corneal layer	19/(79.1%) [d]
Nodule containing mite	1/(4.1%)

[a] For case definition see Materials and Methods [b] Multiple classifications possible. [c] In four cases, the mite was lost directly following the extraction. [d] not visible macroscopically.

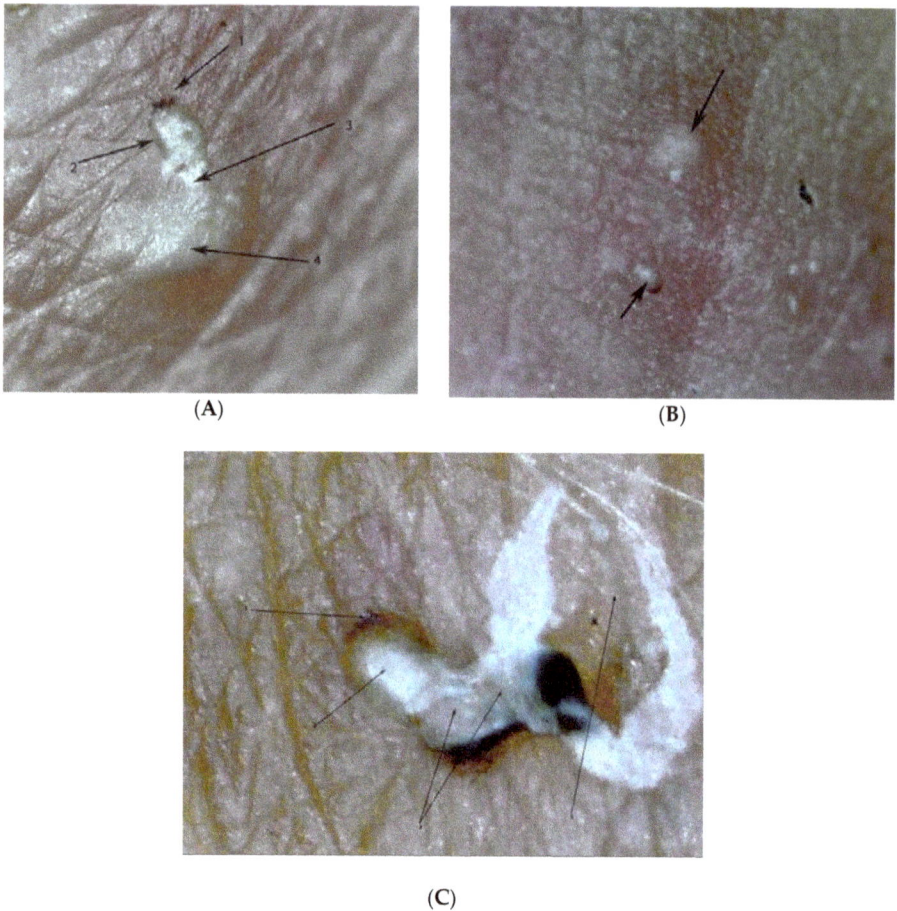

Figure 6. (A) Oval-shaped acarine eminence at the end of the tunnel (2) with the delta-wing sign (1); partially obliterated tunnel (3) connecting the acarine eminence with the pearly vesicle (4); magnification 50-fold. **(B)** Pearly vesicle (top) and acarine eminence (bottom) located at a distance from each other; no tunnel visible; the delta-wing sign is clearly visible (arrow bottom); magnification 15-fold. **(C)** Acarine eminence (3) at the end of an S-shaped tunnel containing a mite (2) with delta-wing sign visible (1); pearly vesicle destroyed by scratching (4); magnification 80-fold.

The microscopic aspect of a mite differed according whether its ventral or dorsal part was turned towards the surface of the skin (Figure 7A,B). Partially or completely obliterated tunnels were observed in 16 patients (Figure 8A,B). Those tunnels did not contain a mite. Tunnels in the process of obliteration showed a circumscript hyperpigmentation, not visible macroscopically (Figure 9). The length of a tunnel varied from less than 1 mm to about 10 mm. In some cases, tunnels showed multiple entry and exit points (Figure 10). In a single case, a mite was detected outside a tunnel moving on the skin. One nodule was identified which contained 2 mites (Figure 11).

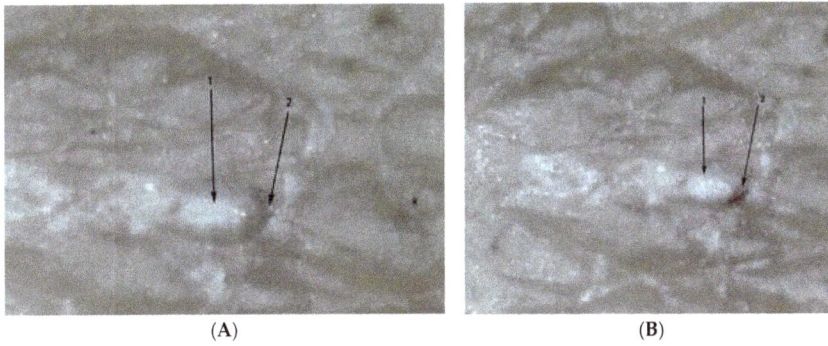

Figure 7. (**A**) Sarcoptes mite inside an acarine eminence with its dorsal part turned towards the surface of the skin (1); delta-wing sign visible (2); magnification 65-fold. (**B**) The same mite after having changed its position (1); now the ventral part is turned towards the surface of the skin (2); delta-wing sign not clearly visible.

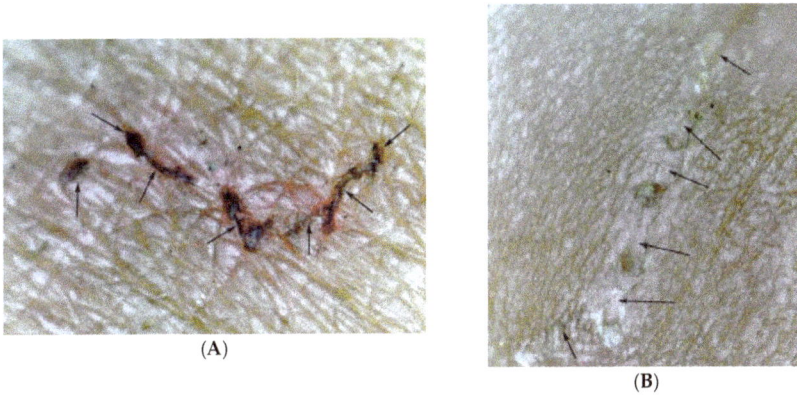

Figure 8. (**A**) Partially obliterated tunnel, obliterated parts show micro-haemorrhages (arrows); magnification 15-fold. (**B**) Totally obliterated tunnel; only residues of micro-haemorrhages visible; magnification 15-fold.

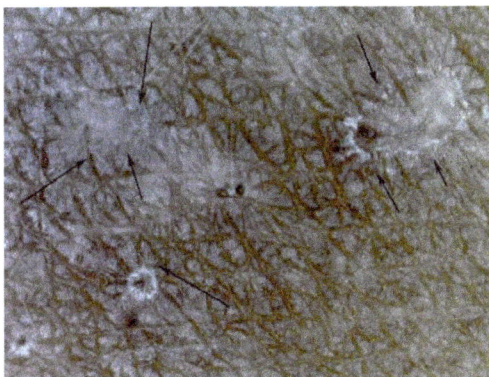

Figure 9. Microscopic circumscribed hyperpigmented areas (arrows) around a sinusoidal tunnel; magnification 30-fold.

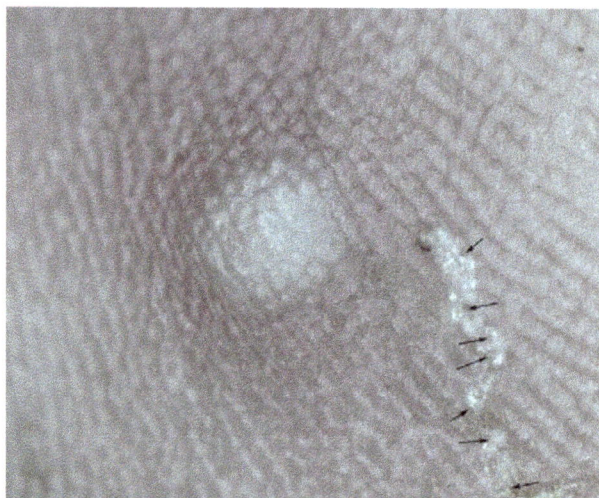

Figure 10. Serpiginous tunnel with multiple entry and exit points (arrows); magnification 15-fold.

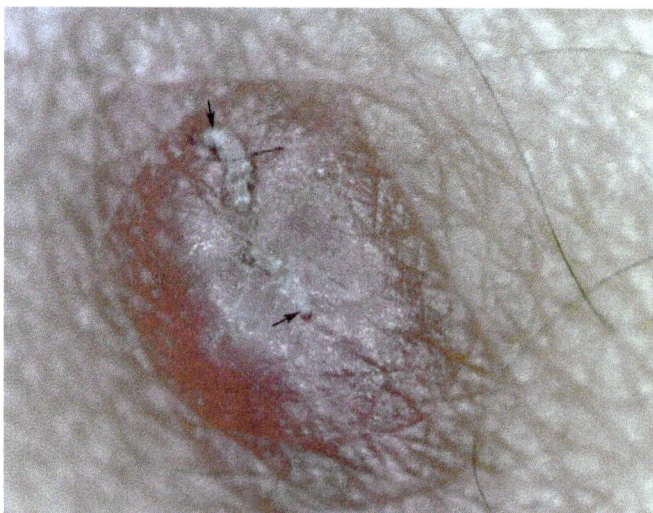

Figure 11. Nodule containing two mites (arrows); magnification 25-fold.

Usually, when excoriations were present macroscopically, micro-hemorrhages were visible microscopically (Figure 8A). Besides, the handheld digital microscope demonstrated the presence of tiny excoriations which were not visible macroscopically (Figure 12).

Lesions caused by *Trombicula alfreddugesi*, a mite endemic in the tropical rain forest of the Amazon and the Orinoco Basin, were ancillary findings by digital microscopy. The morphological characteristics of *T. alfreddugesi* are easily differentiated from those of a *Sarcoptes* (Figure 13).

All participants of the study were at ease with the examination of the skin by digital microscopy. Elder patients found it informative to spot the parasite that caused their disease.

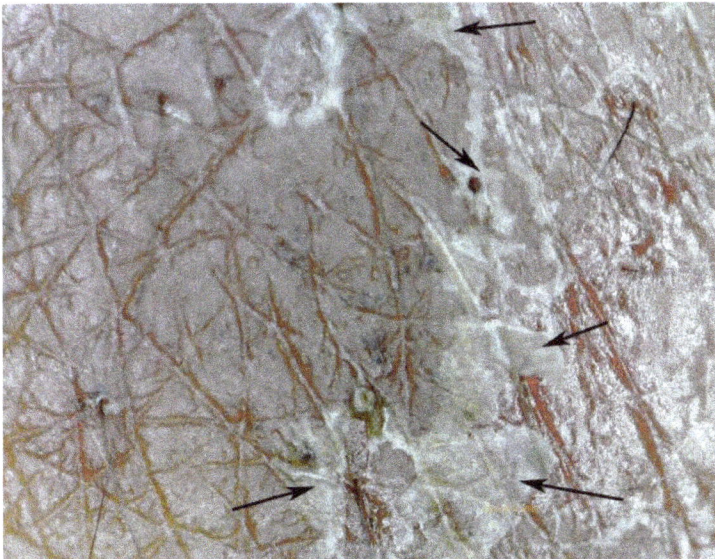

Figure 12. Microscopic excoriations of the stratum corneum not visible microscopically (arrows); magnification 100-fold.

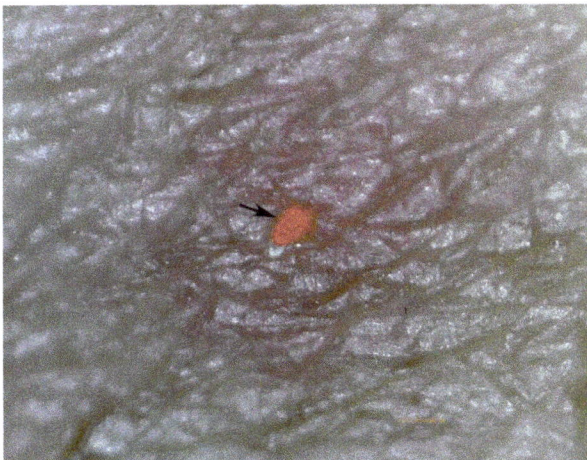

Figure 13. *Trombicula alfreddugesi* identified by the digital handheld microscope (arrow); magnification 10-fold.

4. Discussion

Scabies can mimic a broad range of infectious and non-infectious diseases [12] and the clinical picture is frequently masked by superinfection [13]. Hence, the specificity of clinical diagnosis is low, and its sensitivity depends on the experience of the observer. Since simple and accurate diagnostic techniques do not exist, in resource-poor settings, the diagnosis of scabies is based on the presence of suspicious clinical findings such as itchy papules or on a case definition of which neither sensitivity nor specificity is known [18,24].

Our findings also explain why a diagnosis based solely on the identification of a tunnel, such as by means of a burrow ink test, has a notoriously low sensitivity and specificity [25,26].

Based on our findings in tungiasis, a skin disease where the parasite is embedded in the lower strata of the epidermis and is difficult to identify macroscopically [19], we decided to use a digital handheld microscope for the detection of *Sarcoptes* mites in situ. The application of the digital handheld microscope is totally inoffensive and well tolerated even by small children [19]. The digital microscope is directly placed on the skin and illuminates a circumscript area of the skin of a diameter of 30 mm with 8 LED. The area examined is displayed on a color monitor with a resolution of 5 megapixels. Resolution of pictures can be further enhanced by connecting the microscope with a laptop or a tablet computer and enlarging the picture on the computer in real time. Photos and videos are stored on a Micro-SD card inside the microscope. The price of the handheld digital microscope is in the order of 120 US$. Previously described optical methods for the in vivo detection of mites used highly sophisticated stationary and expensive equipment such as reflectance-mode confocal microscopy or epiluminescence microscopy which are not suitable for resource-poor settings [27–29].

The digital handheld microscope allowed the identification of 24 cases of scabies out of 111 participants who fulfilled the admission criteria. Except for one case, mites were seen in the acarine eminence at the end of the tunnel. We presume that the acarine eminence is caused by a mite feeding on corneal cells and thereby exerting pressure on the surrounding layers of corneal cells. It reflects a dilatation of the upper corneal layer by a biologically active foreign body moving forward in the skin. The pearly vesicle was described first by the French dermatologist Pierre-Antoine-Ernest Bazin in 1862 [22]. We suppose that the pearly vesicle reflects an acute local inflammation at the point where a female mite has penetrated into the stratum corneum. Due to scratching, a pearly vesicle is frequently decapitated and only a residue remains. Ideally, the pearly vesicle and the acarine eminence should be linked by a tunnel. In practice though, pearly vesicles and tunnels are destroyed by scratching or become invisible due to bacterial superinfection [20,23]. The appearances of the pearly vesicle may vary under different environmental conditions and in colder climates and older persons, for instance, the mite entry point is often drier and scaly. This emphasizes the importance of adapting training to suit local conditions and using descriptive words that are easily understandable by local health workers.

An intriguing observation was the finding that the ventral and the dorsal part of an embedded *Sarcoptes* mite showed a different pigmentation pattern: The triangular pigmentation at the anterior part of the mite (the delta-wing sign visible in dermoscopy) being pronounced, when its dorsal part was turned towards the skin. Since the other body areas of a mite are almost translucent and a mite may change its position with regard to the skin's surface, this explains why in dermoscopy the delta-wing sign is not consistently present [24,30–32]. Obviously, even in non-pigmented skin, the delta-wing sign cannot be seen in the dermatoscope when the ventral end of the mite is positioned towards the surface of the skin or when the mite has changed its direction and its rear end is situated towards the end of the tunnel.

Faecal pellets were only inconsistently detectable in the handheld digital microscope and eggs were only seen in a single occasion. Neither faecal pellets nor eggs are reliable indicators of active scabies in digital microscopy and dermoscopy. Actually, it has been previously shown that eggs and faecal pellets need to be stained to become clearly visible [33,34].

The digital microscope also showed that tunnels considerably vary in size and shape and degree of obliteration. Surprisingly, we observed that tunnels may have various entry and exit points and that there are intact tunnels not inhabited by a mite. This confirms previous observations [29]. The presence of a tunnel as such, therefore, cannot be considered pathognomonic for the presence of active scabies and does not allow for a conclusion on the necessity of treatment [28]. Our findings also explain why a diagnosis based solely on the identification of a tunnel, such as by means of a burrow ink test, have a notoriously low sensitivity and specificity [25,26].

Our study corroborates previous findings that dermoscopy is an inappropriate means to diagnose scabies in a resource-poor setting [24]. Although the sensitivity of the technique is rather high (0.85; 95% CI 0.70–0.94), its specificity is low (0.46; 95% CI, 0.34–0.58) [24]. This can be explained by the finding that dermoscopy only yields optimal results when examiners are trained in the diagnosis of scabies [30] and that artefacts induced by scratching, such as crusts, or punctuate bleeding or small particles of dirt can be confounded with a mite [35,36].

Our study has several limitations. First, due to the lack of privacy, we excluded the genital area in both sexes and the peri-mamillary area in women. Since the morphological characteristics of lesions at these topographic areas may differ from those of other parts of the skin, e.g., noduli are very common on the penis, but rare at the abdomen, we cannot exclude that the distribution patterns of acarine eminence and/or the pearly vesicle are the same at all topographic areas of the skin. Second, we used the extraction of a mite from the acarine eminence by the experienced mother as a proof that the morphological characteristics seen in the digital handheld microscope were actually that of a *Sarcoptes* mite. We therefore can only conclude on the specificity of the method, but not on its sensitivity. A study to compare the sensitivity of the digital handheld microscopy with other diagnostic techniques used in resource-poor settings is currently being performed. Third, since all patients presented themselves voluntarily, we cannot rule out that a selection bias towards patients with a severe form of scabies might have occurred.

In conclusion, the proof-of-principle study showed that the digital handheld microscope is an accurate diagnostic instrument to diagnose scabies in resource-poor settings in people with pigmented skin. In addition, the technique allows the detection of micro-pathological alterations of the skin presumably caused by scratching or due to an immune response of the host. If applied in a systematic way, handheld digital microscopy will provide new insights into the biological host-parasite-relationships of *Sarcoptes* mites and eventually lead to the understanding of pathogenesis and pathophysiology of skin alterations caused by *S. scabiei*.

Author Contributions: Study concept and design: H.F. and H.M.; Acquisition of data: H.M. and H.F.; Analysis and interpretation of data: H.M., H.F. and J.T.-T.; Drafting of the manuscript: H.F.; Critical revision of the manuscript for important intellectual content: All authors.

Funding: The study was partially supported by German Doctors e.V. (Frankfurt, Germany). The sponsor undertook no role in the design, execution, or interpretation of the study. Submission of the manuscript was decided by tablerthe authors. The sponsor had no influence in drafting and revising the manuscript.

Acknowledgments: We are very grateful that the experienced mothers Belkis Bernal Rodriguez, Martha Lucia Sanchez Perez, Maria Sanchez Perez and Denia Valenzuela Lima shared their knowledge with us. We are also very grateful for the support by the community health workers, particularly Cesar de Jesus Tamayo Londoño.

Conflicts of Interest: The authors declare no conflict of interest.

Ethical Considerations: The study was performed as part of a routine health care provided by public health personnel of Vaupés Health Department. When the medical team arrived in a community, the procedure was explained to community leaders, community health assistants and study participants. The examination of the skin for the diagnosis of scabies and other dermatological conditions is part of the routine health care and was carried out with the aim to identify and treat patients with scabies. The examination of minors was made with the authorization and in the presence of at least one of their parents. As illiteracy is frequent in indigenous populations, participants—and in the case of minors the respective care-giver—were asked to provide oral informed consent. There was a written authorization from the traditional indigenous authorities. In accordance with Resolution 008430 of 1993 of the Ministry of Health and Social Protection of Colombia which regulates research in humans, the study was classified as risk-free, because the examination with digital microscopy is totally inoffensive. The study was approved by the Ethical Committee of the Universidad del Cauca, certificate 6.1-1.25/021.

References

1. Engelman, D.; Kiang, K.; Chosidow, O.; McCarthy, J.; Fuller, C.; Lammie, P.; Hay, R.; Steer, A. Toward the global control of human scabies: Introducing the international alliance for the control of scabies. *PLoS Negl. Trop. Dis.* **2013**, *7*, e2167. [CrossRef] [PubMed]
2. Feldmeier, H.; Heukelbach, J. Epidermal parasitic skin diseases: A neglected category of poverty-associated plagues. *Bull. World Health Organ.* **2009**, *87*, 152–159. [CrossRef] [PubMed]
3. Heukelbach, J.; Feldmeier, H. Scabies. *Lancet* **2006**, *367*, 1767–1774. [CrossRef]
4. Berrios, X.; Lagomarsino, E.; Solar, E.; Sandoval, G.; Guzman, B.; Riedel, I. Post-streptococcal acute glomerulonephritis in chile—20 years of experience. *Pediatr. Nephrol.* **2004**, *19*, 306–312. [CrossRef] [PubMed]

5. Hay, R.J.; Steer, A.C.; Engelman, D.; Walton, S. Scabies in the developing world—Its prevalence, complications, and management. *Clin. Microbiol. Infect.* **2012**, *18*, 313–323. [CrossRef] [PubMed]
6. Worth, C.; Heukelbach, J.; Fengler, G.; Walter, B.; Liesenfeld, O.; Feldmeier, H. Impaired quality of life in adults and children with scabies from an impoverished community in Brazil. *Int. J. Dermatol.* **2012**, *51*, 275–282. [CrossRef] [PubMed]
7. Feldmeier, H.; Jackson, A.; Ariza, L.; Calheiros, C.M.L.; de Lima Soares, V.; Hengge, U.R.; Heukelbach, J. The epidemiology of scabies in an impoverished community in rural brazil: Presence and severity of disease are associated with poor living conditions and illiteracy. *J. Am. Acad. Dermatol.* **2009**, *60*, 436–443. [CrossRef] [PubMed]
8. Carapetis, J.R.; Connors, C.; Yarmirr, D.; Krause, V.; Currie, B.J. Success of a scabies control program in an australian aboriginal community. *Pediatr. Infect. Dis. J.* **1997**, *16*, 494–499. [CrossRef] [PubMed]
9. Heukelbach, J.; Wilcke, T.; Winter, B.; Feldmeier, H. Epidemioloy and morbidity of scabies and pediculosis capitis in resource-poor communities in Brazil. *Br. J. Dermatol.* **2007**, *153*, 150–156. [CrossRef] [PubMed]
10. Jackson, A.; Heukelbach, J.; Feldmeier, H. Transmission of scabies in an endemic area. *Br. J. Infect. Dis.* **2007**, *11*, 307–308.
11. Currie, B.J.; Connors, C.M.; Krause, V.L. Scabies programs in aboriginal communities. *Med. J. Aust.* **1994**, *161*, 636–637. [PubMed]
12. Feldmeier, H.; Wilcke, T. Scabies in childhood. In *Recent Advances in Pediatrics*; David, T.J., Ed.; The Royal Society of Medicine Press: London, UK, 2007; pp. 25–38.
13. Jackson, A.; Heukelbach, J.; Ferreira da Silva Filho, A.; Barros Campelo Junior, E.; Feldmeier, H. Clinical features and associated morbidity of scabies in a rural community in alagoas, Brazil. *Trop. Med. Int. Health* **2007**, *12*, 493–502. [CrossRef] [PubMed]
14. Cestari, T.F.; Martignago, B.F. Scabies, pediculosis, bedbugs, and stinkbugs: Uncommon presentations. *Clin. Dermatol.* **2005**, *23*, 545–554. [CrossRef] [PubMed]
15. Schmeller, W.; Bendick, C.; Stingl, P. *Dermatosen aus drei Kontinenten—Bildatlas der Vergleichenden Dermatologie*, 1st ed.; Schattauer: Stuttgart, Germany, 2005; p. 238.
16. Feldmeier, H. Diagnosis of parasitic skin diseases. In *Evidence Based Dermatology*, 2nd ed.; Maibach, H., Farzam, G., Eds.; PMPH-USA: Raleigh, NC, USA, 2010; pp. 73–86.
17. Walton, S.F.; Currie, B.J. Problems in diagnosing scabies, a global disease in human and animal populations. *Clin. Microbiol. Rev.* **2007**, *20*, 268–279. [CrossRef] [PubMed]
18. Mahe, A.; Faye, O.; N'Diaye, H.T.; Ly, F.; Konare, H.; Keita, S.; Traore, A.K.; Hay, R. Definition of an algorithm for the management of common skin diseases at primary health care level in sub-saharan africa. *Trans. R. Soc. Trop. Med. Hyg.* **2005**, *99*, 39–47. [CrossRef] [PubMed]
19. Thielecke, M.; Nordin, P.; Ngomi, N.; Feldmeier, H. Treatment of tungiasis with dimeticone: A proof-of-principle study in rural kenya. *PLoS Negl. Trop. Dis.* **2014**, *8*, e3058. [CrossRef] [PubMed]
20. Aguado Taberné, C.; del Pozo Guzmán, R.; García Aranda, J.M. Tratamiento de las infestaciones cutáneas. In *Manual de Terapéutica en Atención Primaria*; Central Publications Service of the Basque Government: Vitoria-Gasteiz, Spain, 2006.
21. Von Humboldt, A. *Südamerikanische Reise*; Ullstein GmbH: Berlin, Germany, 1981.
22. Bazin, E. *Leçons Théoriques et Cliniques sur les Affections Génériques de la Peau*; Adrien Delahaye: Pairs, France, 1862; p. 454.
23. Dorado, J.G.; Fraile, P.A. Sarna, pediculosis y picaduras de insectos. *Pediatríaintegral* **2012**, *16*, 301–320.
24. Walter, B.; Heukelbach, J.; Fengler, G.; Worth, C.; Hengge, U.; Feldmeier, H. Comparison of dermoscopy, skin scraping, and the adhesive tape test for the diagnosis of scabies in a resource-poor setting. *Arch. Dermatol.* **2011**, *147*, 468–473. [CrossRef] [PubMed]
25. Palicka, P.; Mali, L.; Samsinak, K.; Zitek, K.; Vobrazkov, E. Laboratory diagnosis of scabies. *J. Hyg. Epidemiol. Microbiol. Immunol.* **1980**, *24*, 63–70. [PubMed]
26. Woodley, D.; Saurat, J.H. The burrow ink test and the scabies mite. *J. Am. Acad. Dermatol.* **1981**, *6*, 715–722. [CrossRef]
27. Argenziano, G.; Fabbrocini, G.; Delfino, M. Epiluminescence microscopy: A new approach to in vivo detection of sarcoptes scabiei. *Arch. Dermatol.* **1997**, *133*, 751–753. [CrossRef] [PubMed]

28. Lacarrubba, F.; Musumeci, M.L.; Caltabiano, R.; Impallomeni, R.; West, D.P.; Micali, G. High-magnification videodermatoscopy: A new noninvasive diagnostic tool for scabies in children. *Pediatr. Dermatol.* **2001**, *18*, 439–441. [CrossRef] [PubMed]
29. Longo, C.; Bassoli, S.; Monari, P.; Seidenari, S.; Pellacani, G. Reflectance-mode confocal microscopy for the in vivo detection of sarcoptes scabiei. *Arch. Dermatol.* **2005**, *141*, 1336–1337. [CrossRef] [PubMed]
30. Dupuy, A.; Dehen, L.; Bourrat, E.; Lacroix, C.; Benderdouche, M.; Dubertret, L.; Morel, P.; Feuilhade de Chauvin, M.; Petit, A. Accuracy of standard dermoscopy for diagnosing scabies. *J. Am. Acad. Dermatol.* **2007**, *56*, 53–62. [CrossRef] [PubMed]
31. Yoshizumi, J.; Harada, T. "Wake sign": An important clue for the diagnosis of scabies. *Clin. Exp. Dermatol.* **2008**, *34*, 711–714. [CrossRef] [PubMed]
32. S1-Leitlinie zu Diagnostik und Therapie der Skabies. Available online: http://www.awmf.org/leitlinien/detail/ll/013-052.html (accessed on 31 January 2006).
33. Bhutto, A.M.; Honda, M.; Kubo, Y.; Nonaka, S.; Yoshida, H. Introduction of a fluorescense-microscopic technique for the detection of eggs, egg shells, and mites in scabies. *J. Dermatol.* **1993**, *20*, 122–124. [CrossRef] [PubMed]
34. Uenotsuchi, T.; Moroi, Y.; Urabe, K.; Tsuji, G.; Takahara, M.; Furue, M. The scybala (fecal pellets) of *Sacroptes scabiei* var. *Hominis* are obviously stained with chlorazol black E. *J. Dermatol.* **2004**, *31*, 511–512. [PubMed]
35. Neynaber, S.; Wolff, H. Diagnosis of scabies with dermoscopy. *Can. Med. Assoc. J.* **2008**, *178*, 1540–1541. [CrossRef] [PubMed]
36. Prins, C.; Stucki, L.; French, L.; Saurat, J.H.; Braun, R.P. Dermoscopy for the in vivo detection of sarcoptes scabiei. *Dermatology* **2004**, *208*, 241–243. [CrossRef] [PubMed]

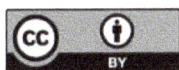

Tropical Medicine and
Infectious Disease

MDPI

Review

Integrated Management of Skin NTDs—Lessons Learned from Existing Practice and Field Research

Rie R. Yotsu [1,2]

[1] School of Tropical Medicine and Global Health, Nagasaki University, Nagasaki 852-8102, Japan; ryotsu@nagasaki-u.ac.jp

[2] Department of Dermatology, National Center for Global Health and Medicine, Tokyo 162-8655, Japan

Received: 26 September 2018; Accepted: 11 November 2018; Published: 14 November 2018

Abstract: Integration of neglected tropical diseases (NTDs) into the public health agenda has been a priority in global health for the last decade. Because a number of these diseases share not only the geographical distribution, but also a common feature which is skin involvement, bringing together a sub-group of 'skin NTDs' is one way forward to promote further integration among NTDs. With these diseases, which include leprosy, Buruli ulcer, yaws, mycetoma, lymphatic filariasis, and leishmaniasis, patients may be left with life-long deformities and disabilities when diagnosis and treatment are delayed. Stigma is another serious consequence of skin NTDs as it places a large barrier on the economic activities and social life of a patient. As a result, this creates a vicious cycle and obstructs a key goal of society, the elimination of poverty. Enhancement in surveillance systems as well as the further development of diagnostic methods, improvement in treatment and management, and identification of preventative measures for skin NTDs are therefore urgently needed. This article summarizes the existing practices and field research on skin NTDs and identifies potential synergies that could be achieved by adopting this integrated approach.

Keywords: case management; integration; mass drug administration; neglected tropical diseases; skin infections; skin NTDs; surveillance; training; tropical skin diseases

1. Introduction

Neglected tropical diseases (NTDs) are a group of infectious diseases that prevail in tropical and sub-tropical regions, affecting impoverished populations living in conditions of poor sanitation and in close contact with infectious vectors and livestock; such communities also have very limited access to adequate healthcare [1]. It is estimated that over one billion people in 149 countries are affected [2]. In May 2013, the World Health Assembly (WHA) adopted resolution WHA66.12, which calls on Member States to intensify and integrate measures against these NTDs to effectively and efficiently enhance the health and social well-being of the affected populations [2].

Successful integration of diagnostic and therapeutic interventions has happened for some NTDs, particularly among those that can be managed at community level by mass drug administration (MDA). This set of diseases forms the basis of a sub-group sometimes known as preventative chemotherapy and transmission control (PCT) NTDs, which includes such diseases as cysticercosis, foodborne trematode infections, lymphatic filariasis, onchocerciasis, schistosomiasis and soil-transmitted helminthiasis. Dracunculiasis (guinea-worm disease) is reaching close to eradication through transmission control; however, the recent transmission seen in dogs is hindering the last drive in Chad, which may show further spread [3]. In contrast, there are other NTDs where early diagnosis and management on an individual basis may be the only workable therapeutic measure, at least at present, and these are categorized as innovative and intensified disease management (IDM) NTDs. As IDM NTDs need considerable resources, including personnel with skills and financial support, and these measures do not produce a dramatic and immediately visible impact, which may lead to lower investment in research and development, the control of this set of diseases is lagging behind the PCT-NTDs [2].

Interestingly, a number of IDM-NTDs share a common feature, which is involvement of the skin, for example, in the forms of nodules, patches, edema, and ulceration (Figure 1). To assist in a breakthrough in the above-mentioned gap in the global health agenda, there is a move designed to improve integrated strategies to group these NTDs with skin manifestations under the banner of skin NTDs [4,5]. Among the skin NTDs are leprosy, Buruli ulcer, yaws, cutaneous and mucocutaneous leishmaniasis, chromoblastomycosis and mycetoma, and ectoparasites including scabies and tungiasis. Human African trypanosomiasis and post Kala-azar dermal leishmaniasis may present with skin signs, which although not the main symptom of the disease, may aid in early detection. Lymphatic filariasis and onchocerciasis are also skin NTDs, which are controlled by MDAs, but as control measures are rolled out across endemic areas there will be a residue of individual cases that have escaped detection or preemptive therapy with MDAs, whose recognition and treatment is essential in order to achieve effective control. Yaws and scabies are skin NTDs that are potentially controlled or eliminated through preventative chemotherapy, and the expansion of this approach on a larger scale is currently under study [6–10].

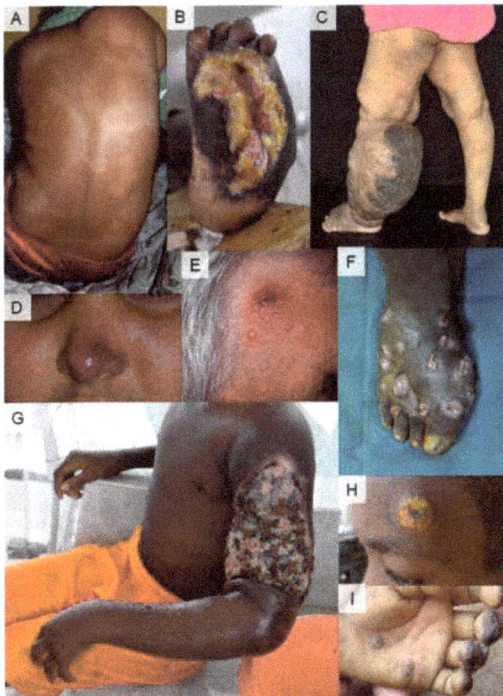

Figure 1. Clinical presentation of skin NTDs. (**A**) Leprosy (borderline tuberculoid leprosy). Ill-defined, multiple hypo-pigmented patches on the back. (**B**) Deformities of the feet and ulcer from peripheral neuropathy in leprosy. (**C**) Lymphatic filariasis. Unilateral lymphedema of the limb. (image: Saravu R. Narahari) (**D**) Mucocutaneous leishmaniasis. Redness and swelling of the nose. Inside: destruction of the nasal mucosa. Same patient as (**A**) (co-infection). (**E**) Cutaneous leishmaniasis. Infiltrated granulomatous lesion with central ulceration on the forehead. (**F**) Mycetoma. Multiple nodules with openings of draining sinuses discharging pus and blood. (image: Ahmed Fahal) (**G**) Buruli ulcer. Ulceration on the arm with extensive edema. Black and yellowish necrotic tissue on wound surface with some traditional remedies at first visit. (**H**) Yaws (primary yaws). Nodule with central ulceration with yellow crust on the forehead. (image: Kingsley Asiedu) (**I**) Tungiasis. Multiple small nodules with central black dot (body part of the adult flea) on the palm and on the finger tips.

In addition, there are other skin diseases that are not formally recognized by WHO as NTDs that contribute a huge disease burden in impoverished populations. These include podoconiosis (a geochemical, non-filarial elephantiasis due to long-term contact with irritant red clay soil), fungal and bacterial skin infections, and tropical ulcers [11,12]. These diseases should also be considered as neglected. However, their management as public health problems may also benefit from this skin NTDs integrative approach.

Surveillance and early detection, MDA, and case and morbidity management are potential areas for integrative initiatives for skin NTDs. This paper is not a systematic review of all skin NTDs, but rather it summarizes the current state of knowledge and lessons learned from existing practice and field research to aid in effective project implementation for managing skin NTDs.

2. Active Surveillance

There are several factors that hinder early detection and treatment of skin NTDs. Skin NTDs are often painless or accompanied by limited discomfort—this feature prevents patients and families from presenting to healthcare facilities at an early stage [13–15]. Low awareness of the disease among the populations at the highest risk also adds to the delay in seeking help, and this is compounded by the consequences of stigma and discrimination often associated with these diseases [13–16]. Many patients tend to seek treatment preferentially with traditional healers rather than at health care centers, as there is easier access and lower cost [15–17]. This health seeking behavior is also linked to the common perception that the diseases may result from mystical causes (witchcraft and curses) [15–17].

In the light of current perceptions among health authorities and communities, and given the lack of mass population measures or field-friendly diagnostic tests, active surveillance is still the most effective measure for early detection and thereby, treatment for most skin NTDs in order to prevent patients from developing disabilities, disfigurement, and comorbidities. Early detection and treatment are also key to cutting further transmission of the diseases, for instance, in leprosy, scabies, and yaws, and this underlines the importance of active surveillance.

As skin diseases can be detected by visual examination—a unique feature in this set of diseases—that if used effectively, for instance by organizing community skin surveys or treatment initiatives, is one simple approach for detection of skin NTDs that would otherwise remain hidden. Outreach skin surveys have been conducted with successful results in the case of leprosy in different parts of the world, for example, in India, Pacific Islands, Malawi, Cameroon, and recently in Brazil [18–25]. The Brazilian project led by the Ministry of Health targeted more than nine million schoolchildren aged between 5–14 years for skin screening of leprosy coupled with de-worming (albendazole for soil-transmitted helminthiases) [25]. In Japan where leprosy is no longer prevalent, school skin surveys played a considerable role in achieving a decline in cases during the 1970s in Okinawa, the most southern island of Japan, which remained as the last pocket during the endemic era [26]. Consecutive surveys at 3–5 year intervals were behind this success.

As part of promoting integration of skin NTDs, in line with the current global approach, there have been newer studies. An observational study in Cameroon reviewed the different means of detection of a total of 815 cases of yaws identified during the three-year period between 2012 and 2015 in one endemic region [27]. They reported that these cases were reported through the synergistic effect of five approaches: passive yaws detection at local clinics after training of local staff on NTDs, small community-based NTD case detection activities, community-based yaws screening immediately following Buruli ulcer outreach programs, school-based screening, and house-to-house searches. Rapid cure of yaws increased the uptake of, and confidence in, the treatment of Buruli ulcers, and thus led to a "win-win" situation for the two diseases.

In Côte d'Ivoire, another West African country, school skin surveys in areas identified as co-endemic for leprosy, Buruli ulcer, and yaws are also in the process of implementation [12]. The project is sometimes coupled with other activities, such as de-worming, if the timing coincides, to achieve resource mobilization as well as increased acceptance by the community. In this project, the latter is also enhanced by targeting all skin diseases, a strategy that also prevents creating unnecessary feelings of stigma and discrimination against skin NTDs. Targeting all skin diseases therefore appears to be a way forward. However, a careful strategy needs to be prepared as there is usually a high prevalence of skin diseases in such communities where skin NTDs are prevalent—ranging from infectious to inflammatory. This may pose a practical challenge in project implementation, i.e., cost of medications and ensuring referral pathways. In communities in African countries where skin NTDs are likely to be endemic, prevalence of skin diseases can range from 26% to 80% [12,28–33].

Key points in implementing integrated surveillance:

1. Selection of the intervention area: try to collect past data and develop mapping methods to identify co-distribution of cases of skin NTDs
2. Training of local healthcare workers both on skin NTDs and common skin diseases
3. Treatment: develop protocols on how to manage the different diseases anticipated; be prepared to treat or to refer
4. Look for opportunities for integration with other community- or school-based activities, e.g., de-worming, vitamin A and micronutrient supplementation, onchocerciasis and/or lymphatic filariasis control, to gain a synergic effect
5. Plan for repeat rounds/follow-up activities, decide on the appropriate intervals.

3. Mass Drug Administration and Prophylaxis

Lymphatic filariasis and onchocerciasis are already operationally covered by active MDA programs. In addition, several other skin NTDs are thought to be controllable using MDAs, and field research is ongoing.

Yaws comes first on that list, and recent studies have shown that high coverage with MDA consisting of single-dose azithromycin may be effective in control of the disease. A study conducted in an island off Papua New Guinea (16,092 residents) showed a rapid reduction in the prevalence of active yaws infection from 1.8% before mass treatment with azithromycin (30 mg/kg) to a minimum of 0.1% at 18 months, with 84% coverage [9,34]. However, with longer follow-up up to 42 months, a significant increase in cases to 0.4% was observed, indicating that a single round of drug administration may not be enough. These cases were mainly found in individuals who had not received the mass treatment or as new infection in residents. This finding suggests the need for repeated intervention to achieve elimination of yaws. In Ghana, a similar study to assess the effectiveness of this MDA strategy in endemic communities surrounded by other yaws-endemic communities is on-going, i.e., non-isolated communities in contrast to the work in Papua New Guinea. In the pilot study report, the prevalence of active and latent yaws in children reduced from 10.9% before mass treatment to 2.2% at 12 months, in 16,287 children with 89% coverage [7]. The best dosage regimen is also under investigation. An additional benefit would be that azithromycin MDA is also active against trachoma allowing for possible integration of the control of these two NTDs [8].

Scabies is also another disease that potentially may be targeted by MDAs, as oral ivermectin, one of the major drugs used in the control of a number of other NTDs, is also highly effective in scabies. Successful mapping and co-administration of mass treatment studies for scabies have been conducted in the Solomon Islands and integrated with existing programs for trachoma and yaws [10,35–37]. In Brazil, selective MDA by targeting communities heavily infected with ectoparasites and enteroparasites using ivermectin considerably reduced the prevalence of a range of coexisting parasitic skin infections, including scabies, pediculosis, cutaneous larva migrans and tungiasis [38]. Similarly, the African Program for Onchocerciasis [39] and the Global Programme to Eliminate Lymphatic Filariasis [40] reported a coincident effect in reducing the number of cases of scabies, an off-target disease. Further integrated activities are planned as part of the assessment of the impact of triple-drug treatment (ivermectin, albendazole, and diethylcarbamazine citrate) for lymphatic filariasis [41]. Use of ivermectin could increase community acceptance of the MDAs through the treatment of skin conditions, particularly if it benefits those severely affected by itching and sores.

Two countries with extensive experience in NTD control, Ethiopia and Fiji are currently developing comprehensive scabies control programs [42]. To further plan on the potential of MDAs for scabies, more studies on dosage and issues related to ivermectin use during pregnancy and in small children are needed. Furthermore, prevalence of scabies is likely to rise again after a certain period of time, and therefore, more operational research is needed to define the best intervals between rounds of MDA. The development of moxidectin, a macrocyclic lactone similar to ivermectin, but with a much longer half-life, for the treatment of human scabies may promote MDAs for scabies [43,44]. Recently in June 2018, the United States Food and Drug Administration (FDA) approved the use of moxidectin for onchocerciasis in patients aged 12 years and older [45].

Although not on the same massive scale as yaws or scabies, there have been attempts to prevent occurrence and interrupt transmission of leprosy using one-dose rifampicin chemoprophylaxis in contact cases (post-exposure prophylaxis). This intervention was tested in Bangladesh in a cluster-randomized controlled trial including 21,711 participants, with successful outcomes at 2-years with a 56.5% reduction in new cases in the intervention group [46]. This protective effect was seen only in the first two years. No additional protective effect was observed after 4 and 6 years, but the total impact of the intervention was still statistically significant after 6 years [47]. A similar result was reported from another study in Indonesia [48]. With the long latent period of leprosy—which can sometimes be more than several decades, long-term follow up is necessary to assess the true effect of interventions for this disease. In the past, chemoprophylaxis (1 to 2 doses of a combination of rifampicin, ofloxacin, and minocycline) has been tested in three Pacific Islands, namely Kiribati, the Federated States of Micronesia, and the Republic of the Marshall Islands, all small islands with a high level of leprosy endemicity [19–21]. Now two decades after this intervention, they remain among the countries with the highest new case detection rates for leprosy per population globally [49]. Short-term reduction in new cases of leprosy was observed during the first few years after the intervention, in which active case detection at baseline could have played a considerable role in enhancing the effect of treating some sub-clinical cases. In other words, chemoprophylaxis alone may not be effective unless it is coupled with well-planned active case finding, and the prophylaxis is delivered in the form of several rounds of medication at adequate intervals [26,50]. Currently, the Leprosy Post-Exposure Prophylaxis [51] study—a joint study between India, Indonesia, Myanmar, Nepal, Sri Lanka, and Tanzania using single dose rifampicin—was designed to accelerate the uptake of the evidence for post-exposure prophylaxis and introduce it into national leprosy programs [51]. Recently published interim analysis show that the program has enrolled 5941 index patients and identified a total of 123,331 contacts [52]. Efficacy results are awaited.

MDAs and prophylaxis may be effective in the control of several skin NTDs, but it is important to note that repeated dosing and other surveillance activities are often needed, as mentioned above. We should also be careful in implementing MDAs/prophylaxis as some drugs may not be safe for use in children, in pregnant women, and in individuals for whom they are contra-indicated. Monitoring for adverse reactions should be carefully done as their occurrence might have a negative impact on the campaigns. How to address these constraints should be elucidated before implementing the strategy on a larger scale. Furthermore, the funds necessary for implementation are not available at the moment, as there is limited interest from donors. Identification of the target populations is also very important not only for the success of the intervention, but also for minimizing cost.

Key points in implementing mass drug administration:

1. Careful identification of target populations or case definition
2. Identifying intervals between rounds and number of rounds; some diseases have long latent periods which may be difficult to assess
3. Obtaining strong, coordinated public-private partnerships, including pharmaceutical companies

4. Assessment of secondary effects on other diseases (e.g., leprosy vs. tuberculosis), including increasing the risk of drug resistance

5. Addressing the issues of stigma and discrimination if implementing for contact cases.

4. Current Status of Diagnosis and Treatment for Skin NTDs

Few skin NTDs can be confirmed with reliable point-of-care diagnostic tests, and therefore a clinical examination remains the cornerstone of diagnosis. This poses a major challenge, not just in case management of individual patients with skin NTDs, but also in understanding the true epidemiology and disease burden in endemic areas.

To take Buruli ulcer as an example, a study in Cameroon has shown that only 27% among the 327 patients with ulcerative lesions suspected as Buruli ulcer seen at one of their tertiary hospital were confirmed to be Buruli ulcer [53]. Other diagnosis ranged from vascular, bacterial infections, post-traumatic, fistulated osteomyelitis, as well as neoplasia. The team used a combination of Ziehl-Neelsen staining, PCR, and culture from either swab or fine-needle aspiration, skin biopsies, and several systemic tests for diagnostic confirmation [53]. In field settings, these tests are not easy to perform, and it is not difficult to imagine that some patients who have been given a diagnosis based solely on clinical appearance are treated unnecessarily or given the wrong drugs.

PCR targeting IS2404 is currently the test most used for confirming Buruli ulcer. However, access to PCR in many places in West Africa where Buruli ulcer is endemic is very limited. Moreover, adequate skills in sample taking and ensuring transportation of samples in good condition adds to the challenge. It sometimes may take weeks and months to reach the laboratory. It is very difficult to rule out the possibility of false negatives under such conditions. It is also noteworthy that some of the PCR positives with IS2404 include other mycobacterial diseases, for example, *M. marinum*, *M. chelonae*, and *M. smegmatis*, whose distribution in these countries is not yet well understood [54]. Some promising studies are underway in order to develop a rapid diagnostic tool for Buruli ulcer, including the loop-mediated isothermal amplification (LAMP) test [55,56], thin layer chromatography for the detection of mycolactone (lipid toxin produced by the causing bacteria of Buruli ulcer) [57], and antigen detection assays [58].

Table 1 provides the list of diagnostic tests and Table 2 provides treatments currently used for each skin NTD. As treatment of many skin NTDs is of long duration, it is important that diagnostic confirmation be made before initiating treatment. Furthermore, some skin NTDs are associated with considerable stigma and discrimination. Labeling a patient with a specific diagnosis unnecessarily is also another issue that needs to be addressed, and development of easier and more reliable diagnostic methods would also improve these important social aspects associated with skin NTDs. Recently, a point-of-care test for syphilis has been used for early detection of yaws, as they are both from the spirochete bacterium group, replacing the traditional laboratory methods such as rapid plasma reagin (RPR) and *Treponema pallidum* hemagglutination assay (TPHA) [59]. However, a positive test does not necessarily mean that the lesion is due to active yaws, as there are also other pathogenic species in this same group [59]. Further studies for the development of diagnostic tools and reliability checking are needed for all skin NTDs.

Treatments used for skin NTDs are also very limited and many are old drugs or combinations [60]. Integrated advocacy among the skin NTDs may aid in the development of better diagnostic tools and treatment options.

Trop. Med. Infect. Dis. **2018**, 3, 120

Table 1. Diagnostic methods and tools for skin NTDs.

	Pathogen	Rapid Diagnostic Test	PCR	Microscopy	Culture	Serology	Others
Buruli ulcer	*Mycobacterium ulcerans*	X	O	O	O	X	LAMP test, thin layer chromatography, antigen detection assays under development
Cutaneous leishmaniasis (CL)/mucocutaneous leishmaniasis (ML)	*Leishmania species*	X	O	O, Skin smears	O	X	LAMP test, antigen detection assays under development (Montenegro skin test)
Lymphatic filariasis (LF)	Microfilaria (*Wuchereria bancrofti; Brugia malayi*, etc.)	O	O	O, Blood smears	X	Δ, Anti-filarial antibodies	Ultrasonography
Onchocerciasis	Microfilaria (*Onchocerca volvulus*)	O	O	O, Skin snips	X	Δ, Anti-filarial antibodies	Direct observation of adult worms from nodule(s), slit-lamp eye exam, serological and antigen tests under development
Leprosy	*Mycobacterium leprae*	X	O	O	X	Δ, Anti-PGL-I antibody	Thickened nerves, loss of muscle strength, anesthetic skin lesion
Mycetoma	Fungal or bacterial species	X	O	Δ	O	X	X-rays, CT, ultrasonography, etc.
Podoconiosis	Irritant alkalic clay soils	N/A	N/A	N/A	N/A	N/A	Location, history, clinical findings; negative results for LF and other lymphedema-causing diseases; genetic susceptibility
Scabies	*Sarcoptes scabiei var. hominis*	X	Δ	O	X	X	Dermatoscopy, burrow ink test
Tungiasis	*Tunga penetrans* (sand fleas)	X	Δ	O	X	X	Direct observation of adult fleas and eggs from skin lesion(s), dermatoscopy
Yaws	*Treponema pallidum* subsp. *pertenue*	O	O	O	O	PRP, TPHA, FTA-ABS, etc.	Diagnostics for differentiation of *Treponema pallidum* species under development

O = available; Δ = available but not confirmatory or standardized; X = unavailable.

Table 2. Treatment and management for skin NTDs.

	Medical Treatment	Surgery	Wound or Lymphedema Management	Self-Morbidity Management	Prevention
Buruli ulcer	**Standard:** Oral rifampicin + clarithromycin for 8 weeks **Other tested regimens:** Oral rifampicin + either 1 or 2 of [ciprofloxacin, ethambutol, moxifloxacin, amikacin, etc.]	Yes	Yes	Yes	Limited, route of transmission unknown (Stay away from contaminated water sources)
Cutaneous leishmaniasis (CL)/mucocutaneous leishmaniasis (ML)	Individualized treatment depending on species (no standard) Amphotericin B deoxycholate, pentavalent antimonials, fluconazole, ketoconazole, miltefosine, paromomycin ointment, etc. **Simple CL** lesion(s) with low ML-risk: natural healing may occur **Complex CL** lesion(s) with high-ML risk, severe lesion(s), immunocompromised persons, etc.: treat all cases	No	Yes	No	Limited (Avoid sand fly bites)
Lymphatic filariasis (LF)	Oral albendazole ± [diethylcarbamazine (DEC) or ivermectin] When long-term treatment is possible: Oral DEC (1–12 days) ± doxycycline for 4 to 6 weeks Note: DEC contraindicated in onchocerciasis endemic sites	Yes	Yes	Yes	Avoid mosquito bites, MDAs, vector control, etc.
Onchocerciasis	Oral ivermectin	Yes	No	No	Avoid blackfly bites, MDAs, vector control, etc.
Leprosy	**Multiple drug therapy (MDT):** Oral rifampicin + dapsone + clofazimine for 6 to 12 months	Yes	Yes	Yes	Contact tracing and early detection; prophylaxis with one-dose rifampicin in trial
Mycetoma	Antibiotics or antifungals depending on species for long-term	Yes	Yes	Yes	Footwear
Podoconiosis	N/A	Yes	Yes	Yes	Footwear
Scabies	Oral ivermectin, 1–2 doses 1 week apart	No	No	No	Early diagnosis and treatment of contacts, possible MDAs in endemic communities
Tungiasis	None (primary treatment: hygienic mechanical removal of fleas), antibiotics if secondary infection is indicated	No	Yes	No	Footwear
Yaws	Single oral azithromycin or injectable benzathine penicillin	No	Yes	No	Contact tracing and early detection, possible MDAs in endemic communities

Key points in diagnosis and treatment of skin NTDs:

1. Training of local healthcare workers on clinical diagnosis
2. Training of local healthcare workers on diagnostic tests, including sample taking; make a routine for performing diagnostic tests
3. Need for the development of new point-of-care diagnostic tools
4. Developments that enhance laboratory confirmation
5. Need for further investigation of new drugs and regimens for skin NTDs.

5. Wound and Lymphedema Management–Cross-Cutting Treatment

Despite the availability of different drugs for systemic treatment, the cross-cutting component in the management of a number of skin NTDs is wound (leprosy, Buruli ulcer, yaws, cutaneous leishmaniasis, tropical ulcers, etc.) and lymphedema (lymphatic filariasis and podoconiosis) management, which can be delivered potentially with the same knowledge, skills, and in the same settings. Integration of wound and lymphedema management for skin NTDs is already happening in the field. In many of the co-endemic areas, leprosy and Buruli ulcers are managed in the same facilities, as well as lymphatic filariasis and podoconiosis (Figure 2).

Wounds are among the most frequently encountered skin problems in rural settings in low- and middle-income countries, where skin NTDs are also endemic [53,61]. The causes can range from trauma, burns, bacterial infections as well as to non-communicable diseases such as diabetes and peripheral arterial diseases [53,61]. A large proportion of wounds are at risk of progressing to a chronic stage when not supported by proper diagnosis and wound care. Skills in evaluating the abnormal signs and symptoms, such as when to stop using topical antiseptics, when to suspect secondary infection, when to suspect malignant alteration, are skills that are lacking as there is limited training and the need for the expertise in wound care is not well recognized. A study conducted in Ghana and in Benin interviewing health care personnel dealing with the wound management of Buruli ulcer patients reported that standard of wound care differed greatly both between personnel and between institutions [62]. Limited accessibility to clean water can lead to prolonged secondary infection, as well as infrequent dressing changes due to poor availability of dressing materials and access to health facilities. Use of traditional medicines, and sometimes use of local folk treatments such as ash and toothpaste, hinder the normal wound healing process.

The most important component in wound management is achieving a clean wound bed with red granulation tissue, protected from infection and trauma [63,64]. Securing clean water to wash the wound surface regularly and thoroughly is the foremost priority; having normal saline solution is ideal, if not, tap water fit for drinking or cooled boiled water can be used for this purpose [65,66] (Figure 2). There is currently a wide range of wound dressing products designed for use in developed countries to keep the wound bed moist. They are often costly, although they may be useful if they shorten the wound healing time [67–70]. Nonetheless, there are good wound care techniques applicable in places where patients with ulcerative skin NTDs reside, using materials that are readily available, e.g., saline, vaseline [65]. The use of honey should not be dismissed although further assessment is needed [71]. Removal of necrotic tissue on the wound surface is another important component in wound management [63,64], which can be achieved through training of the local healthcare providers.

The main pillar in management of lymphedema is also based on hygiene—regular and thorough washing with soap and water—and skin care. A systematic review by Stocks et al., reported that participation in hygiene-based lymphedema management decreased the incidence of acute dermatolymphangioadenitis (ADLA) by one-third [72]. These inflammatory episodes, which are characterized by pain, fever, and swelling of the affected limb create a vicious cycle as they further erode lymphatic function stimulating more fibrosis and it is therefore important to prevent these [73]. Protecting the skin barrier function with simple emollients such as vaseline as well as limb exercise are also key to reducing inflammation and swelling [74,75].

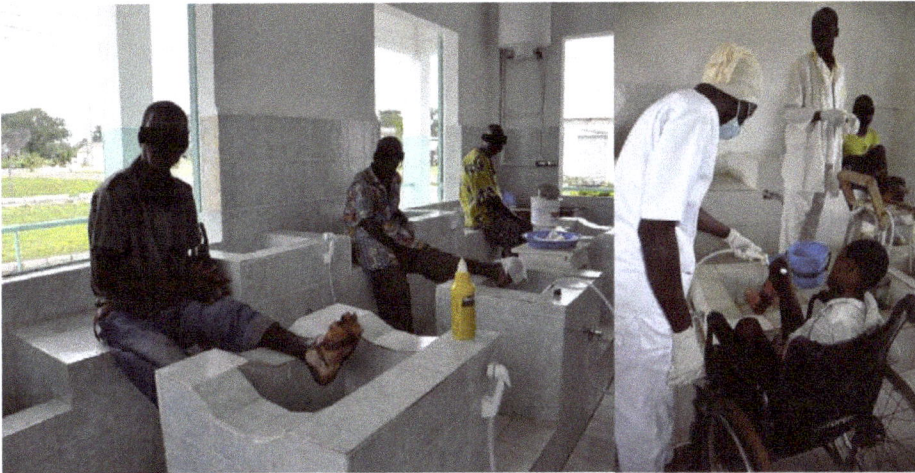

Figure 2. Wound care facility in Côte d'Ivoire for leprosy, Buruli ulcer, and other ulcers.

Studies investigating wound or lymphedema care in resource-limited settings are lacking. The severe impact a wound or a lymphedema can have on the quality of life of those affected is under-recognized [76–82]. Furthermore, findings from some cost analyses carried out in the developed world show a strikingly high cost burden [83,84], and this also needs to be assessed in resource-limited settings. There has been a recent study investigating the cost of wound care for cutaneous leishmaniasis in Afghanistan comparing different methods [85]. More studies of this kind will further improve the efficient management of skin NTDs. There are also other opportunities for integration between skin NTDs and chronic diseases, such as diabetes, in limb care or between other interventions such as clean water, better sanitation and hygiene (WASH) [77], which should be further explored.

Key points in wound and lymphedema management:

1. Implementation of a simple algorithm utilizing inexpensive and easily obtainable products for wound management/lymphedema management
2. Better use of those resources that are available in the local setting
3. Cost-analysis
4. Training and deployment of helpers including both local health care workers and "the expert patient".

6. Self-Morbidity Management to Improve Outcomes and Social Inclusion

Some skin NTDs, when diagnosed late, can lead to life-long disabilities and disfigurement. This may result from diseases with extensive ulceration or lymphedema as listed in the above section (Buruli ulcer, leprosy, tropical ulcers, lymphatic filariasis, podoconiosis, etc.) but there are other causes. For instance, ulceration, disabilities and deformities in a leprosy patient can also occur as a result of peripheral nerve damage—clawing toes, drop hands and feet, etc. Often patients with limb lesions from mycetoma are managed by amputation [80] as is the case with other severe forms of ulceration. Early identification and treatment can reduce this.

As outlined in the above section, the use of locally available methods and materials at low cost, which are also culturally accepted, are key in achieving a sustainable morbidity management program. A good example of this is a study by Narahari et al. in India, where the group developed an integrative treatment protocol for morbidity reduction of lymphatic filariasis by combining Ayurvedic exercises, compression therapy and modern dermatology drugs to treat bacterial entry points [77]. While the treatments for such conditions may include complex procedures such as lymphovascular shunts and debulking surgery, this integrative and non-invasive treatment, widely available in the local Indian settings was strikingly successful in reducing the volume of the limbs and also led to fewer episodes of ADLA.

In Ethiopia, integrated morbidity management for lymphatic filariasis and podoconiosis are in the process of implementation by the health ministry and partners, with some highly successful outcomes. Integration for leprosy and Buruli ulcer are already happening in the field, even in places where the national public health programs are still organized in a vertical pattern. As leprosy and Buruli ulcer share the same goal, which is prevention of disability (POD), the two diseases might be expected to benefit from synergies in management. It is of note that they also share similarities in diagnosis and treatment as the causative organisms come from the same mycobacterial disease group, and advocacy strategies have focused on more integration between the two [86].

As these skin NTDs are chronic, management of individual patients, including skin care and dressing or compression at home are critical in achieving success in treatment outcomes. A systematic review by Douglass et al., reported that intensity of training of patients in self-care practices and frequency of monitoring improved treatment outcomes [87], while similar findings were reported by Sathiaraj et al. for leprosy [88] (Figure 3).

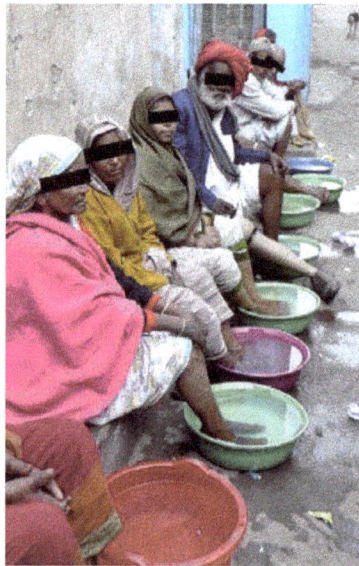

Figure 3. Education on self-skin care for prevention of disabilities (POD) for people affected by leprosy in a village in India.

Better treatment outcomes can be achieved when there is involvement of patients themselves and their carers. Self-care and carer assisted programs are also important in helping to reduce the work burden of local healthcare providers, as without these integrative techniques may even add to their work load. The success of Narahari et al. in their morbidity management for lymphatic filariasis was possible through recruiting patients accompanied by a family member willing to support self-care at home [77]. Carers must be willing and actively take part in the management of the family member, including support in dressing changes and skin care, relief of odor and pain, nourishment, helping with mobility, encouraging them to maintain adequate hygiene by bathing and, above all, making sure that they feel welcome in their society so that they can live full lives, marry, and achieve employment. [89]. As emphasized here, social inclusion is indeed another critical dimension in case management of skin NTDs, which can benefit from a synergized approach to skin NTD integration.

Key points in self-morbidity management to improve outcomes and social inclusion:

1. Use of locally available methods and materials at low cost
2. Patient training for self-care
3. Patient empowerment
4. Carer training
5. Interventions to promote social inclusion.

7. Training and Referrals

No disease control programs can be successful without good training of the local healthcare providers and workers, who are the closest to patients. This is certainly true for skin NTDs as clinical diagnosis remains the most readily available diagnostic measure and an important entry point for disease control of most skin NTDs. Most of the successful projects introduced here have been achieved through good and effective training. One of the major strategies deployed in the Ethiopian lymphatic filariasis-podoconiosis integrated program has been training, guideline development featuring a simple algorithm on clinical assessment, treatment and referral needs, and a defined care package [90]. This initiative also developed and rolled out a teaching video for healthcare workers on integrated morbidity management.

For integration, it is essential to provide suitable training for local healthcare providers on skin NTDs, as well as common skin diseases as these are more frequent and a better knowledge of these diseases will empower them. A well-trained healthcare provider who gains the confidence and acceptance of the population is key to achieving good results. In a study in Côte d'Ivoire during which we conducted screening of schoolchildren with skin NTDs, training was given with this consideration and it was effective in extending the program to a larger population with skilled local healthcare providers [12]. These healthcare providers perceived that the training was very helpful for their daily practices and their involvement in our project has been continuous. WHO and the expert panel group recently developed a training manual "Recognizing neglected tropical diseases through changes on the skin: a training guide for front-line health workers", which was developed with the vision to support such activities [91]. As the endemicity of diseases varies from one place to another, the document can be modified to be country/context-specific.

Along with capacity building at field level, clear referral pathways, e.g., for clinical consultation, referral for hospitalization, sending of samples to laboratories, etc. need to be established or strengthened to ensure better integrative management of skin NTDs, irrespective of disease type. We need to bear in mind that there is a wide range of skin diseases, other than skin NTDs, in which diagnosis are difficult, and some can even be fatal, e.g., acute infections, drug eruptions, and cutaneous malignancies. A study in Brazil where leprosy services have been decentralized has demonstrated the importance of referral centers in support of local health services in treating skin diseases [92].

With increasing availability and accessibility to mobile phones and internet, teledermatology is one way forward for establishing an adequate training, support and referral system. In a comprehensive project for mycetoma management in Sudan, a computer application on computer tablets or smartphones connected house-to-house survey medical teams, regional tertiary center, and experts at national level [80]. In Malawi and Ghana, a community-led SMS reporting tool for the rapid assessment of lymphatic filariasis morbidity burden was successful in involving community-based health surveillance workers/volunteers to participate in reporting and continuous monitoring of patients [93]. A similar approach could be established for other skin NTDs with respect to co-endemicity, and involvement of dermatologists will enable the approach. However, as there is a shortage of dermatologists in these settings, besides mobilization of local dermatologists, establishment of networks extending beyond the country may be necessary [94]. Two examples of such projects are described in this issue [95,96].

8. Next Steps

Integration of programs for skin NTDs is happening at national level. Some of the countries that have integrated their national public health programs for leprosy and Buruli ulcer include Benin, Cameroon, Congo Brazzaville, Gabon, Papua New Guinea and Togo; Nigeria combines leprosy, Buruli ulcer, and tuberculosis (TB). Some countries such as Côte d'Ivoire, Democratic Republic of Congo, and Ghana [86] still have separate control programs. However, these countries are also exploring integration of these skin NTDs, including yaws. Identifying the most appropriate combination of diseases, based on disease control measures and co-endemicity, is the key to successful integration.

Identifying opportunities beyond NTDs, such as integration with TB programs (DOTS), WASH, and non-communicable diseases (NCDs) may open a new door. Recent screening activities in Kiribati for NCDs and TB produced off-target results—identification of new leprosy cases. As the underlying risk factors for skin NTDs are poverty and poor hygiene, integration with poverty reduction programs should also be explored. A systematic review by Tomczyk et al. reported that access to footwear use significantly reduced the incidence of Buruli ulcer, cutaneous larva migrans, tungiasis, hookworm infection, soil-transmitted helminth infection, strongyloidiasis, and leptospirosis [97].

Whatever the case, attention needs to be paid to facilitating a reduction in the workload of front-line healthcare workers. Consideration is also needed as to how well any program can retain workers with skills needed in management of skin NTDs, to improve early detection and treatment outcomes, prevent or minimize disabilities, and ease the burden on governments and NGOs [86].

Establishment of expert working groups for guideline making, training materials, advocacy, etc. could facilitate this process. Recently, WHO and the working group on leprosy and yaws published guidelines for each disease [59,98]. An international alliance for the control of scabies (IACS) has been formed to advance collaboration [42,99]. Further research in the field demonstrating the burden of disease, and the effectiveness and synergies of control strategies, may increase the visibility of skin NTDs within the global health agenda and attract greater attention from international agencies and donors.

9. Conclusions

Many skin NTDs disproportionately affect the world's most disadvantaged people living in the low- and middle-income countries. They are often chronic in nature and may lead to chronic secondary conditions, including life-long disabilities and disfigurement, creating a vicious cycle for individuals, families, and society. Until recently, they were the most neglected among other NTDs as their disease control measures rely mostly on individual case management and any visible impact in the control achievements was limited. The present drive towards integration of skin NTDs together or with other programs has significant potential to reverse this limitation. There is a body of existing practice and field research for each disease among those interested in skin NTDs, which have the potential to further enhance the process of integration. There has also been new research on skin NTDs including approaches to integration that have had encouraging outcomes. It is essential that we build on these good practices and the lessons learned in order to formulate sound strategies for the shared goal of the fight against NTDs.

Funding: This study was supported by the following: (1) Grant-in-Aid for Scientific Research <KAKENHI>, Japan (https://www.jsps.go.jp/english/e-grants/index.html), grant number: 16K21656; and (2) Japan Agency for Medical Research and Development (AMED), Japan (http://www.amed.go.jp/en/), grant number: 18jm0510004h0001. The funders had no role in study design, data collection and analysis, decision to publish, or preparation of the manuscript.

Acknowledgments: The author thanks the Côte d'Ivoire research team for our collaborative work which contributed to enrich the content of this article: National Leprosy Control Program Côte d'Ivoire, National Buruli Ulcer Control Program Côte d'Ivoire, Bamba Vagamon (Raoul Follereau Institute Côte d'Ivoire), Aubin Yao, Landry Koffi Kouadio (MAP International), Kouamé Kouadio, Aka N'Guetta, David Coulibaly N'Golo (Pasteur Institute Côte d'Ivoire), Julien Aké (Effect Hope), Konan N'Guessan (Sightsaver) and Amari Akpa. Thanks also goes to Daisuke Utsumi (Department of Dermatology, University of the Ryukyus, Okinawa, Japan) for his contribution in the wound management section through his experience in Kenya.

Conflicts of Interest: Nothing to declare.

References

1. Hotez, P. *Forgotten People, Forgotten Diseases: The Neglected Tropical Diseaes and Their Impact on Global Health and Development*, 2nd ed.; ASM Press: Washington, DC, USA, 2013.
2. Department of Control of Neglected Tropical Diseases, WHO. *Neglected Tropical Diseases*; WHO: Geneva, Switzerland, 2018; Available online: http://www.who.int/neglected_diseases/diseases/en/ (accessed on 5 August 2018).
3. Eberhard, M.L.; Ruiz-Tiben, E.; Hopkins, D.R.; Farrell, C.; Toe, F.; Weiss, A.; Withers, P.C., Jr.; Jenks, M.H.; Thiele, E.A.; Cotton, J.A.; et al. The peculiar epidemiology of dracunculiasis in Chad. *Am. J. Trop. Med. Hyg.* **2014**, *90*, 61–70. [CrossRef] [PubMed]
4. Engelman, D.; Fuller, L.; Solomon, A.; McCarthy, J.; Hay, R.; Lammie, P.; Steer, A. Opportunities for integrated control of neglected tropical diseases that affect the skin. *Trends Parasitol.* **2016**, *32*, 843–854. [CrossRef] [PubMed]
5. Mitja, O.; Marks, M.; Bertran, L.; Kollie, K.; Argaw, D.; Fahal, A.H.; Fitzpatrick, C.; Fuller, L.C.; Garcia Izquierdo, B.; Hay, R.; et al. Integrated control and management of neglected tropical skin diseases. *PLoS Negl. Trop. Dis.* **2017**, *11*, e0005136. [CrossRef] [PubMed]
6. WHO. Eradication of yaws—The Morges strategy. *Wkly. Epidemiol. Rec.* **2012**, *87*, 189–194.
7. Abdulai, A.A.; Agana-Nsiire, P.; Biney, F.; Kwakye-Maclean, C.; Kyei-Faried, S.; Amponsa-Achiano, K.; Simpson, S.V.; Bonsu, G.; Ohene, S.A.; Ampofo, W.K.; et al. Community-based mass treatment with azithromycin for the elimination of yaws in Ghana-Results of a pilot study. *PLoS Negl. Trop. Dis.* **2018**, *12*, e0006303. [CrossRef] [PubMed]
8. Marks, M.; Mitja, O.; Bottomley, C.; Kwakye, C.; Houinei, W.; Bauri, M.; Adwere, P.; Abdulai, A.A.; Dua, F.; Boateng, L.; et al. Comparative efficacy of low-dose versus standard-dose azithromycin for patients with yaws: A randomised non-inferiority trial in Ghana and Papua New Guinea. *Lancet Glob. Health* **2018**, *6*, e401–e410. [CrossRef]
9. Mitja, O.; Godornes, C.; Houinei, W.; Kapa, A.; Paru, R.; Abel, H.; Gonzalez-Beiras, C.; Bieb, S.V.; Wangi, J.; Barry, A.E.; et al. Re-emergence of yaws after single mass azithromycin treatment followed by targeted treatment: A longitudinal study. *Lancet* **2018**, *391*, 1599–1607. [CrossRef]
10. Romani, L.; Whitfeld, M.J.; Koroivueta, J.; Kama, M.; Wand, H.; Tikoduadua, L.; Tuicakau, M.; Koroi, A.; Andrews, R.; Kaldor, J.M.; et al. Mass drug administration for scabies control in a population with endemic disease. *N. Engl. J. Med.* **2015**, *373*, 2305–2313. [CrossRef] [PubMed]
11. Elson, L.; Wright, K.; Swift, J.; Feldmeier, H. Control of tungiasis in absence of a roadmap: Grassroots and global approaches. *Trop. Med. Infect. Dis.* **2017**, *2*, 33. [CrossRef] [PubMed]
12. Yotsu, R.R.; Kouadio, K.; Vagamon, B.; N'Guessan, K.; Akpa, A.J.; Yao, A.; Ake, J.; Abbet Abbet, R.; Tchamba Agbor Agbor, B.; Bedimo, R.; et al. Skin disease prevalence study in schoolchildren in rural Cote d'Ivoire: Implications for integration of neglected skin diseases (skin NTDs). *PLoS Negl. Trop. Dis.* **2018**, *12*, e0006489. [CrossRef] [PubMed]
13. Atre, S.R.; Rangan, S.G.; Shetty, V.P.; Gaikwad, N.; Mistry, N.F. Perceptions, health seeking behaviour and access to diagnosis and treatment initiation among previously undetected leprosy cases in rural Maharashtra, India. *Lepr. Rev.* **2011**, *82*, 222–234. [PubMed]
14. Nicholls, P.G.; Chhina, N.; Bro, A.K.; Barkataki, P.; Kumar, R.; Withington, S.G.; Smith, W.C. Factors contributing to delay in diagnosis and start of treatment of leprosy: Analysis of help-seeking narratives in northern Bangladesh and in West Bengal, India. *Lepr. Rev.* **2005**, *76*, 35–47. [PubMed]
15. Mulder, A.A.; Boerma, R.P.; Barogui, Y.; Zinsou, C.; Johnson, R.C.; Gbovi, J.; van der Werf, T.S.; Stienstra, Y. Healthcare seeking behaviour for Buruli ulcer in Benin: A model to capture therapy choice of patients and healthy community members. *Trans. R. Soc. Trop. Med. Hyg.* **2008**, *102*, 912–920. [CrossRef] [PubMed]
16. Aujoulat, I.; Johnson, C.; Zinsou, C.; Guedenon, A.; Portaels, F. Psychosocial aspects of health seeking behaviours of patients with Buruli ulcer in southern Benin. *Trop. Med. Int. Health* **2003**, *8*, 750–759. [CrossRef] [PubMed]

17. Stienstra, Y.; van der Graaf, W.T.; Asamoa, K.; van der Werf, T.S. Beliefs and attitudes toward Buruli ulcer in Ghana. *Am. J. Trop. Med. Hyg.* **2002**, *67*, 207–213. [CrossRef] [PubMed]

18. Shetty, V.P.; Pandya, S.S.; Arora, S.; Capadia, G.D. Observations from a 'special selective drive' conducted under National Leprosy Elimination Programme in Karjat taluka and Gadchiroli district of Maharashtra. *Indian J. Lepr.* **2009**, *81*, 189–193. [PubMed]

19. Daulako, E.C. Population screening and mass chemoprophylaxis in Kiribati. *Int. J. Lepr. Mycobact. Dis.* **1999**, *67*, S23–S25.

20. Diletto, C. Elimination of leprosy in the federated states of micronesia by intensive case finding, treatment with WHO/MDT and administration of chemoprophylaxis. *Int. J. Lepr. Mycobact. Dis.* **1999**, *67*, S10–S13.

21. Tin, K. Population screening and chemoprophylaxis for household contacts of leprosy patients in the Republic of the Marshall Islands. *Int. J. Lepr. Mycobact. Dis.* **1999**, *67*, S26–S29.

22. Msyamboza, K.P.; Mawaya, L.R.; Kubwalo, H.W.; Ng'oma, D.; Liabunya, M.; Manjolo, S.; Msiska, P.P.; Somba, W.W. Burden of leprosy in Malawi: Community camp-based cross-sectional study. *BMC Int. Health Hum. Rights* **2012**, *12*, 12. [CrossRef] [PubMed]

23. Nsagha, D.S.; Bamgboye, E.A.; Yediran, A.B.O.O. Childhood leprosy in Essimbiland of Cameroon: Results of chart review and school survey. *Niger. Q. J. Hosp. Med.* **2009**, *19*, 214–219. [CrossRef]

24. Baretto, J.G.; Guimarães, L.D.S.; Frade, M.A.C.; Rosa, P.S.; Salgado, C.G. High rates of undiagnosed leprosy and subclinical infection amongst school children in the Amazon Region. *Mem. Inst. Oswaldo Cruz* **2012**, *107*, 60–67. [CrossRef]

25. WHO. Brazilian School-Based Deworming and Leprosy Case-Finding Campaign Targets More Than 9 Million Chilren. Available online: http://www.who.int/neglected_diseases/brazil_leprosy_sth_2013/en/ (accessed on 20 August 2018).

26. Saikawa, K. Epidemiological implications of school survey in Okinawa (in Japanese). *J. Health Welf. Stat.* **1978**, *25*, 6–23.

27. UmBoock, A.; Awah, P.K.; Mou, F.; Nichter, M. Yaws resurgence in Bankim, Cameroon: The relative effectiveness of different means of detection in rural communities. *PLoS Negl. Trop. Dis.* **2017**, *11*, e0005557. [CrossRef]

28. Ogunbiyi, A.O.; Owoaje, E.; Ndahi, A. Prevalence of skin disorders in school children in Ibadan, Nigeria. *Pediatr. Dermatol.* **2005**, *22*, 6–10. [CrossRef] [PubMed]

29. Hogewoning, A.; Amoah, A.; Bavinck, J.N.; Boakye, D.; Yazdanbakhsh, M.; Adegnika, A.; De Smedt, S.; Fonteyne, Y.; Willemze, R.; Lavrijsen, A. Skin diseases among schoolchildren in Ghana, Gabon, and Rwanda. *Int. J. Dermatol.* **2013**, *52*, 589–600. [CrossRef] [PubMed]

30. Mahe, A.; Prual, A.; Konate, M.; Bobin, P. Skin diseases of children in Mali: A public health problem. *Trans. R. Soc. Trop. Med. Hyg.* **1995**, *89*, 467–470. [CrossRef]

31. Komba, E.V.; Mgonda, Y.M. The spectrum of dermatological disorders among primary school children in Dar es Salaam. *BMC Public Health* **2010**, *10*, 765. [CrossRef] [PubMed]

32. Figueroa, J.I.; Fuller, L.C.; Abraha, A.; Hay, R.J. The prevalence of skin disease among school children in rural Ethiopia—A preliminary assessment of dermatologic needs. *Pediatr. Dermatol.* **1996**, *13*, 378–381. [CrossRef] [PubMed]

33. Murgia, V.; Bilcha, K.D.; Shibeshi, D. Community dermatology in Debre Markos: An attempt to define children's dermatological needs in a rural area of Ethiopia. *Int. J. Dermatol.* **2010**, *49*, 666–671. [CrossRef] [PubMed]

34. Mitja, O.; Houinei, W.; Moses, P.; Kapa, A.; Paru, R.; Hays, R.; Lukehart, S.; Godornes, C.; Bieb, S.V.; Grice, T.; et al. Mass treatment with single-dose azithromycin for yaws. *N. Engl. J. Med.* **2015**, *372*, 703–710. [CrossRef] [PubMed]

35. Lawrence, G.; Leafasia, J.; Sheridan, J.; Hills, S.; Wate, J.; Wate, C.; Montgomery, J.; Pandeya, N.; Purdie, D. Control of scabies, skin sores and haematuria in children in the Solomon Islands: Another role for ivermectin. *Bull. World Health Organ.* **2005**, *83*, 34–42.

36. Kearns, T.M.; Speare, R.; Cheng, A.C.; McCarthy, J.; Carapetis, J.R.; Holt, D.C.; Currie, B.J.; Page, W.; Shield, J.; Gundjirryirr, R.; et al. Impact of an ivermectin mass drug administration on scabies prevalence in a remote australian aboriginal community. *PLoS Negl. Trop. Dis.* **2015**, *9*, e0004151. [CrossRef] [PubMed]

37. Mason, D.S.; Marks, M.; Sokana, O.; Solomon, A.W.; Mabey, D.C.; Romani, L.; Kaldor, J.; Steer, A.C.; Engelman, D. The prevalence of scabies and impetigo in the Solomon islands: a population-based survey. *PLoS Negl. Trop. Dis.* **2016**, *10*, e0004803. [CrossRef] [PubMed]

38. Heukelbach, J.; Winter, B.; Wilcke, T.; Muehlen, M.; Albrecht, S.; de Oliveira, F.A.; Kerr-Pontes, L.R.; Liesenfeld, O.; Feldmeier, H. Selective mass treatment with ivermectin to control intestinal helminthiases and parasitic skin diseases in a severely affected population. *Bull. World Health Organ.* **2004**, *82*, 563–571.

39. Krotneva, S.P.; Coffeng, L.E.; Noma, M.; Zoure, H.G.; Bakone, L.; Amazigo, U.V.; de Vlas, S.J.; Stolk, W.A. African program for onchocerciasis control 1995–2010: Impact of annual ivermectin mass treatment on off-target infectious diseases. *PLoS Negl. Trop. Dis.* **2015**, *9*, e0004051. [CrossRef] [PubMed]

40. Ottesen, E.A.; Hooper, P.J.; Bradley, M.; Biswas, G. The global programme to eliminate lymphatic filariasis: Health impact after 8 years. *PLoS Negl. Trop. Dis.* **2008**, *2*, e317. [CrossRef] [PubMed]

41. Thomsen, E.K.; Sanuku, N.; Baea, M.; Satofan, S.; Maki, E.; Lombore, B.; Schmidt, M.S.; Siba, P.M.; Weil, G.J.; Kazura, J.W.; et al. Efficacy, safety, and pharmacokinetics of coadministered diethylcarbamazine, albendazole, and ivermectin for treatment of bancroftian filariasis. *Clin. Infect. Dis.* **2016**, *62*, 334–341. [CrossRef] [PubMed]

42. Engelman, D.; Kiang, K.; Chosidow, O.; McCarthy, J.; Fuller, C.; Lammie, P.; Hay, R.; Steer, A.; Members of the International Alliance for the Control of Scabies. Toward the global control of human scabies: Introducing the International Alliance for the Control of Scabies. *PLoS Negl. Trop. Dis.* **2013**, *7*, e2167. [CrossRef] [PubMed]

43. Mounsey, K.E.; Bernigaud, C.; Chosidow, O.; McCarthy, J.S. Prospects for moxidectin as a new oral treatment for human scabies. *PLoS Negl. Trop. Dis.* **2016**, *10*, e0004389. [CrossRef] [PubMed]

44. Mounsey, K.E.; Walton, S.F.; Innes, A.; Cash-Deans, S.; McCarthy, J.S. In vitro efficacy of moxidectin versus Ivermectin against *Sarcoptes scabiei*. *Antimicrob. Agents Chemother.* **2017**, *61*, e00381-17. [CrossRef] [PubMed]

45. Administration, U.S.F.A.D. Drugs@FDA: FDA Approved Drug Products. 2018. Available online: https://www.accessdata.fda.gov/scripts/cder/daf/index.cfm?event=BasicSearch.process (accessed on 31 August 2018).

46. Moet, F.J.; Pahan, D.; Oskam, L.; Richardus, J.H.; Group, C.S. Effectiveness of single dose rifampicin in preventing leprosy in close contacts of patients with newly diagnosed leprosy: Cluster randomised controlled trial. *BMJ* **2008**, *336*, 761–764. [CrossRef] [PubMed]

47. Feenstra, S.G.; Pahan, D.; Moet, F.J.; Oskam, L.; Richardus, J.H. Patient-related factors predicting the effectiveness of rifampicin chemoprophylaxis in contacts: 6 year follow up of the COLEP cohort in Bangladesh. *Lepr. Rev.* **2012**, *83*, 292–304. [PubMed]

48. Bakker, M.I.; Hatta, M.; Kwenang, A.; Van Benthem, B.H.; Van Beers, S.M.; Klatser, P.R.; Oskam, L. Prevention of leprosy using rifampicin as chemoprophylaxis. *Am. J. Trop. Med. Hyg.* **2005**, *72*, 443–448. [CrossRef] [PubMed]

49. WHO. Global leprosy update, 2016: Accelerating reduction of disease burden. *Wkly. Epidemiol. Rec.* **2017**, *35*, 501–520.

50. Tiwari, A.; Dandel, S.; Djupuri, R.; Mieras, L.; Richardus, J.H. Population-wide administration of single dose rifampicin for leprosy prevention in isolated communities: A three year follow-up feasibility study in Indonesia. *BMC Infect. Dis.* **2018**, *18*, 324. [CrossRef] [PubMed]

51. Barth-Jaeggi, T.; Steinmann, P.; Mieras, L.; van Brakel, W.; Richardus, J.H.; Tiwari, A.; Bratschi, M.; Cavaliero, A.; Vander Plaetse, B.; Mirza, F.; et al. Leprosy Post-Exposure Prophylaxis (LPEP) programme: Study protocol for evaluating the feasibility and impact on case detection rates of contact tracing and single dose rifampicin. *BMJ Open* **2016**, *6*, e013633. [CrossRef] [PubMed]

52. Steinmann, P.; Cavaliero, A.; Aerts, A.; Anand, S.; Arif, M.; Ay, S.S.; Aye, T.M.; Barth-Jaeggi, T.; Banstola, N.L.; Bhandari, C.M.; et al. The Leprosy Post-Exposure Prophylaxis (LPEP) programme: Update and interim analysis. *Lepr. Rev.* **2018**, *89*, 102–116.

53. Toutous Trellu, L.; Nkemenang, P.; Comte, E.; Ehounou, G.; Atangana, P.; Mboua, D.J.; Rusch, B.; Njih Tabah, E.; Etard, J.F.; Mueller, Y.K. Differential diagnosis of skin ulcers in a *Mycobacterium ulcerans* endemic area: Data from a prospective study in cameroon. *PLoS Negl. Trop. Dis.* **2016**, *10*, e0004385. [CrossRef] [PubMed]

54. Nguetta, A.; Coulibaly, N.D.; Kouamé-Elogne, N.C.; Acquah, K.J.R.; Christiane, A.A.; Kouamé, K.; N'Guessan, K.; Aboa, K.; Aubin, Y. Phenotypic and genotypic characterization of mycobacteria isolates from Buruli ulcer suspected patients reveals the involvement of several mycobacteria in chronic skin lesions. *Am. J. Microbiol. Res.* **2018**, *6*, 79–87. [CrossRef]

55. Ablordey, A.; Amissah, D.A.; Aboagye, I.F.; Hatano, B.; Yamazaki, T.; Sata, T.; Ishikawa, K.; Katano, H. Detection of *Mycobacterium ulcerans* by the loop mediated isothermal amplification method. *PLoS Negl. Trop. Dis.* **2012**, *6*, e1590. [CrossRef] [PubMed]

56. Beissner, M.; Phillips, R.O.; Battke, F.; Bauer, M.; Badziklou, K.; Sarfo, F.S.; Maman, I.; Rhomberg, A.; Piten, E.; Frimpong, M.; et al. Loop-mediated isothermal amplification for laboratory confirmation of buruli ulcer disease-towards a point-of-care test. *PLoS Negl. Trop. Dis.* **2015**, *9*, e0004219. [CrossRef] [PubMed]

57. Wadagni, A.; Frimpong, M.; Phanzu, D.M.; Ablordey, A.; Kacou, E.; Gbedevi, M.; Marion, E.; Xing, Y.; Babu, V.S.; Phillips, R.O.; et al. Simple, rapid *Mycobacterium ulcerans* disease diagnosis from clinical samples by fluorescence of mycolactone on thin layer chromatography. *PLoS Negl. Trop. Dis.* **2015**, *9*, e0004247. [CrossRef] [PubMed]

58. Dreyer, A.; Roltgen, K.; Dangy, J.P.; Ruf, M.T.; Scherr, N.; Bolz, M.; Tobias, N.J.; Moes, C.; Vettiger, A.; Stinear, T.P.; et al. Identification of the Mycobacterium ulcerans protein MUL_3720 as a promising target for the development of a diagnostic test for Buruli ulcer. *PLoS Negl. Trop. Dis.* **2015**, *9*, e0003477. [CrossRef] [PubMed]

59. WHO. *Eradication of Yaws: A Guide for Programme Managers*; WHO: Geneva, Switzerland, 2018.

60. Yotsu, R.; Richardson, M.; Ishii, N. *Drugs for Treating Buruli Ulcer*; Cochrane Systematic Review: London, UK, 2018.

61. Ryan, T.J. Public health dermatology: Regeneration and repair of the skin in the developed transitional and developing world. *Int. J. Dermatol.* **2006**, *45*, 1233–1237. [CrossRef] [PubMed]

62. Velding, K.; Klis, S.A.; Abass, K.M.; Tuah, W.; Stienstra, Y.; van der Werf, T. Wound care in Buruli ulcer disease in Ghana and Benin. *Am. J. Trop. Med. Hyg.* **2014**, *91*, 313–318. [CrossRef] [PubMed]

63. Attinger, C.E.; Janis, J.E.; Steinberg, J.; Schwartz, J.; Al-Attar, A.; Couch, K. Clinical approach to wounds: Debridement and wound bed preparation including the use of dressings and wound-healing adjuvants. *Plast. Reconstr. Surg.* **2006**, *117*, 72s–109s. [CrossRef] [PubMed]

64. Lee, J.C.; Kandula, S.; Sherber, N.S. Beyond wet-to-dry: A rational approach to treating chronic wounds. *Eplasty* **2009**, *9*, e14. [PubMed]

65. Fernandez, R.; Griffiths, R. Water for wound cleansing. *Cochrane Database Syst. Rev.* **2012**. [CrossRef] [PubMed]

66. Cooper, D.D.; Seupaul, R.A. Is water effective for wound cleansing? *Ann. Emerg. Med.* **2012**, *60*, 626–627. [CrossRef] [PubMed]

67. Anandan, V.; Jameela, W.A.; Saraswathy, P.; Sarankumar, S. Platelet rich plasma: Efficacy in treating trophic ulcers in leprosy. *J. Clin. Diagn. Res.* **2016**, *10*, WC06–WC09. [CrossRef] [PubMed]

68. Conde-Montero, E.; Horcajada-Reales, C.; Clavo, P.; Delgado-Sillero, I.; Suarez-Fernandez, R. Neuropathic ulcers in leprosy treated with intralesional platelet-rich plasma. *Int. Wound J.* **2016**, *13*, 726–728. [CrossRef] [PubMed]

69. Murase, C.; Kono, M.; Nakanaga, K.; Ishii, N.; Akiyama, M. Buruli ulcer successfully treated with negative-pressure wound therapy. *JAMA Dermatol.* **2015**, *151*, 1137–1139. [CrossRef] [PubMed]

70. Jebran, A.F.; Schleicher, U.; Steiner, R.; Wentker, P.; Mahfuz, F.; Stahl, H.C.; Amin, F.M.; Bogdan, C.; Stahl, K.W. Rapid healing of cutaneous leishmaniasis by high-frequency electrocauterization and hydrogel wound care with or without DAC N-055: A randomized controlled phase IIa trial in Kabul. *PLoS Negl. Trop. Dis.* **2014**, *8*, e2694. [CrossRef] [PubMed]

71. Jull, A.B.; Walker, N.; Deshpande, S. Honey as a topical treatment for wounds. *Cochrane Database Syst. Rev.* **2013**. [CrossRef]

72. Stocks, M.E.; Freeman, M.C.; Addiss, D.G. The effect of hygiene-based lymphedema management in lymphatic filariasis-endemic areas: A systematic review and meta-analysis. *PLoS Negl. Trop. Dis.* **2015**, *9*, e0004171. [CrossRef] [PubMed]

73. Dreyer, G.; Medeiros, Z.; Netto, M.J.; Leal, N.C.; de Castro, L.G.; Piessens, W.F. Acute attacks in the extremities of persons living in an area endemic for bancroftian filariasis: Differentiation of two syndromes. *Trans. Roy. Soc. Trop. Med. Hyg.* **1999**, *93*, 413–417. [CrossRef]

74. Brooks, J.; Ersser, S.J.; Cowdell, F.; Gardiner, E.; Mengistu, A.; Matts, P.J. A randomized controlled trial to evaluate the effect of a new skincare regimen on skin barrier function in those with podoconiosis in Ethiopia. *Br. J. Dermatol.* **2017**, *177*, 1422–1431. [CrossRef] [PubMed]

75. Negussie, H.; Molla, M.; Ngari, M.; Berkley, J.A.; Kivaya, E.; Njuguna, P.; Fegan, G.; Tamiru, A.; Kelemework, A.; Lang, T.; et al. Lymphoedema management to prevent acute dermatolymphangioadenitis in podoconiosis in northern Ethiopia (GoLBeT): A pragmatic randomised controlled trial. *Lancet Glob. Health* **2018**, *6*, e795–e803. [CrossRef]

76. Effah, A.; Ersser, S.J.; Hemingway, A. Support needs of people living with *Mycobacterium ulcerans* (Buruli ulcer) disease in a Ghana rural community: A grounded theory study. *Int. J. Dermatol.* **2017**, *56*, 1432–1437. [CrossRef] [PubMed]

77. Narahari, S.R.; Bose, K.S.; Aggithaya, M.G.; Swamy, G.K.; Ryan, T.J.; Unnikrishnan, B.; Washington, R.G.; Rao, B.P.; Rajagopala, S.; Manjula, K.; et al. Community level morbidity control of lymphoedema using self care and integrative treatment in two lymphatic filariasis endemic districts of South India: A non randomized interventional study. *Trans. R. Soc. Trop. Med. Hyg.* **2013**, *107*, 566–577. [CrossRef] [PubMed]

78. Bartlett, J.; Deribe, K.; Tamiru, A.; Amberbir, T.; Medhin, G.; Malik, M.; Hanlon, C.; Davey, G. Depression and disability in people with podoconiosis: A comparative cross-sectional study in rural Northern Ethiopia. *Int. Health* **2016**, *8*, 124–131. [CrossRef] [PubMed]

79. Bennis, I.; De Brouwere, V.; Belrhiti, Z.; Sahibi, H.; Boelaert, M. Psychosocial burden of localised cutaneous Leishmaniasis: A scoping review. *BMC Public Health* **2018**, *18*, 358. [CrossRef] [PubMed]

80. Bakhiet, S.M.; Fahal, A.H.; Musa, A.M.; Mohamed, E.S.W.; Omer, R.F.; Ahmed, E.S.; El Nour, M.; Mustafa, E.R.M.; Sheikh, A.R.M.E.; Suliman, S.H.; et al. A holistic approach to the mycetoma management. *PLoS Negl. Trop. Dis.* **2018**, *12*, e0006391. [CrossRef] [PubMed]

81. Wiese, S.; Elson, L.; Feldmeier, H. Tungiasis-related life quality impairment in children living in rural Kenya. *PLoS Negl. Trop. Dis.* **2018**, *12*, e0005939. [CrossRef] [PubMed]

82. Walker, S.L.; Lebas, E.; De Sario, V.; Deyasso, Z.; Doni, S.N.; Marks, M.; Roberts, C.H.; Lambert, S.M. The prevalence and association with health-related quality of life of tungiasis and scabies in schoolchildren in southern Ethiopia. *PLoS Negl. Trop. Dis.* **2017**, *11*, e0005808. [CrossRef] [PubMed]

83. Guest, J.F.; Ayoub, N.; McIlwraith, T.; Uchegbu, I.; Gerrish, A.; Weidlich, D.; Vowden, K.; Vowden, P. Health economic burden that different wound types impose on the UK's National Health Service. *Int. Wound J.* **2017**, *14*, 322–330. [CrossRef] [PubMed]

84. Tchero, H.; Kangambega, P.; Lin, L.; Mukisi-Mukaza, M.; Brunet-Houdard, S.; Briatte, C.; Retali, G.R.; Rusch, E. Cost of diabetic foot in France, Spain, Italy, Germany and United Kingdom: A systematic review. *Ann. Endocrinol.* **2018**, *79*, 67–74. [CrossRef] [PubMed]

85. Stahl, H.C.; Ahmadi, F.; Nahzat, S.M.; Dong, H.J.; Stahl, K.W.; Sauerborn, R. Health economic evaluation of moist wound care in chronic cutaneous leishmaniasis ulcers in Afghanistan. *Infect. Dis. Poverty* **2018**, *7*, 12. [CrossRef] [PubMed]

86. Walsh, D.S.; De Jong, B.C.; Meyers, W.M.; Portaels, F. Leprosy and Buruli ulcer: Similarities suggest combining control and prevention of disability strategies in countries endemic for both diseases. *Lepr. Rev.* **2015**, *86*, 1–5. [PubMed]

87. Douglass, J.; Graves, P.; Gordon, S. Self-care for management of secondary lymphedema: A systematic review. *PLoS Negl. Trop. Dis.* **2016**, *10*, e0004740. [CrossRef] [PubMed]

88. Sathiaraj, Y.; Norman, G.; Richard, J. Long term sustainability and efficacy of self-care education on knowledge and practice of wound prevention and management among leprosy patients. *Indian J. Lepr.* **2010**, *82*, 79–83. [PubMed]

89. Ryan, T. Wound healing in the developing world. *Dermatol. Clin.* **1993**, *11*, 791–800. [CrossRef]

90. Deribe, K.; Kebede, B.; Tamiru, M.; Mengistu, B.; Kebede, F.; Martindale, S.; Sime, H.; Mulugeta, A.; Kebede, B.; Sileshi, M.; et al. Integrated morbidity management for lymphatic filariasis and podoconiosis, Ethiopia. *Bull. World Health Organ.* **2017**, *95*, 652–656. [CrossRef] [PubMed]

91. WHO. *Recognizing Neglected Tropical Diseases through Changes on the Skin: A Training Guide for Front-Line Health Workers*; WHO: Geneva, Switzerland, 2018.

92. Barbieri, R.R.; Sales, A.M.; Hacker, M.A.; Nery, J.A.; Duppre, N.C.; Machado, A.M.; Moraes, M.O.; Sarno, E.N. Impact of a reference center on leprosy control under a decentralized public health care policy in Brazil. *PLoS Negl. Trop. Dis.* **2016**, *10*, e0005059. [CrossRef] [PubMed]

93. Stanton, M.C.; Mkwanda, S.Z.; Debrah, A.Y.; Batsa, L.; Biritwum, N.K.; Hoerauf, A.; Cliffe, M.; Best, A.; Molineux, A.; Kelly-Hope, L.A. Developing a community-led SMS reporting tool for the rapid assessment of lymphatic filariasis morbidity burden: Case studies from Malawi and Ghana. *BMC Infect. Dis.* **2015**, *15*, 214. [CrossRef] [PubMed]

94. Hay, R.; Estrada, R.; Grossmann, H. Managing skin disease in resource-poor environments—The role of community-oriented training and control programs. *Int. J. Dermatol.* **2011**, *50*, 558–563. [CrossRef] [PubMed]

95. Faye, O.; Bagayoko, C.O.; Dicko, A.; Ciseé, L.; Berthé, S.; Traoré, B.; Fofana, Y.; Niang, M.; Traoré, S.T.; Karabinta, Y.; et al. A teledermatology pilot programme for the management of skin diseases in primary health care centres: Experiences from a Resource-Limited Country (Mali, West Africa). *Trop. Med. Infect. Dis.* **2018**, *3*, 88. [CrossRef] [PubMed]

96. Mieras, L.F.; Taal, A.T.; Post, E.B.; Ndeve, A.G.Z.; van Hees, C.L.M. The development of a mobile application to support peripheral health workers to diagnose and treat people with skin diseases in resource-poor settings. *Trop. Med. Infect. Dis.* **2018**, *3*, 102. [CrossRef] [PubMed]

97. Tomczyk, S.; Deribe, K.; Brooker, S.J.; Clark, H.; Rafique, K.; Knopp, S.; Utzinger, J.; Davey, G. Association between footwear use and neglected tropical diseases: A systematic review and meta-analysis. *PLoS Negl. Trop. Dis.* **2014**, *8*, e3285. [CrossRef] [PubMed]

98. WHO. *Guidelines for the Diagnosis, Treatment and Prevention of Leprosy*; WHO, Regional Office for South-East Asia: New Delhi, India, 2018.

99. Engelman, D.; Fuller, L.C.; Steer, A.C.; International Alliance for the Control of Scabies. Consensus criteria for the diagnosis of scabies: A Delphi study of international experts. *PLoS Negl. Trop. Dis.* **2018**, *12*, e0006549. [CrossRef] [PubMed]

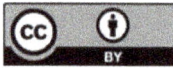

Tropical Medicine and Infectious Disease

MDPI

Article

The Mite-Gallery Unit: A New Concept for Describing Scabies through Entodermoscopy

Gaetano Scanni [ORCID]

MD Dermatologist, Dipartimento di Medicina dei Servizi ASL Bari, Via Vico Traversa 11, 70127 Bari, Italy; gaetano.scanni@alice.it

Received: 16 January 2019; Accepted: 11 March 2019; Published: 16 March 2019

Abstract: Scabies has always represented a diagnostic challenge for dermatologists, especially in subclinical cases or in atypical ones due to the coexistence of other diseases. Fortunately, dermatoscopy has enabled easier and faster in situ diagnosis. The aim of this study is to examine old and new dermatoscopic signs that *Sarcoptes scabiei* produces on the skin during its whole life cycle through *entodermoscopy* (dermatoscopy with an entomological focus) which, unlike traditional optical microscope examination, allows the local micro-environment to be preserved intact. Patients were enrolled during outbreaks of scabies from hospitals or nursing homes for the elderly in Bari (Italy). The study was performed applying both immersion and polarized dry dermatoscopy. The systematic use of dermatoscopy highlighted the morphological complexity of the *Sarcoptes* tunnel that had been described previously as a simple unitary structure. On the contrary, it is possible to distinguish three separate segments of the burrow that introduce a new anatomo-functional concept called the Mite-Gallery Unit (MGU). This approach, based on the mite life cycle and local skin turnover (the latter usually being ignored), allows the dermatologist to recognize not only *Sarcoptes* using the gallery, but also new descriptors including tunnels without *Sarcoptes*, those with acari alone, and those with associated signs of inflammation. The diagnosis of scabies using optical microscopy until recently has always involved demonstrating the mite and its products outside the human body (on a glass slide) without taking into account exactly what happens within the epidermis. Entodermoscopy is a term used to encapsulate both the presence of the parasite, the usual target of microscopy, and the changes produced in the superficial layers of the epidermis in situ. Thus, the scabies tunnel or burrow can be shown to be composed of three parts, the Head, Body, and Tail, in which different events affecting both mite and host develop. The Mite-Gallery Unit provides a new anatomical and functional explanation of scabies because it provides a more comprehensive in vivo and in situ dermatoscopic diagnosis. In this respect, dermatoscopy takes into account the behavior of the mite in addition to its interaction with its habitat, the human skin.

Keywords: Mite-Gallery Unit (MGU); Entodermoscopy (EDS); Dry Dermatoscopy (d-DS); Wet Dermatoscopy (w-DS); Enhanced Dermatoscopy (e-DS)

---

1. Introduction

Diagnosis of scabies, even in the presence of objective and subjective epidemiological evidence, requires the detection of mites and their products. In clinical variants or in forms complicated by co-morbidities (diabetes, senile pruritus, neurological syndromes) or side effects of therapy (cortisone, acaricides), the detection of mites is absolutely essential for diagnosis because other clinical clues are unreliable or misleading [1]. The purpose of this article is to demonstrate that, by using entodermoscopy, it is possible to obtain direct and indirect evidence which may improve diagnostic reliability in both ordinary and atypical cases of scabies.

2. Materials and Methods

Two types of dermatoscope were used. The Delta 20 (Heine Optotechnik GmbH & Co. KG Kientalstraße 7, 82211 Herrsching, Germany) uses a glass plate and mineral oil at the skin interface in a mode that will be referred to as wet dermatoscopy (w-DS). The DermLite Pro II (Dermlite, 3Gen, San Juan Capistrano, CA, USA) is a dermatoscope without plate and liquid as it uses a polarized light that blocks the reflections from the epidermis; a side button allows the operator to switch alternately between polarized and normal light. This mode of observation will be referred to as dry dermatoscopy (d-DS). Pictures were obtained using two compact digital cameras: a Minolta G850 (5 Mp 3× optical, Minolta Corp., Osaka, Japan) for the Delta 20 (w-DS) and a Sony W70 (7 Mp 3× optical, Sony Corp., Tokyo, Japan) for the Dermlite (d-DS). The method using a dermatoscope with a digital camera is commonly referred to as digital dermatoscopy. The clinical observations herein are based on 63 patients examined in nursing homes for the elderly or public hospitals in the city of Bari (Italy) during contained outbreaks of scabies over the period 2011–2014.

Photographic documentation was generated after receiving patients' informed consent.

Entodermoscopy as a Diagnostic Tool

Entodermoscopy is a neologism proposed in 2006 by Scanni and Bonifazi for the dermoscopic diagnosis of ectoparasitosis [2], subsequently extended to superficial skin infections by Zalaudek et al. [3]. Entodermoscopy is not only a new term, but, importantly, it represents a different approach to the observation of the relationship between host and parasite for which a deeper knowledge of microbiology, entomology, and behaviour is required. Epiluminescence microscopy can be compared to traditional microscopic examination in which the instrument is resting on the patient to look directly at the skin. Consequently, the mite and its burrow can be observed in situ and in vivo, two conditions that together allow the observer to preserve the local microhabitat which is disassembled by more traditional methods (e.g., optical microscopy). As a tool, entodermoscopy has two major requirements. First, it requires magnifications higher than 10×, which can be achieved in digital dermatoscopy by extending the camera's optical zoom (generally about 3–5×) and in post-production by examining the image (jpg file) in full format. Thanks to the combination of these two steps (maximum optical zoom + full-frame jpg file), sufficient detail is obtained to capture all the features of the tunnel in a mode that can be referred to as enhanced digital dermatoscopy (e-DS). This approach can help the dermatologist when videodermatoscopy is not available. Digital zoom is generally avoided because artifacts (pixelation/noise) are incompatible with a true and reliable image. The second requirement of entodermoscopy is the type of illumination and mode of contact between instrument and skin. The differences between wet contact and dry non-contact dermatoscopy in the case of melanocytic lesions are already known [4]. In the case of parasitosis, polarized dermatoscopes offer the advantage of leaving the microhabitat intact without the need to wet or crush the field of observation. This option is essential with, for example, pathogens such as lice or ticks.

In addition, the alternate switching from normal to polarized light allows a quick comparison between skin texture and structures below it, respectively, as well as the insect's cuticle and internal organs, accurately completing the morphological and topographical reconstruction. The new findings described in this article derive from the comparative use of different dermatoscopes and light sources.

3. Results

In health facilities where scabies has already been diagnosed and treated, the main objective is often to understand if persistent itching is caused by the side effects of acaricides (e.g., benzyl benzoate), pre-existing co-morbidities, failure of therapy, or re-infestation. Since direct examination is not always sufficient to resolve these questions and optical microscopy is time consuming, any other instrumental help, including dermatoscopy, is worthy of attention and investigation. The methodical use of dermatoscopes has led to the introduction of a list of eight points, some already known and others previously undescribed, as an innovative morphological/functional key.

3.1. Definition of the Mite-Gallery Unit (MGU)

Generally, the burrow of scabies is described as a linear formation a few millimeters in length that has always been considered a unitary structure (Figure 1).

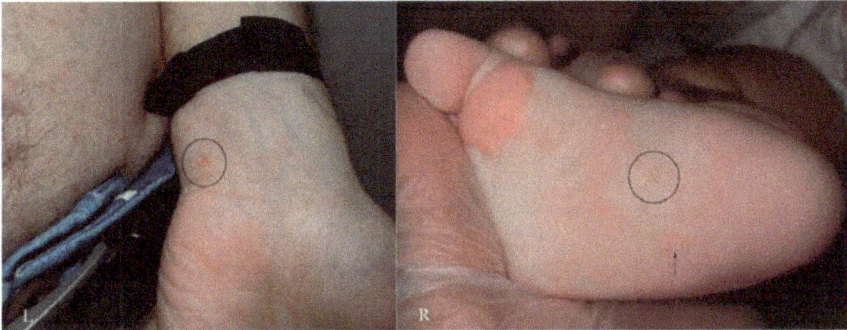

Figure 1. Objective examination of scabies in adults (L) and children (R).

An intact burrow is a whitish, slightly raised linear structure with a tortuous path a few millimeters long set against a variably erythematous background (circles, L-R). The appearance is pathognomonic. However, scratching that partially or completely destroys it can change its macroscopic and dermatoscopic appearance (arrow, R).

Dermatoscopy reveals different *anatomical and functional* sections determined by both the mite life cycle and host epidermal turnover usually not taken into consideration but, none the less, able to affect the morphology of the tunnel itself. The gallery can be divided into three contiguous segments—Head, Body, and Tail—that together provide a new set of diagnostic markers called the Mite-Gallery Unit (MGU) (Figure 2).

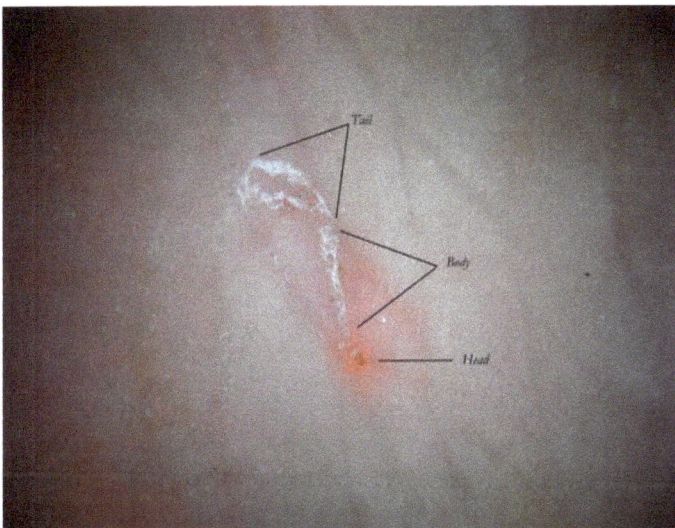

Figure 2. The Mite-Gallery Unit (MGU) in non-polarized dry dermatoscopy (d-DS).

The Mite-Gallery Unit (MGU) structure can be divided into three parts: the *Head* hosting the mite; the *Body*, which represents what is clinically defined as the burrow containing the eggs and feces of the parasite; and the *Tail* at the end of the tunnel, which provides an incomplete structure as it is without a roof but is made of keratin collarettes, visible only in d-DS. Erythema may be present in the background around and immediately behind the mite.

The dermatoscopic observation should preferably be conducted at magnifications between 10 and 30× with different results depending on whether a liquid interface (wet dermatoscopy) or dry skin surface free from the compression of the plate (dry dermatoscopy) are used.

The MGU Head houses the mite which is visible due to its refractile area located anteriorly between the buccal apparatus (*gnatosoma*) and the second pair of legs. It appears as a dark "V" formation with the vertex that indicates the point of progression of the tunnel towards the healthy skin. In this segment, the roof of the tunnel is intact.

The MGU Body represents the longest part of the entire tunnel and appears white if observed with wet dermatoscopy. In this segment, the roof of the tunnel is no longer intact because it is interrupted by holes at roughly regular intervals.

The MGU Tail is the terminal segment of the tunnel even if the roof is completely absent. This part can only be identified in dry dermatoscopy as this is able to define the edges of the tunnel in the form of small desquamatory collarettes. In w-DS the liquid medium prevents these from being visible, which explains why in previous studies this morphological variation was not reported.

The first description of the tunnel compared its appearance to that of a jet plane with delta wings followed by a white trail as a result of observation under wet dermatoscopy [5]. The observation of this phenomenon, however, was not accompanied by any functional interpretation. Entodermoscopy by studying the microstructure of the three components of the tunnel explains the "jet trail" effect as the interaction between the liquid interface and air contained in the tunnel that, due to the pressure of the dermatoscope, emerges from the small holes of the roof, forming a strip of small reflective bubbles under the optical plate.

In fact, if dry dermatoscopy is used, the white trail is no longer visible and only a tunnel can be observed whose roof is interrupted by several openings from which air escapes if compressed (Figure 3).

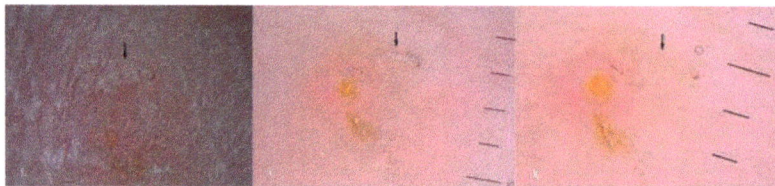

Figure 3. Dry dermatoscopy vs. wet dermatoscopy (w-DS) of the same Mite-Gallery Unit.

When viewed using d-DS, the roof of the tunnel appears to be interrupted by several holes that allow air to exit (L). The first description of an MGU resembling a white jet trail was due to trapped air between the tunnel and the glass plate used in the w-DS (C). Under continued pressure, this picture disappears as all of air bubbles are pushed away and the liquid medium passes inside (R). Beneath there is a collection of serum that reflects the LEDs of the dermatoscope (L).

Another consequence of these holes, not previously described in the literature, is that the microbubble trail is by no means a persistent sign as it disappears when MGU observation is repeated several times or for excessive time in the wet modality. After the first contact with the dermatoscope, all the air inside the tunnel will be largely dispersed on the surface and replaced by the interface fluid; this makes the roof indistinguishable from the surrounding skin (Figure 3 R). In this situation, the tunnel body can only be recognized because of the head that houses the *Sarcoptes*, reducing the local diagnostic sensitivity which relies on the tunnel's refractability. Therefore, in order to obtain good photographic documentation in w-DS of an intact MGU, it is necessary to keep the microbubbles under the plate without breaking off skin contact and to avoid repeating the viewing session. However, if air leakage decreases the dermatoscopic sensitivity as regards the external structure of the MGU, it provides ideal conditions to better observe the internal components of the tunnel (local diagnostic specificity).

3.2. Content of the Gallery and Other Markers of the Mite

Thanks to the higher magnifications (e-DS) and to the fact that the roof of the tunnel in w-DS becomes transparent when liquid medium is inside, it is possible to distinguish, with sufficient clarity, the eggs of the *Sarcoptes* located behind the mite. The oval eggs are grouped at a short distance from each other with a major axis that is generally at right angles to that of the MGU, which also allows the edges of the embryo inside to be glimpsed, if enlarged further. In this part of the gallery there are also the parasite's feces derived by the digestion of keratin and cellular fluids; under the optical microscope, feces usually appear as dark refractile dots (stercoraceous bullets), whereas under dermatoscopy, they appear as small white-gray spheres (Figure 4).

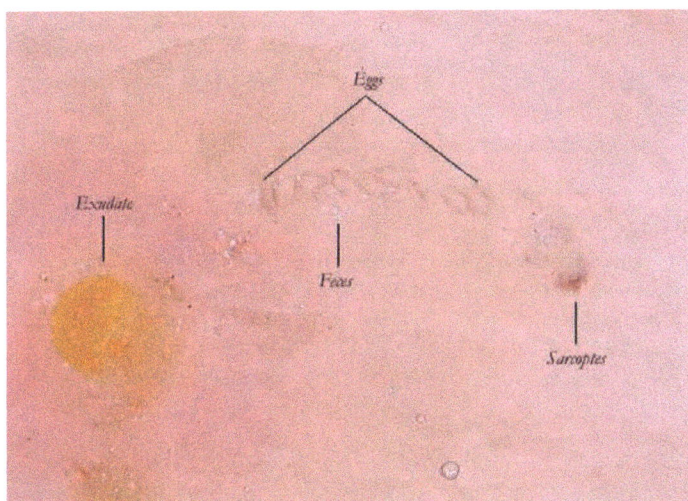

Figure 4. Content of the gallery. An MGU in enhanced wet dermatoscopy mode.

The absence of bubbles and the penetration of the liquid film into the tunnel makes the roof transparent and allows one to glimpse the row of eggs, which is otherwise not easily visible. The white dots are the feces of the mite. A seropurulent exudate is located to the left.

If the examiner is interested in studying the inside of the tunnel, he/she must use wet dermatoscopy and make sure that all the air in the tunnel is extruded, pushing the dermatoscope plate several times onto the skin to ensure entry of the liquid medium.

It is commonly thought that the only visible part of the mite in w-DS is the front end, in the shape of a "V" which corresponds to the *gnatosoma* and the first pair of legs. But enhanced dermatoscopy allows the identification of novel structures on the body of the *Sarcoptes scabiei* that, under conditions of optimal magnification, show some visible refraction. These are mechano-sensory structures [6] located on the back of the mite called "bristles" (*spine-like type*) whose thicker bases (*sockets*) appear under a dermatoscope as fine brown dots (*ladybird sign*). This feature, not yet reported in the literature, is a good example of convergence between dermatoscopy and entomology. Even the body of the mite, which is usually transparent, can be distinguished by the slight opalescence of its cuticle under enhanced wet dermatoscopy (Figure 5).

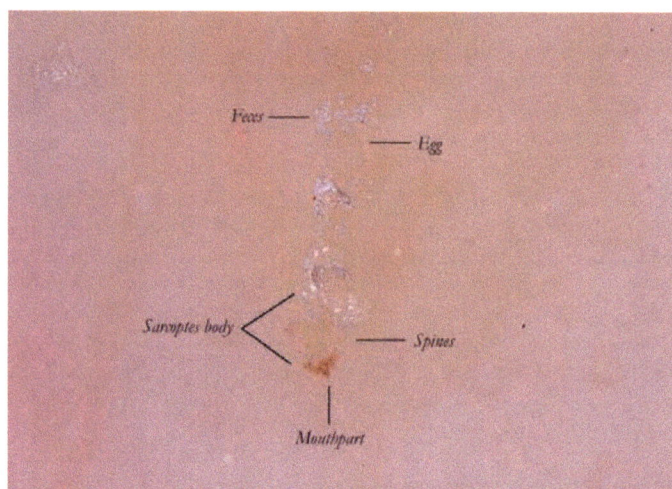

Figure 5. The Body of the mite. Enhanced wet dermatoscopy of an MGU in w-DS mode. In addition to refraction of its anterior part, *Sarcoptes scabiei* shows an opalescent body with several scattered dark dots (*ladybird sign*). These structures correspond to the "bristles" on the body that enable, amongst other things, the adherence of the mite within the tunnel.

3.3. Spatio-Temporal Evolution of the Mite-Gallery Unit

The MGU is not a static structure. This concept is not usually explored further because it is irrelevant to clinical diagnosis. On the contrary, patterns change if we access the microscopic details that are appreciable only in situ and in vivo in the context of the entodermoscopy.

The MGU is a dynamic structure because its morphology derives from a reciprocal interference of two different movements: the horizontal one of the mite and the vertical one of the epidermis. The epidermis has an estimated turnover time of around 45 days [7] during which the cellular layers are pushed upwards, ending with desquamation. In the presence of local inflammation (e.g., psoriasis) the upwards growth rate is greatly accelerated.

Histologically, the scabies burrow was always thought to be allocated in the *stratum corneum* even though confocal microscopy has recently revealed that the *Sarcoptes* mite is located closer to the *stratum spinosum* [8].

The integrity of the tunnel is therefore subordinate to the mite's ability to maintain the same height in the epidermis to resist the tangential (rubbing) and elastic (contraction and distension) forces that act on the skin during the natural movements of the human body. The mite must out of necessity compensate for the direction of growth of the epidermis [9] in order to protected itself, but especially to ensure that the eggs can hatch just inside the tunnel. It follows that the tunnel represents two different time sequences depending on the point being observed, with the head being the newest part and the tail the initial and oldest part.

Therefore, as a dynamic structure the gallery moves closer to the skin surface with the passing of time and is at its most superficial at the tail where the roof becomes thin enough to collapse under the effect of the forces acting on it [10]. For this reason, near the tail there is no longer an intact tunnel but, rather, the borders of its base as collarettes visible only with dry dermatoscopy. Entodermoscopy, through linking the local factors of the host to the biology of the parasite, highlights an anatomic and functional difference of the MGU not previously appreciated under conditions of ordinary optical microscopy which cannot provide a detailed view of the mite's whole microenvironment. Dermatoscopy instead reveals that the MGU is a dynamic entity in terms of both space (elongation phase) and time (maturation phase).

The collapsed roof is the result of an autonomous phenomenon and cannot be attributed to the scratching by the host as that would also destroy the other parts of the gallery rather than a very small part of it (the tail). This is further confirmed by the fact that the skin immediately around and adjacent to the tail remains intact (Figure 2).

3.4. MGU Perforated Roof

As mentioned above, the roof of the MGU body is interrupted by holes (Figure 6). At the moment, the reason for these openings has not been precisely identified [11]. It is possible that they represent the exit sites for the larvae to leave the tunnel, but other explanations cannot be ruled out. The possibility exists that the *Sarcoptes* mite itself pierces the roof to guarantee exchange of air and humidity necessary for hatching the eggs. Another possibility is that the tunnel intercepts the ostia of the sweat glands by separating them from the rest of the duct. In any case, these holes cause the strip of microbubbles under the plate used in wet dermatoscopy to show the pathognomonic appearance of a "jet trail" [5].

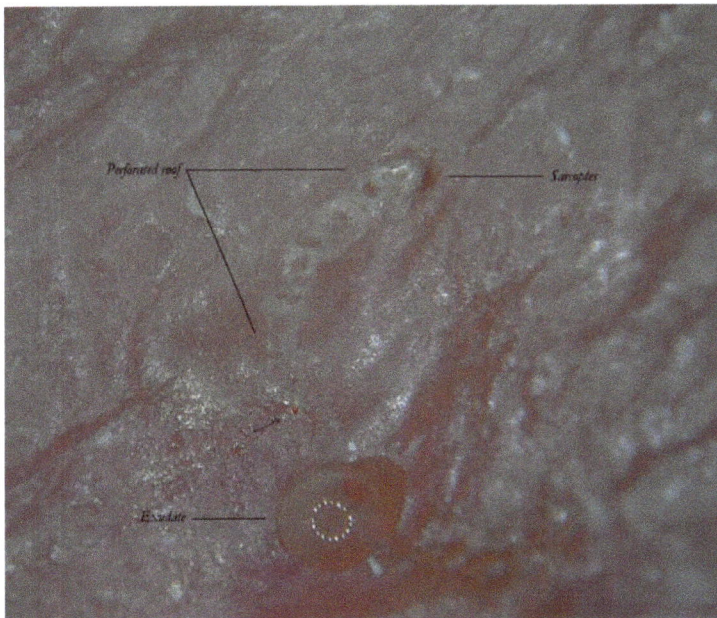

Figure 6. Enhanced dermatoscopy of the MGU's roof in non-polarized dry mode (d-DS). The body of the gallery is not completely intact due to numerous holes which give it a riddled aspect. From these openings the larvae of the *Sarcoptes* are believed to exit. On the right, one can see the reflective front part of the mite. At the bottom, dermatoscope LEDs are reflected on the serous exudate.

3.5. Moulting and Coupling Pockets

The greater part of the MGU consists of the tunnel body where the most important events of the mite life cycle take place. In this segment, eggs are collected and hatch. After about four days, these eggs produce six-legged larvae morphologically similar to a miniature adult [12]. The larvae must undergo two more moults to the eight legged stage (proto/trito nymph) before becoming an adult; this process appears to take place mainly outside the mother tunnel in small niches, called "moulting pockets", dug in order to provide limited shelter. Only when fully developed and after fertilization does the female mite dig a new definitive tunnel as it is known in temperate climates [13].

The moulting pockets, well known to entomologists, present as small dimples in the most superficial layer of the *stratum corneum*; in these, the larvae remain attached, maturing into nymphs and then into the adult [12].

Mating is also performed in a pocket in which the adult female is found by a male whose track is lost afterwards. Normally, these niches are not described in dermatological textbooks because they have no diagnostic relevance and are of dimensions invisible to the naked eye. However, their significance increases if we return to dermatoscopic examination in which they appear as an incomplete MGU composed only of a head without a body and a tail (Figure 7), regardless of the dermatoscope used. The preferred mode of observation is still the d-DS with normal or polarized light.

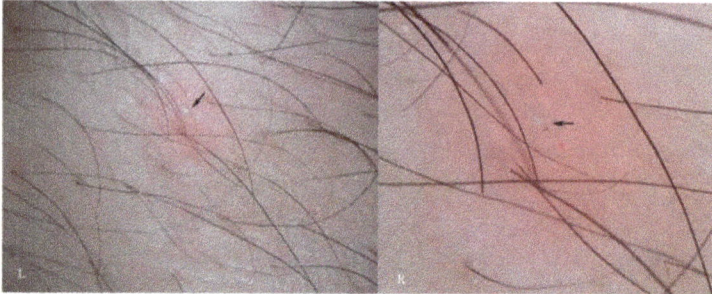

Figure 7. Moulting pocket in dry dermatoscopy with non-polarized (L) and polarized light (R). In this structure the complete Mite-Gallery Unit does not develop because the mite remains stationary until the moulting process is completed or mating happens. There is instead only a small whitish raised area (arrows, L-R), corresponding to the whole body of the *Sarcoptes*, behind which a real tunnel is not visible (R). Around the pocket, an area of erythema with blurred borders is easily recognizable

According to another report, the immature forms, besides digging a niche or pocket from scratch, can also take refuge in the openings of hair follicles [14]. A rash of pseudo-folliculitis is traditionally considered to be a secondary, non-specific symptom in the course of scabies (Figure 8). Assuming that the juvenile mite may shelter in human follicles, too, then the erythematous change associated with them may be regarded as a new "specific" sign. At the moment, personal observations and those of other authors have not been able to identify any traces of immature forms as features of in vivo refraction in these forms are unknown. It is possible that under higher magnification (>200×) these forms may become appreciable if present and visible.

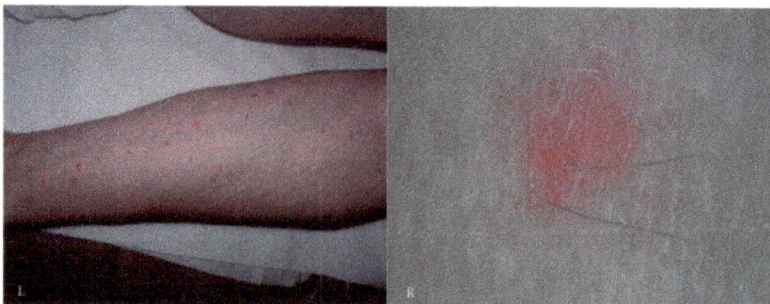

Figure 8. Scabies pseudo-follicular exanthema observed in non-polarized dry dermatoscopy. Folliculitis-like lesions (L) are commonly considered to be a non-specific sign of scabies (L). In dermatoscopy, only a peri-ostial erythematous halo is appreciated with some pinpoint-like vessels inside it (R). There are no signs of a complete or atypical MGU.

3.6. Inflammatory Response Induced By the MGU

In a primary infestation, the host's immunity to scabies develops after about four weeks. If we consider only the skin around the MGU, using dermatoscopy we can distinguish different types of response over time and depending on the anatomical sites involved. Generally, there is erythema around the head of the gallery where the mite is located or along the entire length of the MGU.

A vesicular or free exudate appears when the spongiotic inflammatory process [15] reaches the skin surface. If an infection coexists, this phenomenon is more pronounced. Where the skin is thicker, as on the palm of the hand and on the wrist, the exudate remains trapped in the superficial epidermis, forming semitransparent (*dyshidrotic-like*) circular areas [16] that, over time, become superficial as yellowish desquamations (Figure 9). The mite, the feces, and the eggs activate a different humoral and cellular immune response, probably depending on the time of exposure to the antigens that gradually accumulate over the course of the infestation. This reflects the life cycle of the mite.

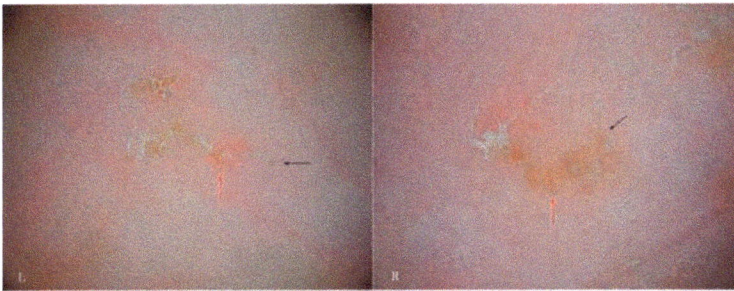

Figure 9. Inflammatory response to an MGU observed under polarized light dry dermatoscopy of a hand lesion. Next to the mite (black arrows, L-R) the skin is normal, while in the central part of the gallery an erythematous halo (red arrow, L) is evident. Immediately behind the mite, inflammation can also occur in microvesicles trapped in the epidermis (red arrow, R). The tail of the gallery is characterized by keratin collarettes.

In other cases, the inflammatory response may be nodular as in the buttocks, genital, and flexural regions. This phenomenon, known for its resistant pruritic symptoms, is interpreted as the effect of cell-mediated hyperreactivity to mite antigens [17] even if scrapings for mites are generally negative. Dermatoscopy, however, can identify the parasite, especially in the initial phases of the formation of nodules compared to the older lesions (Figure 10). Serial dermatoscopic observations could clarify the exact progression of the host's local immune response, probably stimulated by deeper penetration of antigens (intradermal) in areas undergoing physical pressure.

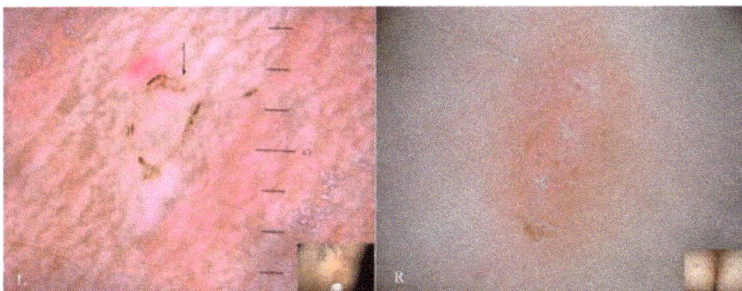

Figure 10. Nodular scabies observed in wet (L) and dry polarized light (R) dermatoscopy. A mite is easily recognizable in one of the axillary (insert) papules of a subject of African ethnicity (arrow, L). A buttock (insert) nodule present for a few weeks appears uninhabited instead (R).

3.7. Morphological Variants of the MGU

The linear MGU is not the only expression of the mite in the host skin–parasite interaction. There are forms of "atypical MGUs" in which only the head of the gallery is recognizable but not the body because it is partly or completely replaced by erosions or polycyclic scales (Figures 11 and 12). These morphological variants develop in areas where local exudative or hyperkeratotic inflammatory reactions have occurred; this fact must be kept in mind because, although they appear clinically to be secondary lesions, this can be excluded by the dermatoscopic examination. The preferred mode of observation is dry dermatoscopy because it is more sensitive to the surface texture. In fact, as it misses the tunnel, wet dermatoscopy would not show any trail of bubbles and the wet scales could become slightly refractive.

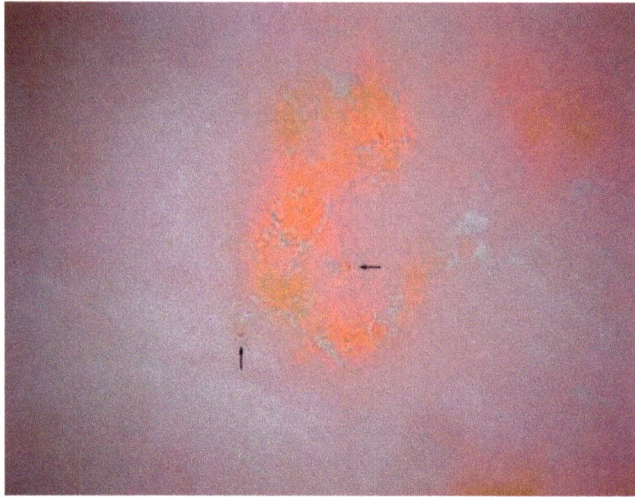

Figure 11. Dry dermatoscopy with polarized light of an atypical MGU. Two mites (arrows) can be recognized behind which there is no tunnel but an erythematous area with polycyclic borders.

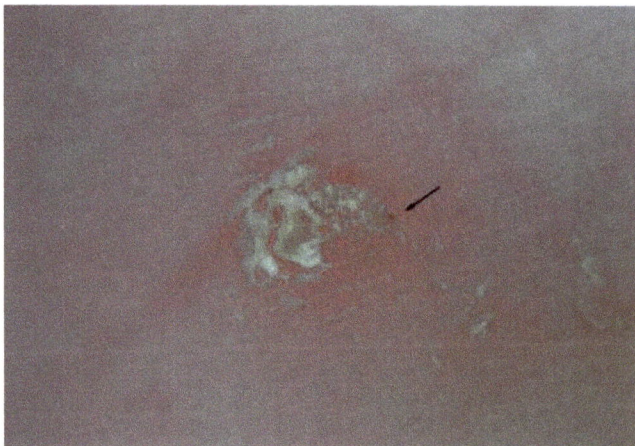

Figure 12. Dry dermatoscopy with non-polarized light of an atypical MGU. The refractive part of the mite (arrow) is evident, behind which there is an aggregate of scales rather than an ordinary gallery.

3.8. MGU Evolution at the End of the Mite Life Cycle or After Therapy

When the formation of new parts of the tunnel ceases, due to therapy or termination of the mite's life cycle, after a few days, all the MGUs will be remodeled and replaced only by traces in the form of polycyclic keratinised outlines appearing like a *"ghost gallery"*. Post-inflammatory phenomena and local superinfection can also contribute to their formation. Detection of phantom galleries might be useful in assessing scabies when the therapeutic outcome is uncertain, or in the absence of active MGUs, to confirm the success of a therapy, itching being a subjectively variable criterion (Figure 13).

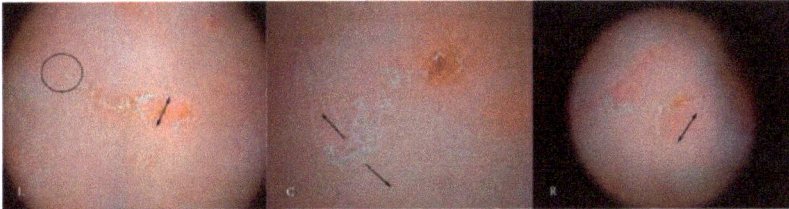

Figure 13. Evolution of an MGU towards a "ghost gallery" under polarized dry dermatoscopy. Three different examples. A mature MGU ends with a tail made up of keratinised collarettes that progressively move away from each other (black arrow, L). *Sarcoptes* is identifiable in the front part of the burrow (circle, L). When the mite is at the end of its life cycle or after therapy, the other parts of the tunnel undergo the normal processes of remodelling of the skin (C), forming the thin and polycyclic keratinic edges of a ghost gallery (C/R).

4. Discussion and Conclusions

Since dermatoscopy provides the description of the only pathognomonic sign of scabies (the burrow) as "delta wing plane + jet trail" [5], dermatologists have tried to replace the traditional scraping test with a faster dermatoscopic diagnosis which is more patient friendly [18].

The mite together with its tunnel is an important high diagnostic feature, but the global diagnostic sensitivity remains low because burrows, during clinical examination, are visible in only about 20% of patients [19]. In this article, the effect of *Sarcoptes* on and within the skin is described as an anatomical and functional entity, that is dynamic in both space and time. This is called the Mite-Gallery Unit (MGU), which consists of a head, body, and tail that take on a definable role in the production of the earlier and later dermatoscopic semeiotics of the insect's life cycle.

This setting allows us to add new diagnostic descriptors in which *Sarcoptes* can be recognized in exudative, hyperkeratotic, and nodular lesions clinically considered to be non-specific but which, on the contrary, are useful sites for dermatoscopic examination.

To detect these signs, it is necessary to use both dry polarized and wet dermatoscopy helped by specific maneuvers to make the outside and inside of the tunnel visible (local diagnostic specificity).

Thanks to entodermoscopy, two other parts of the mite (spines and body cuticle) can be identified, making the diagnosis more reliable even when the *acarus* is not associated with a visible tunnel. The juvenile forms hitherto excluded from the diagnosis can be detected in superficial epidermal *pockets* whose pathological effects are still unknown. Considering human skin turnover is an integral element in the diagnosis it is possible to follow the fate of the MGU even when, at the end of its life cycle, the mite no longer forms new parts of the tunnel but a "phantom" imprint remains nonetheless.

No traditional microscopic examination has ever produced a detailed anatomical and functional description of the tunnel such as the one obtained via entodermoscopy. The principles and rationale of entodermoscopy are very close to a behavioural approach as they involve the study of the acari, while taking care not to modify the local habitat—something that is a feature of traditional optical microscope examinations in scabies and other ectoparasitoses.

A new instrument (*entodermoscope*) with higher magnification (>200×), different light source options (normal/polarized/tangential), and micromanipulators operating in the field of examination

Trop. Med. Infect. Dis. **2019**, *4*, 48

could add valuable information as yet unknown. Meanwhile, entodermoscopy provides a new vision of the host–parasite relationship which will benefit diagnosis and as seems likely, in the future, our understanding of transmission and the assessment of innovative preventive or therapeutic strategies.

Funding: This research received no external funding.

Conflicts of Interest: The author declares no conflict of interest.

References

1. Richey, H.K.; Fenske, N.A.; Cohen, L.E. Scabies: Diagnosis and management. *Hosp. Pract.* **1986**, *21*, 124. [CrossRef]
2. Scanni, G.; Bonifazi, E. Viability of the head louse eggs in pediculosis capitis. A dermoscopy study. *Eur. J. Pediat. Dermatol.* **2006**, *16*, 201–204.
3. Zalaudek, I.; Giacomel, J.; Cabo, H.; Di Stefani, A.; Ferrara, G.; Hofmann-Wellenhof, R.; Malvehy, J.; Puig, S.; Stolz, W.; Argenziano, G. Entodermoscopy: A new tool for diagnosing skin infections and infestations. *Dermatology* **2008**, *216*, 14–23. [CrossRef] [PubMed]
4. Benvenuto-Andrade, C.; Dusza, S.W.; Agero, A.L.; Scope, A.; Rajadhyaksha, M.; Halpern, A.C.; Marghoob, A.A. Differences between polarized light dermoscopy and immersion contact dermoscopy for the evaluation of skin lesions. *Arch. Dermatol.* **2007**, *143*, 329–338. [CrossRef] [PubMed]
5. Argenziano, G.; Fabbrocini, G.; Delfino, M. Epiluminescence microscopy. A new approach to in vivo detection of Sarcoptes scabiei. *Arch. Dermatol.* **1997**, *133*, 751–753. [CrossRef] [PubMed]
6. Yoshimura, H.; Ohigashi, T.; Uesugi, M.; Uesugi, K.; Higashikawa, T.; Nakamura, R.; Mori, Y.; Shinohara, K. Sarcoptes scabiei var. hominis: Three-dimensional structure of a female imago and crusted scabies lesions by X-ray micro-CT. *Exp. Parasitol.* **2009**, *122*, 268–272. [CrossRef] [PubMed]
7. Weinstein, G.D.; McCullough, J.L.; Ross, P. Cell Proliferation in Normal Epidermis. *J. Investig. Dermatol.* **1984**, *82*, 623–628. [CrossRef] [PubMed]
8. Levi, A.; Mumcuoglu, K.Y.; Ingber, A.; Enk, C.D. Detection of living Sarcoptes scabiei larvae by reflectance mode confocal microscopy in the skin of a patient with crusted scabies. *J. Biomed. Opt.* **2012**, *17*, 060503. [CrossRef] [PubMed]
9. Arlian, L.G.; Morgan, M.S. A review of Sarcoptes scabiei: Past, present and future. *Parasites Vectors* **2017**, *10*, 297. [CrossRef] [PubMed]
10. Mellanby, K. *Biology of the Parasite in: Scabies*; Oxford University Press: London, UK, 1943; Chapter 2; p. 9.
11. Fimiani, M.; Mazzatenta, C.; Alessandrini, C.; Paccagnini, E.; Andreassi, L. The behaviour of Sarcoptes scabiei var. hominis in human skin: An ultrastructural study. *J. Submicrosc. Cytol. Pathol.* **1997**, *29*, 105–113. [PubMed]
12. Arlian, L.G. Biology, host relations, and epidemiology of Sarcoptes scabiei. *Annu. Rev. Entomol.* **1989**, *34*, 139–161. [CrossRef] [PubMed]
13. Meinking, T.L. Infestations. *Curr. Probl. Dermatol.* **1999**, *11*, 106–107. [CrossRef]
14. Varma, M.R.G. Ticks and mites. In *Medical Insects and Arachnids*; Lane, R.P., Crosskey, R.W., Eds.; Springer: Dordrecht, The Netherlands, 1993; pp. 597–658.
15. Falk, E.S.; Eide, T.J. Histologic and clinical findings in human scabies. *Int. J. Dermatol.* **1981**, *20*, 600–605. [CrossRef] [PubMed]
16. Lyell, A. Diagnosis and treatment of scabies. *Br. Med. J.* **1967**, *2*, 223–225. [CrossRef] [PubMed]
17. Bauer, J.; Blum, A.; Sönnichsen, K.; Metzler, G.; Rassner, G.; Garbe, C. Nodular scabies detected by computed dermatoscopy. *Dermatology* **2001**, *203*, 190–191. [CrossRef] [PubMed]
18. Dupuy, A.; Dehen, L.; Bourrat, E.; Lacroix, C.; Benderdouche, M.; Dubertret, L.; Morel, P.; Feuilhade de Chauvin, M.; Petit, A. Accuracy of standard dermoscopy for diagnosing scabies. *J. Am. Acad. Dermatol.* **2007**, *56*, 53–62. [CrossRef] [PubMed]
19. Hewitt, K.A.; Nalabanda, A.; Cassell, J.A. Scabies outbreaks in residential care homes: Factors associated with late recognition, burden and impact. A mixed methods study in England. *Epidemiol. Infect.* **2015**, *143*, 1542–1551. [CrossRef] [PubMed]

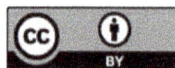

Tropical Medicine and Infectious Disease

MDPI

Article

Diagnosis and Management of Fungal Neglected Tropical Diseases In Community Settings—Mycetoma and Sporotrichosis

Roberto Estrada-Castañón [1], Guadalupe Estrada-Chávez [2] and María de Guadalupe Chávez-López [3],*

[1] Community Dermatology Mexico C.A.; Health Secretary Guerrero, 39355 Acapulco, Guerrero, Mexico; restrada_13@hotmail.com

[2] Department of Dermatology and Dermato-Oncology, Instituto Estatal de Cancerología "Dr. Arturo Beltrán Ortega", Health Secretary Guerrero, Faculty of Medicine, Universidad Autónoma de Guerrero Mexico, Community Dermatology Mexico C.A., 39850 Acapulco, Guerrero, Mexico; estradaguadalupe@hotmail.com

[3] Department of Dermatology and Mycology Acapulco General Hospital, Health Secretary Guerrero, Community Dermatology Mexico C.A., 39355 Acapulco, Guerrero, Mexico

* Correspondence: chavezg13@live.com.mx; Tel.: +52-744-4463882

Received: 19 March 2019; Accepted: 26 April 2019; Published: 16 May 2019

Abstract: Background: This is a retrospective, analytic observational study where we describe cases of sporotrichosis and mycetoma from Acapulco General Hospital and Community Dermatology Mexico C.A. over 25 years. Analysis of environmental features that favour the development of such diseases has been made, as well as the limitations in the study and treatment of such diseases in resource poor settings. Methods: We reviewed the information on 76 sporotrichosis and 113 mycetoma patients out of a total of 14,000 consultations at Acapulco General Hospital and from Community Dermatology clinics. We analysed the epidemiological and mycological characteristics and the investigations used for diagnosis such as direct examination, culture, intradermal test reactions, and biopsy. Results: In total 91 confirmed cases of actinomycetoma, 22 of eumycetoma and 76 of sporotrichosis have been identified including diagnostic studies for both diseases and their treatment. Discussion: The results obtained have been analysed and interpreted in patients with mycetoma and sporotrichosis in the state of Guerrero, México, along with limitations in their management in areas with limited economic and logistical resources. The prevalence of mycetoma in our setting is compared with other centres where patients from all over the country are seen. The possible causes for variations in prevalence in specific areas has been looked for, in one of the poorest states of the Mexican Republic.

Keywords: subcutaneous mycosis; actinomycetoma; eumycetoma; sporotrichosis Community dermatology

---

1. Introduction

Mycetoma and sporotrichosis are two of the most widely distributed implantation (subcutaneous) mycoses worldwide. Mycetoma is a chronic infectious disease, which can be caused by different species of fungus (eumycetoma) or by aerobic filamentous bacteria (actinomycetoma). Clinical characteristics include, local swelling, and draining sinuses with serosanguinous or purulent exudates (Figure 1), which contains the infective forms known as "grains" (Figure 2) Climatic and geographic conditions have been described previously and the main endemic zone identified as between the Tropic of Cancer at lattitudes 15° south and 30° north; this has been referred to as the "Mycetoma belt" by the World Health Organisation (WHO). It includes countries like Chad, Ethiopia, India, Mauritania, Senegal, Somalia, Sudan, Yemen, and in the Americas: Mexico and Venezuela [1].

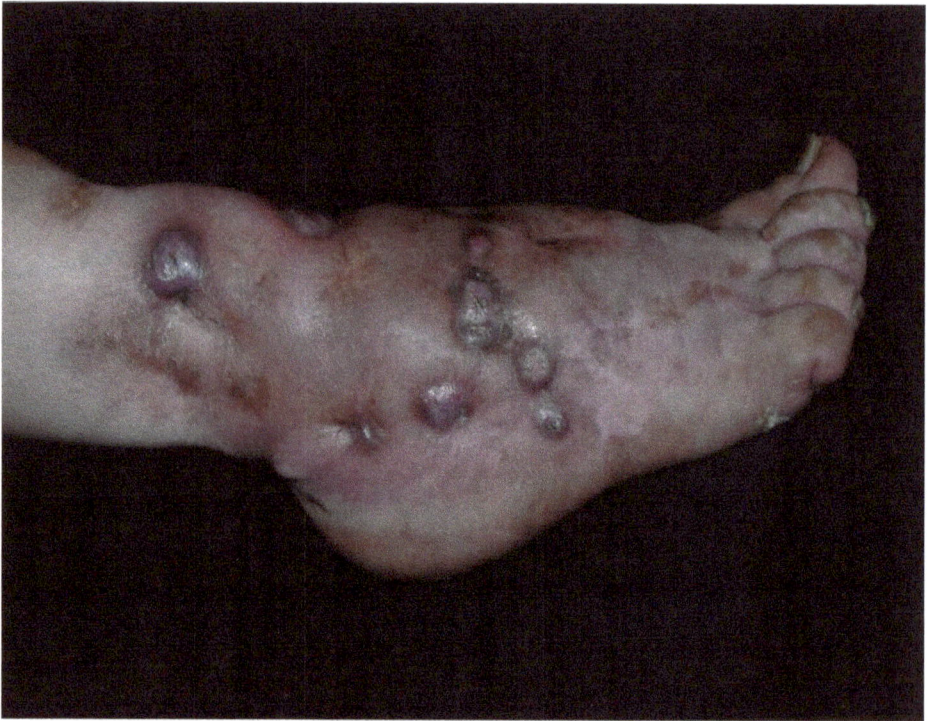

Figure 1. Eumycetoma of the foot.

Mexico has been identified as the country with the highest incidence of mycetoma in Latin America [2] and one of the most endemic countries around the world [3]. Mycetoma has been recognised by the WHO, as a neglected tropical disease (NTD) in 2016 in a WHA 69.21 resolution [4].

Even though sporotrichosis does not have the same morbidity patterns, except in disseminated or systemic forms, as mycetoma, because of its capacity for dissemination, its severity and neglect; it accounts for significant disability, morbidity, and reduction in the quality of life of affected individuals, who are mostly peasants; these are mainly farmers living in remote areas where diagnosis and treatment is frequently delayed due to lack of experience of local health personal working in the communities. Sporotrichosis is a chronic granulomatous implantation mycosis, caused by a group of dimorphic fungi belonging to the genus, *Sporothrix* . It affects either humans or some animal species [5] It is considered, in some cases, to be an occupational disease, not only in farmers, but also in florists, carpenters, and workers using hay for packing or building. Latin America has reported a high incidence of the infection, particularly in Brazil and Mexico [6], although in the former most cases, in the most recent outbreak, are caused by the zoonotic species *Sporothrix brasiliensis*, spread by cats, unlike the disease in Mexico.

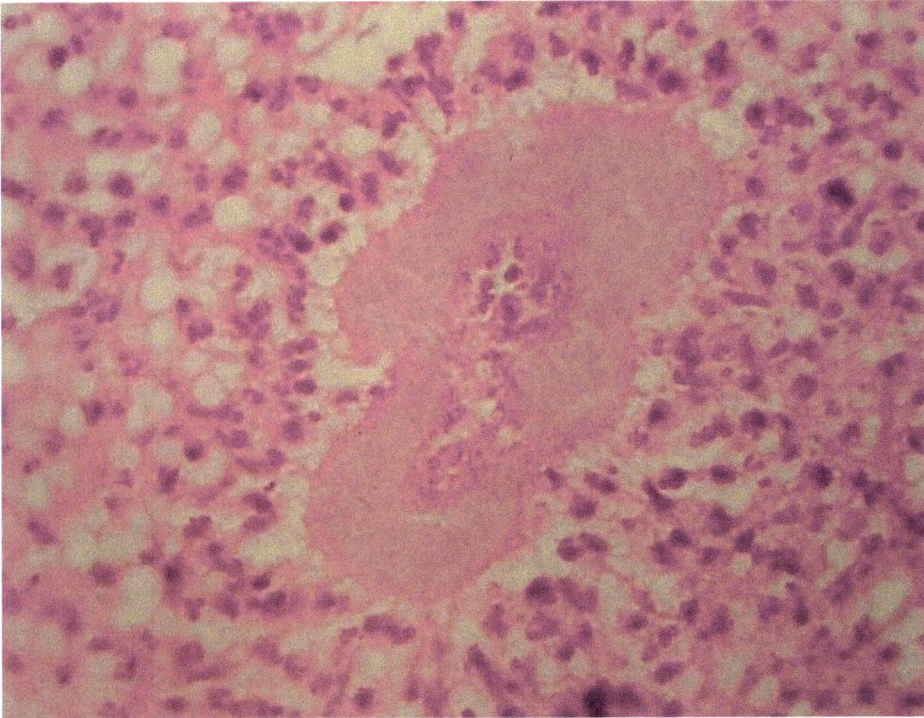

Figure 2. Grain histopathology (actinomycetoma) Haematoxylin and Eosin 100X.

Guerrero State in Mexico, is located at the south west of the Mexican Republic, on the coast of the Pacific Ocean between the coordinates 17°36′47″N 99°57′00″O with a territory of 63,794 km^2; to the West it is crossed by the mountain chain, the Sierra Madre del Sur, which provides very wide climatic and environmental diversity, with valleys and hills suitable for the development of different deep and subcutaneous mycoses. It is divided into seven natural regions, which determined its political division (Figure 3): The North and Mountain areas "Norte" and "Montaña" are arid and with difficult terrain, rich in mining and caves that are frequently visited by cave explorers and tourists, in whom cases of histoplasmosis have been reported [7], the "Tierra Caliente" (warm earth) area, has a wide valley crossed by the Balsas river and very high daily temperatures which provides the name to the region, cases of coccidioidomycosis [8] have been reported from there. A mountain chain divides the central region "Centro" into the other two regions, which are the small and big coastal areas, "Costa chica" and "Costa Grande", these are rich in vegetation, with coffee and palm plantations, where cases of paracoccidioidomycosis [9] and chromoblastomycosis [10] have been reported. Nevertheless, as in other areas of the world, mycetoma and sporotrichosis are the most frequent subcutaneous mycoses in Mexico [3] and in Guerrero State [11], making it the country with second or third highest prevalence of these disesases [1,2].

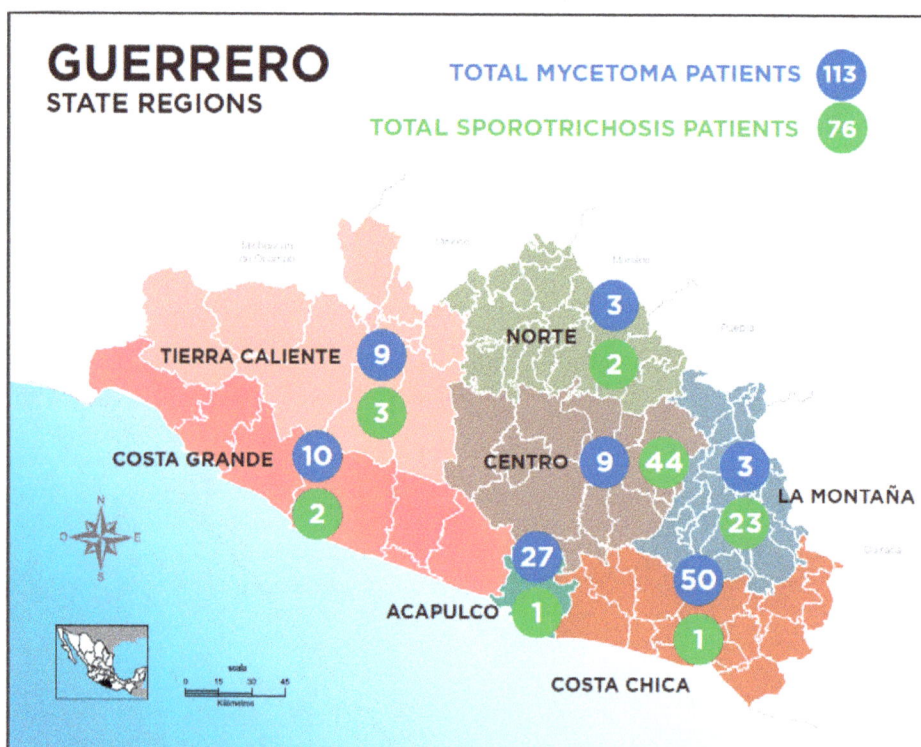

Figure 3. Map of Guerrero State showing cases of mycetoma and sporotrichosis.

Mycetoma is more frequent in the Coastal and Tierra Caliente areas. Sporotrichosis is more frequent in the Mountain and Central areas (Figure 3). Affected farmers live in conditions of poverty that can be severe in isolated regions.

Community Dermatology Mexico (CDM) is a 28 year old programme whose goal is to assist people in need or without access to specialized dermatological care, by teaching basic dermatology to health workers working in remote areas where there is less opportunity for continuous medical education and to identify, refer, and/or treat patients with both simple and complicated dermatological problems and to carry out research [12,13], the reason for this communication.

2. Methods

We report an analytical, retrospective, observational study in which we reviewed 14,000 consultations at the Acapulco General Hospital and records of the Community Dermatology program over the last 20 years. The information obtained in the communities was the result of visits to the areas with a high marginality index amongst the seven regions of Guerrero state, with the support of the State health programme called Desarollo Integral de la Familia or DIF and the Secretary of Health. Of the mycetoma and sporotrichosis cases that were identified clinically, all were referred to our Dermatology Department at the Acapulco General Hospital for further studies and treatment.

Due to limitations associated with field work and the logistics needed for transportation of basic material and equipment, the studies, that were feasible, were restricted to mycological scrapings for direct examination, punch biopsies, and occasionally the inoculation of samples of lesional exudate onto media for subsequent culture, which were subsequently completed in the mycology facility in our institution. All organisms that were speciated in this study were identified by culture.

In order to facilitate and assist the management of affected patients, we provided financial support for transportation and food during their trip to Acapulco city, where after having any ancillary studies such as imaging including Computer Assisted Tomography (CAT) scans in specific cases, culture, or further mycological studies, free treatment for their specific health conditions was provided after evaluation; this included: Trimethoprim sulfamethoxazole and dapsone (DDS) for patients with actinomycetoma, itraconazole (100–200mg daily), and terbinafine (250 mg daily) for eumycetoma patients and potassium iodide for sporotrichosis; the use of the latter medication is due to cost constraints.

Despite the support given to the patients, 38% did not attend subsequent consultations because of economic, language, personal reasons or sometimes because family members or friends, raised the spectre of unnecessary amputation. Distance and poverty were constant barriers to consent, study, and treatment.

In order to review cases we developed a basic recording format including, patient information, in Excel and graphics were made with statistics analysis SPSS.9

3. Results

Table 1 shows the results from 113 confirmed mycetomas studied. For logistical reasons not all mycological studies could be carried out on all patients. There were more actinomycetomas than eumycetomas with scattered anatomical distributions

Table 1. Mycetoma Patients.

VARIABLE	VALUES	
GENDER	Male	= 85 (75.2%)
	Female	= 28 (24.8%)
AGE	Adults > 18a	= 104 (92.0%)
	Children < 18a	= 9 (8.0%)
OCCUPATION	Farmers	= 53 (48.6%)
	Housewives	= 23 (21.1%)
	Others	= 37 (30.3%)
AFFECTED AREA	Feet	= 34 (30.1%)
	Legs	= 11 (9.7%)
	Upper limbs	= 22 (19.5%)
	Pelvic area	= 19 (16.8%)
	Abdomen	= 6 (5.3%)
	Trunk	= 17 (15.1%)
	Cervical column	= 4 (3.5%)
MYCOLOGY	Cultures (+)	= 82
	Direct Exam (+)	= 101
	Biopsy	= 79
	X ray	= 75
	CT	= 7
TYPE OF MYCETOMA	Actinomycetoma	= 81 (78.6%)
	Eumycetoma	= 22 (21.4%)
ACTINOMYCETES	*Nocardia brasiliensis*	= 64 (70.4%)
	Nocardia spp	= 19 (20.9%)
	Actinomadura madurae	= 6 (6.6%)
	N. otitidis caviarum	= 2 (2.1%)
FUNGI	*Madurella mycetomatis*	= 16 (72.8%)
	Trematosphaeria grisea	= 3 (13.7%)
	Scedosporium boydii	= 2 (9.0%)
	Phomopsis longicola	= 1 (4.5%)
EVOLUTION	<five years	= 84 (74.3%)
	>five years	= 29 (25.7%)
REGION	Costa Chica	= 50 (44.2%)
	Acapulco	= 27 (23.9%)
	Costa Grande	= 10 (8.8%)
	Tierra Caliente	= 9 (8.0%)
	Centro	= 9 (8.0%)
	Norte	= 5 (4.4%)
	Montaña	= 3 (2.7%)

Studies made for confirmation of the diagnosis were: Biopsy in 79 cases, direct examination in 101 and culture in 82 cases. Actinomycetoma cases were caused by *Nocardia brasiliensis* in 64 cases, *Nocardia sp* 19 cases, *Actinomadura madurae* 6, *Nocardia otitidis caviarum* 2. The causative agents in eumycetomas were in most of the cases *Madurella mycetomatis* 16, *Trematosphaeria grisea* 3, *Scedosporium apiospermum* 2, and *Phomopsis longicolla* 1 case.

Table 2 shows the 76 cases of sporotrichosis studied, of which 43 were of the lymphangitic clinical pattern, fixed type 24 and cutaneous disseminated 8. 35 were male, 40 female; 39 adults and 36 children. Most of these patients were farmers; men, women or children work, or are partially involved, in field activities.

Table 2. Sporotrichosis Patients.

VARIABLE	VALUES	
GENDER	Male	= 35 (46.0%)
	Female	= 41 (54.0%)
AGE	Adults > 18	= 39 (51.3%)
	Children < 18	= 37 (48.7%)
OCCUPATION	Farmers	= 62 (81.6%)
	Students	= 2 (2.6%)
	Children not working	= 12 (15.8%)
AFFECTED AREA	Upper limbs	= 32 (42.1%)
	Lower limbs	= 16 (21.1%)
	Face	= 16 (21.1%)
	Trunk	= 4 (5.3%)
	Other	= 8 (10.4%)
MYCOLOGY	Cultures	= 52 (+)
	IDR (Skin Test) [1]	= 45 (+)
	Biopsy	= 31
CLINICAL FORM	Lymphangitic	= 43 (56.8%)
	Fixed	= 24 (32.2%)
	Disseminated	= 8 (11.0%)
EVOLUTION	<1 year	= 18 (23.7%)
	<5 years	= 41 (53.9%)
	>5 years	= 17 (22.4%)
REGION	Centre	= 44 (57.9%)
	High Mountain	= 23 (30.3%)
	Others	= 9 (11.8%)
TREATMENT	Treated	= 56 (73.7%)
	Not treated	= 20 (26.3%)

The sporotrichin used was prepared by the Laboratory of Basic Mycology, Universidad Nacional Autonoma de Mexico.

The most commonly affected area was the upper limb in 32 cases, 16 in lower limbs, 16 on the face, 4 on the thorax and 3 in other localizations. All cases studied included auxiliary laboratory methods such as culture 52 cases, biopsy in 31 cases, intradermal skin test reaction with mycelial sporotrichin of which 45 cases had positive reactions (one was negative). Of diagnosed cases 56 received treatment with saturated solution of potassium iodide (at full dose 4–6 mls three times daily) with complete healing of the clinical lesions. The rest of the patients did not attend consultation for treatment. Almost 60% of cases occurred in patients in the "Central area" adjacent to the "Mountain area" - for this reason often referred to as the "low mountain" zone—but the other 30% were in the "high Mountain" zone; the remaining 11% were from other areas of the state.

4. Discussion

Neglected diseases in developing countries are usually located in remote, isolated areas with limited access, and communication. This means that health systems are limited, and there is a high level of ignorance and malnutrition all of which are reasons why these diseases develop without intervention and reach extremes of severity, leading to severe morbidity and even death amongst affected patients. One of the main and persistent obstacles to care and further research is the lack of properly trained health personnel to identify patients or to perform studies [14]. Additionally personal safety of staff is a further obstacle to investigation and care, imposing a risk in visits to isolated communities. Even though, encounters with criminal groups have been few and without severe consequences during work in the communities, the potential risk for personnel, has now forced us to adapt our working methods to include the use of teledermatology and telemedicine in order to continue the work of teaching, research, and advice for the health personnel based in remote areas [15].

In 1988, Lavalle and Padilla described in a communication [16] that Guerrero was the second commonest source in the country of mycetoma cases attending the "Centro Dermatológico Pascua" (CDP), which is a referral centre for treatment of dermatological problems. In another review of mycetomas by Bonifaz et al., Guerrero was rated 3rd in incidence (1). In comparing our data with that of Lavalle and Bonifaz for patients coming from Guerrero, but diagnosed and treated in the Department of Mycology at the Hospital General de Mexico (HGM), patient parameters were similar: male predominance in 70%, mostly middle aged, foot involvement, though in our studies uncommon areas such as the perianal region [17] or the neck, a source of considerable morbidity, have also been seen to be involved [18]. Causal agents reported in these other studies are also similar with a predominance of actinomycetes in 97% (Lavalle), 82% (Bonifaz), and 81% (Current study). It is worth mentioning that both centres in Mexico city are among the main primary mycology referral laboratories where patients are seen from every part of the country.

Our studies have also found that there are regional variations in disease prevalence for both mycoses in our environment. Eumycetomas are predominantly found in the Costa Chica area where they account for a much higher proportion of cases (30%) compared with the 2–3% reported nationally. Most sporotrichosis cases originate from the Central and Montaña regions (Figure 3). In explanation, besides the environmental characteristics–in the Costa Chica there is pastureland and cattle farming in commo—it is possible that there is a higher genetic predisposition, related to a high proportion of indigenous Mexican groups, for some mycoses. In the Costa Chica there is also a well established population of individuals of African Mexican origin. It has also been suggested in cases of sporotrichosis, in patients of indigenous origin in the Central Mountain areas carry alleles of Class II [19].

Madurella mycetomatis is the most important causal agent found in our series which is similar to studies reported in patients from other areas with high endemicity [20–22]; these isolates have not been subject to molecular identification, therefore the presence of other *Madurella* species is possible. Mycetomas per se have a low mortality, except those cases with neck and dorsal spine involvement [18], nevertheless they do have severe morbidity, which has a serious impact on the earning capacity of the affected patients as they are usually farmers with reduced economic resources and depend directly on their ability to work in the fields. The high cost of the treatment and the long term course of the disease, have a critical impact on the family's health and financial well-being [21].

Histopathological studies are a very valuable diagnostic auxiliary method used to differentiate the actinomycetomas and eumycetomas, for which treatment is completely different. Samples can be easily obtained even in remote areas and together with direct examination and culture can be accessible in areas where resources are extremely limited. Molecular diagnostic techniques are usually out of the reach of decentralized institutions where mycetoma patients are studied and treated [22] and even though simple imaging studies and ultrasound are accessible in order to identify bone involvement, other studies like CAT scan or MRI, can be unaffordable for patients of low income, which represent most of the patients studied in our group [23].

We firmly believe that mycetoma treatment should be as integrated or "holistic" [24]. In our opinion this should include (1) training of the local health personnel, providing the basic knowledge to identify and refer mycetoma cases to centres where they can be properly diagnosed, studied and treated, (2) facilitating the means for patients to attend for consultation, (3) provide appropriate tests for identification of causal agents, together with estimation of the severity index in order to determine the best available treatment for each case, (4) provide free medications throughout treatment duration, and (5) register of every case in order to contribute with information on the epidemiology of mycetoma worldwide (6) establishing a robust system for early detection, and ultimately, prevention of cases in collaboration with local health workers. In the case of sporotrichosis further work needs to be carried out, in order to establish the specific molecular identification of the causative *Sporothrix* species and the reasons for small outbreaks in specific areas, although feline sources of infection are not suspected. As with mycetoma, improving early case recognition is an important goal.

We should point out that even though the number of suspected mycetoma cases diagnosed in Community Dermatology over the last 28 years of work exceeds 240 patients, the diagnosis in many cases has been mainly determined on clinical grounds with some laboratory tests, as discussed previously; in these patients other essential laboratory studies could not be done in order to establish the causal species. Hence, the clinically diagnosed cases have not been included in the analysis.

Finally it is important to mention that 2019 is the year when the Community Dermatology Centre "Dr. Ramon Ruiz Maldonado" (CDM) has been opened in Acapulco in order to treat patients of low and very low incomes from the urban, and especially, rural areas where access to specialized attention is limited or absent.

Author Contributions: All participated in reviewing patients, planning the study and writing the manuscript.

Funding: This research received no external funding.

Acknowledgments: We would like to mention our sincere appreciation to Alexandro Bonifaz MSc for the data from the laboratory of mycology regarding patients from Guerrero State. As well we would like to acknowledge Roderick Hay for the very valuable help, orientation and his participation during the activities of Community Dermatology Mexico and constant encouragement for this communication. To the Secretary of State Health and the DIF Guerrero for the support given to the activities of Community Dermatology Mexico through which fundamental information for this study was obtained. Also to the International Foundation for Dermatology, the American Academy of Dermatology, Galderma Skin Pact Awards and Vaseline Direct Relief for their contributions in order to purchase medicaments and for providing resources to mycetoma and sporotrichosis patients for their study and treatment.

Conflicts of Interest: Authors have no relevant conflicts of interest for the elaboration of this work

References

1. Bonifaz, A.; Tirado Sánchez, A.; Calderón, L.; Saul, A.; Araiza, J.; Hernández, M.; González, G.M.; Ponce, R.M. Mycetoma: Experience of 482 cases in a single center in Mexico. *PLoS Negl. Trop. Dis.* **2014**, *8*. [CrossRef] [PubMed]

2. Lopez-Mtnez, R.; Mendez-Tovar, L.J.; Bonifaz, A.; Arenas, R.; Mayorga, J.; Welsh, O.; Vera-Cabrera, L.; Padilla-Desgarennes, M.C.; Contreras Pérez, C.; Chávez, G. Update on the epidemiology of Mycetoma in Mexico. A review of 3933 cases. *Gac. Med. Mex.* **2013**, *149*, 586–592.

3. Van de Sande, W. Global burden of human mycetoma: A systemic review and metanalisis. *PLoS Negl. Trop. Dis.* **2013**, *7*. [CrossRef]

4. WHO. Available online: https://www.who.int/neglected_diseases/mediacentre/WHA_69.21_Eng.pdf?ua=1 (accessed on 2 February 2019).

5. Werner, A.; Werner, B. Sporotrichosis in man and animals. *Int. J. Dermatol.* **1994**, *33*, 692–700. [CrossRef] [PubMed]

6. Conti, A.D. Sporotrichosis in Latin America. *Mycopath* **1989**, *108*, 113–116.

7. Corcho-Berdugo, A.; Muñoz Hndez, B.; Palma-Cortes, G.; Ramirez Hndez, A.; Martínez-Rivera, M.; Frías-de León, M.; Reyes-Montes, M.; Martínez-Valadez, E.; Manjarrez-Zavala, M.; Alfaro-Ramos, L.; et al. Brote inusual de histoplasmosis en residentes del estado de México. *Gaceta Med. Mex.* **2011**, *5*, 377–384.

8. Mayorga, P.; Epinoza, H. Coccidioidomycosis in México and Central America. *Mycopathol. Mycol. Appl.* **1970**, *41*, 13–23. [CrossRef] [PubMed]

9. Lopez-Martinez, R.; Hernandez-Hernandez, F.; Mendez-Tovar, LJ.; Manzano-Gayosso, P.; Bonifaz, A.; Arenas, R.; Padilla-Desgarennes Mdel, C.; Estrada, R.; Chávez, G. Paracoccidioidomycosis en Mexico. Clinical and epidemiological data from 93 new cases (1972–2012). *Mycoses* **2014**, *57*, 525–530. [CrossRef]

10. Chavez, L.G.; Estrada, C.R.; Estrada, C.G.; Moreno, C.G. Cromoblastomicosis y micetoma. Informe de un caso por presentación simultanea de Fonseca pedrosoi y Nocardia brasiliensis. *Dermatol. Cosm. Med. Quir.* **2014**, *12*, 268–271.

11. Estrada, C.R.; Chavez, L.G.; Estrada, C.G.; Bonifaz, A. Report of 73 cases of cutaneous sporotrichosis in Mexico. *An. Bras. Dermatol.* **2018**, *93*, 907–909. [CrossRef]

12. Estrada, C.R.; Chavez-Lopez, M.G.; Estrada-Chavez, G.; Paredes-Solis, S. Specialized dermatological care for marginalized populations and education at primary care level: Is community dermatology a feasible proposal? *Int. J. Dermatol.* **2012**, *51*, 1345–1350. [CrossRef]

13. Hay, R.J.; Estrada, C.R.; Grossmann, H. Managing skin disease in resource-poor environments- the role of community oriented training and control programs. *Int. J. Dermatol.* **2011**, *50*, 558–563. [CrossRef]

14. El-Safi, S.; Chappuis, F.; Boelaert, M. The Challenges of Conducting Clinical Research on neglected tropical diseases in remote endemic áreas of Sudan. *PLoS Negl. Trop. Dis.* **2016**, *10*. [CrossRef] [PubMed]

15. Chávez, L.G.; Estrada, C.G.; Orozco, F.M.; Solis, R.A.; Solchaga-Rosas, J.; Armendariz-Valle, F.; Estrada-Castañón, R.A. Teledermatología, un modelo de enseñanza y asistencia en atención primaria a la salud. *Gac. Med. Mex.* **2018**, *154*, 1–5.

16. Lavalle, P.; Padilla, M.C.; Perez, J.; Reynoso, S. Contribución al conocimiento de los micetomas en el estado de Guerrero, México. Origen disctribución geográfica y evolución de 100 casos de micetomas. *Dermatol. Rev. Mex.* **1988**, *42*, 232–238.

17. Chávez, G.; Estrada, R.; Bonifaz, A. Perianal actinomycetoma, experience of 20 cases. *Int. J. Dermatol.* **2002**, *41*, 491–493. [CrossRef] [PubMed]

18. Estrada-Chavez, G.; Estrada, R.; Fernandez, R.; Arenas, R.; Reyes, A.; Guevara, C.; Chávez-López, G. Cervical and middle actinomycetomas from Guerrero State, Mexico. *Int. J. Dermatol.* **2017**, *56*, 1146–1149. [CrossRef] [PubMed]

19. Estrada-Chavez, G.; Estrada, R.; Chavez, G.; Vega Memije, M.; Guzmán, R.; García-Lechuga, M.; Granados, J.; Rangel-Gamboa, L. HLA Class II alleles in human sporotrichosis in Mexican Amerindians. *Asia-Pacif. J. Blood Types Genes* **2018**, *2*, 183–190.

20. Ahmed, A.O.; Van-Leeuwen, W.; Fahal, A.; Van de Sande, W. Mycetoma caused by Madurella mycetomatis: A neglected infectious burden. *Lancet Infect. Dis.* **2004**, *4*, 566–574. [CrossRef]

21. Torres, G.E.; Niebla, M.A. *Mycetoma. Clinical and Microbiological Monograph*; Scholar Press: Brivibas gatve, Riga, 2015.

22. Mehantappa, H.; Sruthi, P.; Kusuma, V.; Niveditha, S.R.; Kumar, S.A. Cytological diagnosis of actinomycosis. and eumycetoma. A report of two cases. *Diagn. Cytopathol.* **2010**, *38*, 918–920.

23. Fahal, A.H.; Sjeikh, H.E.; Lider, M.A.; Homeida, M.A.; El Arabi, Y.E.; Mahgoub, E.S. Ultrasonic imaging in mycetoma. *Br. J. Surg.* **1997**, *78*, 765–766.

24. Mubarak, B.S.; Fahal, A.H.; Mudawi, M.A.; El Samani, W.M.; Fathelrahman, R.O.; Eiman, S.A.; El Nour, M.; El Rayah, M.M.; El Sheikh Rahman, M.A.; Suliman, H.S.; et al. A holistic approach to the mycetoma management. *PLoS Negl. Trop. Dis.* **2018**, *12*. [CrossRef]

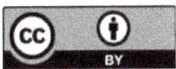

MDPI

St. Alban-Anlage 66

4052 Basel

Switzerland

Tel. +41 61 683 77 34

Fax +41 61 302 89 18

www.mdpi.com

Tropical Medicine and Infectious Disease Editorial Office

E-mail: tropicalmed@mdpi.com

www.mdpi.com/journal/tropicalmed

www.ingramcontent.com/pod-product-compliance
Lightning Source LLC
Chambersburg PA
CBHW051844210326

41597CB00033B/5770